ENVIRONMENTAL HAZARDS AND NEURODEVELOPMENT
Where Ecology and Well-Being Connect

ENVIRONMENTAL HAZARDS AND NEURODEVELOPMENT
Where Ecology and Well-Being Connect

Edited by
Cindy Croft

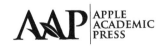

APPLE ACADEMIC PRESS

Apple Academic Press Inc.	Apple Academic Press Inc.
3333 Mistwell Crescent	9 Spinnaker Way
Oakville, ON L6L 0A2	Waretown, NJ 08758
Canada	USA

© 2015 by Apple Academic Press, Inc.

First issued in paperback 2021

Exclusive worldwide distribution by CRC Press, a member of Taylor & Francis Group

No claim to original U.S. Government works

ISBN 13: 978-1-77463-370-0 (pbk)
ISBN 13: 978-1-77188-093-0 (hbk)

Library of Congress Control Number: 2014948303

Library and Archives Canada Cataloguing in Publication

Environmental hazards and neurodevelopment: where ecology and well-being connect/ edited by Cindy Croft.

Includes bibliographical references and index.
ISBN 978-1-77188-093-0 (bound)
1. Pediatric toxicology. 2. Environmental toxicology. 3. Environmental health.
4. Developmental disabilities--Etiology. 5. Child mental health. I. Croft, Cindy, editor

RA1225.E58 2015   618.92'98   C2014-905750-4

Apple Academic Press also publishes its books in a variety of electronic formats. Some content that appears in print may not be available in electronic format. For information about Apple Academic Press products, visit our website at **www.appleacademicpress.com** and the CRC Press website at **www.crcpress.com**

ABOUT THE EDITOR

CINDY CROFT

Cindy Croft, MA in Education, is Director of the Center for Inclusive Child Care, Concordia University, St. Paul, Minnesota. She teaches for the Center for Early Education and Development at the University of Minnesota and in the early childhood program at Concordia University. She has authored two books, *The Six Keys: Promoting Children's Mental Health* and *Children and Challenging Behavior: Making Inclusion Work*, and she provides training and consultation to educators of children with various disabilities. She is a member of the National Association for the Education of Young Children, the Early Childhood and School-Age Trainers Association, the Minnesota Association for Children's Mental Health, and the Minnesota Association for Infant and Early Childhood Mental Health Division.

CONTENTS

ACKNOWLEDGMENT AND HOW TO CITE

The editor and publisher thank each of the authors who contributed to this book, whether by granting their permission individually or by releasing their research as open source articles or under a license that permits free use, provided that attribution is made. The chapters in this book were previously published in various places in various formats. To cite the work contained in this book and to view the individual permissions, please refer to the citation at the beginning of each chapter. Each chapter was read individually and carefully selected by the editor; the result is a book that provides a nuanced study of the effects of the environment on children's development. The chapters included examine the following topics:

- Chapter 1 provides a comprehensive overview of the connections between neurodevelopmental disorders and the environment, which forms the foundation of the chapters that follow. Please note that as of August 2014, the CDC most recently estimates a higher percentage of children who have been identified with autism spectrum disorder (ASD), now currently about 1 in 68. (http://www.cdc.gov/ncbddd/autism/facts.html)
- Although the connection between environmental toxins and neurodevelopment is well-established, Chapter 2 describes the need of researchers for a method that more accurately accesses the prevalence and impact of various risk factors.
- Chapter 3 looks at "why?" environmental exposure has such an impact on the brain's development.
- Chapter 4 provides an inclusive look at the way a particular pesticide contributes to a range of neurodevelopmental issues.
- Chapter 5 provides a description of how endocrine disrupters are some of the most dangerous environmental toxins, contributing to a range of neurodevelopmental conditions.
- Belief in the connection between autism and the environment has become a part of our culture. Chapter 6 argues that researchers need defined strategies for sorting through the extreme claims often made by advocacy groups.
- The most recent edition of the DSM defines autism as a spectrum disorder, with degrees of severity. Chapter 7 investigates the etiological mechanism that contributes to where a child falls on the spectrum.

- Again, many claims are made in popular culture connecting nutrition and autism. Chapter 8 gives insight into the epigenetics of this connection.
- By examining the urine of neurotypical children as compared to the urine of children with autism, the authors of Chapter 9 confirm the connections between mercury exposure and this form of neurodisability.
- Chapter 10 fills out a multi-perspective section on autism with research that indicates that children with autism spectrum disorder may be more sensitive to environmental toxins than their siblings who are not on the spectrum.
- The overview in Chapter 11 gives the research foundation for investigating the connections between environmental toxins and other forms of neurodevelopmental disorder.
- The authors of Chapter 12 take the known connection between PAHs and neurodevelopment a step further, into the specific connections with ADHD (as well as learning disabilities), and then an additional step interfacing school identification of special needs with students' exposure to PAHs in the environment.
- Chapter 13 provides another cross-sectional look at the interface between ADHD and the presence of another environmental toxin, PFCs. The authors reach no firm conclusions, but the basis for further research is established.
- Chapter 14 provides a tragic example of the correlation between learning disabilities and exposure to endocrine disrupters found in ordinary household materials
- Chapter 15 is the essential conclusion to this compendium, offering compelling arguments that as scientists we have a moral and practical duty to do all that we can to act on behalf of our children's well-being.

LIST OF CONTRIBUTORS

Z. Abid
Department of Environmental Health Sciences, Yale School of Public Health, New Haven, CT 06520, USA.

Andréa Aguiar
Department of Comparative Biosciences, College of Veterinary Medicine, University of Illinois at Urbana-Champaign, Urbana, Illinois, USA

Altaf Alabdali
Biochemistry Department, Science College, King Saud University, P.O box 22452, Zip code 11495 Riyadh, Saudi Arabia

Laila Al-Ayadhi
Autism Research and Treatment Center, Riyadh, Saudi Arabia, Shaik AL-Amodi Autism Research Chair, King Saud University, Riyadh, Saudi Arabia, and Department of Physiology, Faculty of Medicine, King Saud University, Riyadh, Saudi Arabia

Jason Allen
Department of Environmental and Occupational Health Sciences, University of Washington, Seattle, Washington, USA

Sarah E. Armel
Department of Environmental and Occupational Health Sciences, University of Washington, Seattle, Washington, USA

Srikesh Arunajadai
Department of Biostatistics, Mailman School of Public Health, Columbia University, New York, New York, USA

Dana B. Barr
Emory University, Atlanta, Georgia, USA

David S. Baskin
Department of Neurosurgery, The Methodist Neurological Institute, 6560 Fannin Street, Scurlock Tower No. 944, Houston, TX 77030, USA

David C. Bellinger
Children's Hospital Boston, Harvard Medical School, Boston, Massachusetts, USA

Linda S. Birnbaum
Children's Environmental Health Center, Mount Sinai School of Medicine, New York, New York

Asa Bradman
Center for Environmental Research and Children's Health, School of Public Health, University of California at Berkeley, Berkeley, California, USA

J. Jeffrey Bradstreet
International Child Development Resource Center, Melbourne, Florida, USA

Atilla Büyükgebiz
Bilim University Faculty of Medicine, Department of Pediatric Endocrinology, İstanbul, Turkey

Jonathan Chevrier
Center for Environmental Research and Children's Health, School of Public Health, University of California at Berkeley, Berkeley, California, USA

Diana Echeverria
Department of Environmental and Occupational Health Sciences, University of Washington, Seattle, Washington, USA and Battelle Centers for Public Health Research and Evaluation, Seattle, Washington, USA

Afaf El-Ansary
Biochemistry Department, Science College, King Saud University, P.O box 22452, Zip code 11495 Riyadh, Saudi Arabia, Autism Research and Treatment Center, Riyadh, Saudi Arabia, Shaik AL-Amodi Autism Research Chair, King Saud University, Riyadh, Saudi Arabia, and Medicinal Chemistry Department, National Research Centre, Dokki, Cairo, Egypt

Brenda Eskenazi
Center for Environmental Research and Children's Health, School of Public Health, University of California at Berkeley, Berkeley, California, USA

A. S. Ettinger
Department of Chronic Disease Epidemiology, Yale School Public Health, New Haven, CT 06520, USA; Yale Center for Perinatal, Pediatric, and Environmental Epidemiology, 1 Church Street, 6th floor, New Haven, CT 06510, USA.

Paul A. Eubig
Department of Comparative Biosciences, College of Veterinary Medicine, University of Illinois at Urbana-Champaign, Urbana, Illinois, USA

Denise I. Fulton
Autism Research Institute, Lacey, Washington, USA

Taylor L. Gist
Department of Neurosurgery, The Methodist Neurological Institute, 6560 Fannin Street, Scurlock Tower No. 944, Houston, TX 77030, USA

Doreen Granpeesheh
Center for Autism and Related Disorders, Tarzana, California, USA

Kim G. Harley
Center for Environmental Research and Children's Health, School of Public Health, University of California at Berkeley, Berkeley, California, USA

J. B. Herbstman
Department of Environmental Health Sciences, Columbia Mailman School of Public Health, New York, NY 10032, USA.

Nicholas J. Heyer
Battelle Centers for Public Health Research and Evaluation, Seattle, Washington, USA

Lori Hoepner
Columbia Center for Children's Environmental Health, Mailman School of Public Health, Columbia University, New York, New York, USA

Megan Horton
Sergievsky Center and Columbia Center for Children's Environmental Health, Mailman School of Public Health, Columbia University, New York, New York, USA

Caroline Johnson
Center for Environmental Research and Children's Health, School of Public Health, University of California at Berkeley, Berkeley, California, USA

Katherine Kogut
Center for Environmental Research and Children's Health, School of Public Health, University of California at Berkeley, Berkeley, California, USA

Luca Lambertini
Children's Environmental Health Center, Mount Sinai School of Medicine, New York, New York

Philip J. Landrigan
Children's Environmental Health Center, Mount Sinai School of Medicine, New York, New York

Elizabeth Mumper
Autism Research Institute and The Rimland Center for Integrative Medicine, Lynchburg, Virginia, USA

Frederica Perera
Columbia Center for Children's Environmental Health, Mailman School of Public Health, Columbia University, New York, New York, USA

Stephen A. Rauch
Center for Environmental Research and Children's Health, School of Public Health, University of California at Berkeley, Berkeley, California, USA

Virginia Rauh
Heilbrunn Center for Population and Family Health, Mailman School of Public Health, Columbia University, New York, New York, USA

James P. K. Rooney
Department of Pharmaceutical and Medicinal Chemistry, Royal College of Surgeons in Ireland, Dublin, Ireland

A. Roy
Department of Chronic Disease Epidemiology, Yale School Public Health, New Haven, CT 06520, USA.

David A. Savitz
Department of Community Health, and Department of Obstetrics and Gynecology, Brown University, Providence, Rhode Island, USA

Susan L. Schantz
Department of Comparative Biosciences, College of Veterinary Medicine and Neuroscience Program, University of Illinois at Urbana-Champaign, Urbana, Illinois, USA

Martyn A. Sharpe
Department of Neurosurgery, The Methodist Neurological Institute, 6560 Fannin Street, Scurlock Tower No. 944, Houston, TX 77030, USA

Kristin Shrader-Frechette
Department of Biological Sciences, University of Notre Dame, Notre Dame, IN, 46556, USA and Department of Philosophy, 100 Malloy Hall, University of Notre Dame, Notre Dame, IN, 46556, USA

P. Lynne Simmonds
Department of Environmental and Occupational Health Sciences, University of Washington, Seattle, Washington, USA

Andreas Sjödin
Division of Laboratory Sciences, National Center for Environmental Health, Centers for Disease Control and Prevention, Atlanta, Georgia, USA

Cheryl R. Stein
Department of Preventive Medicine, Mount Sinai School of Medicine, New York, New York, USA

Angela Spivey
Angela Spivey writes from North Carolina about medicine, environmental health, and personal finance.

Celina Trujillo
Center for Environmental Research and Children's Health, School of Public Health, University of California at Berkeley, Berkeley, California, USA

Toyoharu Tsutsui
La Belle Vie Research Laboratory, 8-4 Nihonbashi-Tomizawacho, Chuo-ku, Tokyo 103-0006, Japan

Tolga Ünüvar
T.C. Ministry of Health, İstanbul Kanuni Sultan Süleyman, Training and Research Hospital, Department of Pediatric Endocrinology, İstanbul, Turkey

Kristine Wessels
Autism Society of Washington, Spokane, Washington, USA

Robin Whyatt
Columbia Center for Children's Environmental Health, Mailman School of Public Health, Columbia University, New York, New York, USA

James S. Woods
Department of Environmental and Occupational Health Sciences, University of Washington, Seattle, Washington, USA

Hiroshi Yasuda
La Belle Vie Research Laboratory, 8-4 Nihonbashi-Tomizawacho, Chuo-ku, Tokyo 103-0006, Japan

INTRODUCTION

The rate of identification of children with neurobiological disabilities has been on the increase in recent years. Millions of dollars in research, funded both privately and publicly, are being spent to understand the factors influencing these increases. Numerous studies have confirmed that the environment in which we are raising our children is influencing their brain development and impacting other developmental outcomes. The Scientific Consensus Statement on Environmental Agents Associated with Neurodevelopmental Disorders speaks to the vulnerability of infants prenatally to agents in our environment (http://www.healthychildrenproject. org/pdfs/080801_Scientific-Concensus-Statement-LDDI.pdf). Direct and indirect causal relationships between environmental toxins and neurological disorders is being recognized as early childhood assessment rates of disabilities rise.

In this compilation of articles within Environmental Hazards and Neurodevelopment: Assessing the Connections, researchers show linkages between what is occurring in the environment that surrounds infants and young children and resulting developmental outcomes. Research points to connections between some neurobiologically based disabilities and early environmental exposures. For instance, autism is being identified in children at a rate of 1 in 77, and the research articles within the second section of this book call attention to environmental factors influencing the neurobiology of autism.

It is critically important for all of us to pay attention to what is happening to our children because of what they are being exposed to early in life. Not only are millions of dollars in funding needed to support early and ongoing interventions when disabilities occur but human potential is undermined when we ignore the risks. This book is important for researchers and professionals working with families and young children but it is also important for policy makers and corporate leaders who make decisions about environmental exposure. We all have a responsibility to protect the brain development of our most vulnerable population, our children.

Cindy Croft

Chapter 1 is an excerpt from the United States Environmental Protection Agency's report titled "America's Children and the Environment" (ACE). The report as a whole presents data from a variety of sources on the topic of children's environmental health, with the aims of compiling data, serving as a resource for policy makers and other public discussions, and attempting to track environmental impacts on children. The section presented here details trends in neurodevelopmental disorders.

The impact of environmental chemicals on children's neurodevelopment is sometimes dismissed as unimportant because the magnitude of the impairments are considered to be clinically insignificant. Such a judgment reflects a failure to distinguish between individual and population risk. The population impact of a risk factor depends on both its effect size and its distribution (or incidence/prevalence). Bellinger's objective in Chapter 2 was to develop a strategy for taking into account the distribution (or incidence/prevalence) of a risk factor, as well as its effect size, in order to estimate its population impact on neurodevelopment of children. The total numbers of Full-Scale IQ points lost among U.S. children 0–5 years of age were estimated for chemicals (methylmercury, organophosphate pesticides, lead) and a variety of medical conditions and events (e.g., preterm birth, traumatic brain injury, brain tumors, congenital heart disease). Although the data required for the analysis were available for only three environmental chemicals (methylmercury, organophosphate pesticides, lead), the results suggest that their contributions to neurodevelopmental morbidity are substantial, exceeding those of many nonchemical risk factors. A method for comparing the relative contributions of different risk factors provides a rational basis for establishing priorities for reducing neurodevelopmental morbidity in children.

In Chapter 3, Spivey details several key discoveries by investigators at the National Institute of Environmental Health Sciences (NIEHS) about some of the basic mechanisms involved in synaptic plasticity, and work by other investigators that explores the hypothesis that environmental toxicants that disrupt synaptic plasticity at critical periods play a role in disorders that have roots in early brain development, such as autism spectrum disorders (ASDs), attention deficit/hyperactivity disorder, and schizophrenia.

In a longitudinal birth cohort study of inner-city mothers and children (Columbia Center for Children's Environmental Health), the authors of Chapter 4, Rauh and colleagues, previously reported that prenatal exposure to chlorpyrifos (CPF) was associated with neurodevelopmental problems at 3 years of age. The goal of the current study was to estimate the relationship between prenatal CPF exposure and neurodevelopment among cohort children at 7 years of age. In a sample of 265 children, participants in a prospective study of air pollution, the authors measured prenatal CPF exposure using umbilical cord blood plasma (picograms/gram plasma) and 7-year neurodevelopment using the Wechsler Intelligence Scale for Children, 4th edition (WISC-IV). Linear regression models were used to estimate associations, with covariate selection based on two alternate approaches. On average, for each standard deviation increase in CPF exposure (4.61 pg/g), Full-Scale intelligence quotient (IQ) declined by 1.4% and Working Memory declined by 2.8%. Final covariates included maternal educational level, maternal IQ, and quality of the home environment. The authors found no significant interactions between CPF and any covariates, including the other chemical exposures measured during the prenatal period (environmental tobacco smoke and polycyclic aromatic hydrocarbons). The article reports evidence of deficits in Working Memory Index and Full-Scale IQ as a function of prenatal CPF exposure at 7 years of age. These findings are important in light of continued widespread use of CPF in agricultural settings and possible longer-term educational implications of early cognitive deficits.

Endocrine disruptors are substances commonly encountered in every setting and condition in the modern world. It is virtually impossible to avoid the contact with these chemical compounds in our daily life.

Molecules defined as endocrine disruptors constitute an extremely heterogeneous group and include synthetic chemicals used as industrial solvents/lubricants and their by-products. Natural chemicals found in human and animal food (phytoestrogens) also act as endocrine disruptors. Different from adults, children are not exposed only to chemical toxins in the environment but may also be exposed during their intrauterine life. Hundreds of toxic substances, which include neuro-immune and endocrine toxic chemical components that may influence the critical steps of hormonal, neurological and immunological development, may affect the fetus via the placental cord and these substances may be excreted in the meconium. Children and especially newborns are more sensitive to environmental toxins compared to adults. Metabolic pathways are immature, especially in the first months of life. The ability of the newborn to metabolize, detoxify and eliminate many toxins is different from that of the adults. Although exposures occur during fetal or neonatal period, their effects may sometimes be observed in later years. Chapter 5, by Ünüvar and Büyükgebiz, aregues that further studies are needed to clarify the effects of these substances on the endocrine system and to provide evidence for preventive measures.

In Chapter 6, Landrigan and colleagues argue that researchers need defined strategies for sorting through the extreme claims often made by advocacy groups. The authors outline some of the future research that needs to be done.

Autism Spectrum Disorders (ASD) is a syndrome with a number of etiologies and different mechanisms that lead to abnormal development. The identification of autism biomarkers in patients with different degrees of clinical presentation (i.e., mild, moderate and severe) will give greater insight into the pathogenesis of this disease and will enable effective early diagnostic strategies and treatments for this disorder. In Chapter 7, Alabdali and colleagues measure the concentration of two toxic heavy metals, lead (Pb) and mercury (Hg), in red blood cells, while glutathione-s-transferase (GST) and vitamin E, as enzymatic and non-enzymatic antioxidants, respectively, were measured in the plasma of subgroups of autistic patients with different Social Responsiveness Scale (SRS) and Childhood Autism Rating Scale (CARS) scores. The results were compared to age- and gender-matched healthy controls. The obtained data showed that the patients with autism spectrum disorder had significantly higher Pb and Hg levels and lower GST activity and vitamin E concentrations compared with the controls. The levels of heavy metals (Hg and Pb), GST and vitamin E were correlated with the severity of the social and cognitive impairment measures (SRS and CARS). Receiver Operating Characteristics (ROC) analysis and predictiveness curves indicated that the four parameters show satisfactory sensitivity, very high specificity and excellent predictiveness. Multiple regression analyses confirmed that higher levels of Hg and Pb, together with lower levels of GST and vitamin E, can be used to predict social and cognitive impairment in patients with autism spectrum disorders. This study confirms earlier studies that implicate toxic metal accumulation as a consequence of impaired detoxification in autism and provides insight into the etiological mechanism of autism.

The interactions between genes and the environment are now regarded as the most probable explanation for autism. In Chapter 8, Yasuda and Tsutsui summarize the results of a metallomics study in which scalp hair concentrations of 26 trace elements were examined for 1,967 autistic children (1,553 males and 414 females aged 0–15 years-old), and discuss recent advances in our understanding of epigenetic roles of infantile mineral imbalances in the pathogenesis of autism. In the 1,967 subjects, 584 (29.7%) and 347 (17.6%) were found deficient in zinc and magnesium, respectively, and the incidence rate of zinc deficiency was estimated at 43.5% in male and 52.5% in female infantile subjects aged 0–3 years-old. In contrast, 339 (17.2%), 168 (8.5%) and 94 (4.8%) individuals were found to suffer from high burdens of aluminum, cadmium and lead, respectively, and 2.8% or less from mercury and arsenic. High toxic metal burdens were more frequently observed in the infants aged 0–3 years-old, whose incidence rates were 20.6%, 12.1%, 7.5%, 3.2% and 2.3% for aluminum, cadmium, lead, arsenic and mercury, respectively. These findings suggest that infantile zinc- and magnesium-deficiency and/or toxic metal burdens may be critical and induce epigenetic alterations in the genes and genetic regulation mechanisms of neurodevelopment in the autistic children, and demonstrate that a time factor "infantile window" is also critical for neurodevelopment and probably for therapy. Thus, early metallomics analysis may lead to early screening/estimation and treatment/prevention for the autistic neurodevelopment disorders.

Increased urinary concentrations of pentacarboxyl-, precopro- and copro-porphyrins have been associated with prolonged mercury (Hg) exposure in adults, and comparable increases have been attributed to Hg exposure in children with autism (AU). The study performend in Chapter 9 by Woods and colleagues was designed to measure and compare urinary porphyrin concentrations in neurotypical (NT) children and same-age children with autism, and to examine the association between porphyrin levels and past or current Hg exposure in children with autism. This exploratory study enrolled 278 children 2–12 years of age. The authors evaluated three groups: AU, pervasive developmental disorder-not otherwise specified (PDD-NOS), and NT. Mothers/caregivers provided information at enrollment regarding medical, dental, and dietary exposures. Urine samples from all children were acquired for analyses of porphyrin, creatinine, and Hg. Differences between groups for mean porphyrin and Hg levels were evaluated. Logistic regression analysis was conducted to determine whether porphyrin levels were associated with increased risk of autism. Mean urinary porphyrin concentrations are naturally high in young children and decline by as much as 2.5-fold between 2 and 12 years of age. Elevated copro- ($p < 0.009$), hexacarboxyl- ($p < 0.01$) and pentacarboxyl- ($p < 0.001$) porphyrin concentrations were significantly associated with AU but not with PDD-NOS. No differences were found between NT and AU in urinary Hg levels or in past Hg exposure as determined by fish consumption, number of dental amalgam fillings, or vaccines received. These findings identify disordered porphyrin metabolism as a salient characteristic of autism. Hg exposures were comparable between diagnostic groups, and a porphyrin pattern consistent with that seen in Hg-exposed adults was not apparent.

The role of thimerosal containing vaccines in the development of autism spectrum disorder (ASD) has been an area of intense debate, as has the presence of mercury dental amalgams and fish ingestion by pregnant mothers. In Chapter 10, Sharpe and colleagues studied the effects of thimerosal on cell proliferation and mitochondrial function from B-lymphocytes taken from individuals with autism, their nonautistic twins, and their nontwin siblings. Eleven families were examined and compared to matched controls. B-cells were grown with increasing levels of thimerosal, and various assays (LDH, XTT, DCFH, etc.) were performed to examine the effects on cellular proliferation and mitochondrial function. A subpopulation of eight individuals (4 ASD, 2 twins, and 2 siblings) from four of the families showed thimerosal hypersensitivity, whereas none of the control individuals displayed this response. The thimerosal concentration required to inhibit cell proliferation in these individuals was only 40% of controls. Cells hypersensitive to thimerosal also had higher levels of oxidative stress markers, protein carbonyls, and oxidant generation. This suggests certain individuals with a mild mitochondrial defect may be highly susceptible to mitochondrial specific toxins like the vaccine preservative thimerosal.

Attention deficit/hyperactivity disorder (ADHD) is the most frequently diagnosed childhood neurobehavioral disorder. Much research has been done to identify genetic, environmental, and social risk factors for ADHD; however, we are still far from fully understanding its etiology. In Chapter 11, Agular and colleagues provide an overview of diagnostic criteria for ADHD and what is known about its biological basis. The authors also review the neuropsychological functions that are affected in ADHD. The goal is to familiarize the reader with the behavioral deficits that are hallmarks of ADHD and to facilitate comparisons with neurobehavioral deficits associated with environmental chemical exposures. Relevant literature on ADHD is reviewed, focusing in particular on meta-analyses conducted between 2004 and the present that evaluated associations between measures of neuropsychological function and ADHD in children. Meta-analyses were obtained through searches of the PubMed electronic database using the terms "ADHD," "meta-analysis," "attention," "executive," and "neuropsychological functions." Although meta-analyses are emphasized, nonquantitative reviews are included for particular neuropsychological functions where no meta-analyses were available. The meta-analyses indicate that vigilance (sustained attention), response inhibition, and working memory are impaired in children diagnosed with ADHD. Similar but somewhat less consistent meta-analytic findings have been reported for impairments in alertness, cognitive flexibility, and planning. Additionally, the literature suggests deficits in temporal information processing and altered responses to reinforcement in children diagnosed with ADHD. Findings from brain imagining and neurochemistry studies support the behavioral findings. Behavioral, neuroanatomical, and neurochemical data indicate substantial differences in attention and executive functions between children diagnosed with ADHD and non-ADHD controls. Comparisons of the neurobehavioral deficits associated with ADHD and those associated with exposures to environmental chemicals may help to identify possible environmental risk factors for ADHD and/or reveal common underlying biological mechanisms.

Exposure to polycyclic aromatic hydrocarbons (PAHs) adversely affects child neurodevelopment, but little is known about the relationship between PAHs and clinically significant developmental disorders. In Chapter 12, Abid and colleagues examined the relationship between childhood measures of PAH exposure and prevalence of attention deficit/ hyperactivity disorder (ADHD), learning disability (LD), and special education (SE) in a nationally representative sample of 1,257 U.S. children 6-15 years of age. Data were obtained from the National Health and Nutrition Examination Survey (NHANES) 2001-2004. PAH exposure was measured by urinary metabolite concentrations. Outcomes were defined by parental report of (1) ever doctor-diagnosed ADHD, (2) ever doctor- or school representative-identified LD, and (3) receipt of SE or early intervention services. Multivariate logistic regression accounting for survey sampling was used to determine the associations between PAH metabolites and ADHD, LD, and SE. Children exposed to higher levels of fluorine metabolites had a 2-fold increased odds (95% C.I. 1.1, 3.8) of SE, and this association was more apparent in males (OR 2.3; 95% C.I. 1.2, 4.1) than in females (OR 1.8; 95% C.I. 0.6, 5.4). No other consistent pattern of developmental disorders was associated with urinary PAH metabolites. However, concurrent exposure to PAH fluorine metabolites may increase use of special education services among U.S. children.

Perfluorinated compounds (PFCs) are persistent environmental pollutants. Toxicology studies demonstrate the potential for perfluorooctanoic acid (PFOA) and other PFCs to affect human growth and development. Attention deficit/hyperactivity disorder (ADHD) is a developmental disorder with suspected environmental and genetic etiology. Chapter 13, by Stein and Savitz, examined the cross-sectional association between serum PFC concentration and parent or self-report of doctor-diagnosed ADHD with and without current ADHD medication. The authors used data from the C8 Health Project, a 2005–2006 survey in a Mid-Ohio Valley community highly exposed to PFOA through contaminated drinking water, to study non-Hispanic white children 5–18 years of age. Logistic regression models were adjusted for age and sex. Of the 10,546 eligible children, 12.4% reported ADHD and 5.1% reported ADHD plus ADHD medication use. We observed an inverted J-shaped association between PFOA and ADHD, with a small increase in prevalence for the second quartile of exposure compared with the lowest, and a decrease for the highest versus lowest quartile. The prevalence of ADHD plus medication increased with perfluorohexane sulfonate (PFHxS) levels, with an adjusted odds ratio of 1.59 (95% confidence interval, 1.21–2.08) comparing the highest quartile of exposure to the lowest. The authors observed a modest association between perfluorooctane sulfonate and ADHD with medication. The most notable finding for PFOA and ADHD, a reduction in prevalence at the highest exposure level, is unlikely to be causal, perhaps reflecting a spurious finding related to the geographic determination of PFOA exposure in this population or to unmeasured behavioral or physiologic correlates of exposure and outcome. Possible positive associations between other PFCs and ADHD, particularly PFHxS, warrant continued investigation.

California children's exposures to polybrominated diphenyl ether flame retardants (PBDEs) are among the highest worldwide. PBDEs are known endocrine disruptors and neurotoxicants in animals. In Chapter 14, Eskenazi and colleagues investigate the relation of in utero and child PBDE exposure to neurobehavioral development among participants in CHAMACOS (Center for the Health Assessment of Mothers and Children of Salinas), a California birth cohort. The authors measured PBDEs in maternal prenatal and child serum samples and examined the association of PBDE concentrations with children's attention, motor functioning, and cognition at 5 (n = 310) and 7 years of age (n = 323). Maternal prenatal PBDE concentrations were associated with impaired attention as measured by a continuous performance task at 5 years and maternal report at 5 and 7 years of age, with poorer fine motor coordination—particularly in the nondominant—at both age points, and with decrements in Verbal and Full-Scale IQ at 7 years. PBDE concentrations in children 7 years of age were significantly or marginally associated with concurrent teacher reports of attention problems and decrements in Processing Speed, Perceptual Reasoning, Verbal Comprehension, and Full-Scale IQ. These associations were not altered by adjustment for birth weight, gestational age, or maternal thyroid hormone levels. Both prenatal and childhood PBDE exposures were associated with poorer attention, fine motor coordination, and cognition in the CHAMACOS cohort of school-age children. This study, the largest to date, contributes to growing evidence suggesting that PBDEs have adverse impacts on child neurobehavioral development.

Although adaptation and proper biological functioning require developmental programming, pollutant interference can cause developmental toxicity or DT. The commentary in Chapter 15, by Shrader-Frechette, assesses whether it is ethical for citizens/physicians/scientists to allow avoidable DT. Using conceptual, economic, ethical, and logical analysis, the commentary assesses what major ethical theories and objectors would say regarding the defensibility of allowing avoidable DT. The commentary argues that (1) none of the four major ethical theories (based, respectively, on virtue, natural law, utility, or equity) can consistently defend avoidable DT because it unjustifiably harms, respectively, individual human flourishing, human life, the greatest good, and equality. (2) Justice also requires leaving "as much and as good" biological resources for all, including future generations possibly harmed if epigenetic change is heritable. (3) Scientists/physicians have greater justice-based duties, than ordinary/average citizens, to help stop DT because they help cause it and have greater professional abilities/opportunities to help stop it. (4) Scientists/physicians likewise have greater justice-based duties, than ordinary/average citizens, to help stop DT because they benefit more from it, given their relatively greater education/consumption/income. The paper shows that major objections to (3)-(4) fail on logical, ethical, or scientific grounds, then closes with practical suggestions for implementing its proposals. Because allowing avoidable DT is ethically indefensible, citizens---and especially physicians/scientists---have justice-based duties to help stop DT.

PART I

OVERVIEW

CHAPTER 1

AMERICA'S CHILDREN AND THE ENVIRONMENT: NEURODEVELOPMENTAL DISORDERS (EXCERPT FROM THE THIRD EDITION)

UNITED STATES ENVIRONMENTAL PROTECTION AGENCY

Neurodevelopmental disorders are disabilities associated primarily with the functioning of the neurological system and brain. Examples of neurodevelopmental disorders in children include attention-deficit/hyperactivity disorder (ADHD), autism, learning disabilities, intellectual disability (also known as mental retardation), conduct disorders, cerebral palsy, and impairments in vision and hearing. Children with neurodevelopmental disorders can experience difficulties with language and speech, motor skills, behavior, memory, learning, or other neurological functions. While the symptoms and behaviors of neurodevelopmental disabilities often change or evolve as a child grows older, some disabilities are permanent. Diagnosis and treatment of these disorders can be difficult; treatment often involves a combination of professional therapy, pharmaceuticals, and home- and school-based programs.

U.S. Environmental Protection Agency. Neurodevelopmental Disorders. In: America's Children and the Environment: Third Edition. *EPA 240-R-13-001. http://www.epa.gov/ace/pdfs/Health-Neurodevelopmental.pdf. Published January 2013. Accessed 15 July, 2014.*

Based on parental responses to survey questions, approximately 15% of children in the United States ages 3 to 17 years were affected by neurodevelopmental disorders, including ADHD, learning disabilities, intellectual disability, cerebral palsy, autism, seizures, stuttering or stammering, moderate to profound hearing loss, blindness, and other developmental delays, in 2006–2008. [1] Among these conditions, ADHD and learning disabilities had the greatest prevalence. Many children affected by neurodevelopmental disorders have more than one of these conditions: for example, about 4% of U.S. children have both ADHD and a learning disability. [2] Some researchers have stated that the prevalence of certain neurodevelopmental disorders, specifically autism and ADHD, has been increasing over the last four decades. [3-7] Longterm trends in these conditions are difficult to detect with certainty, due to a lack of data to track prevalence over many years as well as changes in awareness and diagnostic criteria. However, some detailed reviews of historical data have concluded that the actual prevalence of autism seems to be rising. [4,8-10] Surveys of educators and pediatricians have reported a rise in the number of children seen in classrooms and exam rooms with behavioral and learning disorders. [11-13]

Genetics can play an important role in many neurodevelopmental disorders, and some cases of certain conditions such as intellectual disability are associated with specific genes. However, most neurodevelopmental disorders have complex and multiple contributors rather than any one clear cause. These disorders likely result from a combination of genetic, biological, psychosocial and environmental risk factors. A broad range of environmental risk factors may affect neurodevelopment, including (but not limited to) maternal use of alcohol, tobacco, or illicit drugs during pregnancy; lower socioeconomic status; preterm birth; low birthweight; the physical environment; and prenatal or childhood exposure to certain environmental contaminants. [14-21]

Lead, methylmercury, and PCBs are widespread environmental contaminants associated with adverse effects on a child's developing brain and nervous system in multiple studies. The National Toxicology Program (NTP) has concluded that childhood lead exposure is associated with reduced cognitive function, including lower intelligence quotient (IQ) and reduced academic achievement. [22] The NTP has also concluded that childhood lead exposure is associated with attention-related behavioral problems (including inattention, hyperactivity, and diagnosed attention-deficit/hyperactivity disorder) and increased incidence of problem behaviors (including delinquent, criminal, or antisocial behavior). [22]

EPA has determined that methylmercury is known to have neurotoxic and developmental effects in humans. [23] Extreme cases of such effects were seen in people prenatally exposed during two high-dose mercury poisoning events in Japan and Iraq, who experienced severe adverse health effects such as cerebral palsy, mental retardation, deafness, and blindness. [24-26] Prospective cohort studies have been conducted in island populations where frequent fish consumption leads to methylmercury exposure in pregnant women at levels much lower than in the poisoning incidents but much greater than those typically observed in the United States. Results from such studies in New Zealand and the Faroe Islands suggest that increased prenatal mercury exposure due to maternal fish consumption was associated with adverse effects on intelligence and decreased functioning in the areas of language, attention, and memory. [26-32] These associations were not seen in initial results reported from a similar study in the Seychelles Islands. [33] However, further studies in the Seychelles found associations between prenatal mercury exposure and some neurodevelopmental deficits after researchers had accounted for the developmental benefits of fish consumption. [34-36] More recent studies conducted in the United States have found associations between neurodevelopmental effects and blood mercury levels within the range typical for U.S. women, after accounting for the beneficial effects of fish consumption during pregnancy. [32,37,38]

Several studies of children who were prenatally exposed to elevated levels of polychlorinated biphenyls (PCBs) have suggested linkages between these contaminants and neurodevelopmental effects, including lowered intelligence and behavioral deficits such as inattention and impulsive behavior. [39-44] Studies have also reported associations between PCB exposure and deficits in learning and memory. [39,45] Most of these studies found that the effects are associated with exposure in the womb resulting from the mother having eaten food contaminated with PCBs, [46-51] although some studies have reported relationships between adverse effects and PCB exposure during infancy and childhood. [45,51-53]

Although there is some inconsistency in the epidemiological literature, several reviews of the literature have found that the overall evidence supports a concern for effects of PCBs on children's neurological development. [52,54-58] The Agency for Toxic Substances and Disease Registry has determined that "Substantial data suggest that PCBs play a role in neurobehavioral alterations observed in newborns and young children of women with PCB burdens near background levels." [59] In addition, adverse effects on intelligence and behavior have been found in children of women who were highly exposed to mixtures of PCBs, chlorinated dibenzofurans, and other pollutants prior to conception. [60-63]

A wide variety of other environmental chemicals have been identified as potential concerns for childhood neurological development, but have not been as well studied for these effects as lead, mercury, and PCBs. Concerns for these additional chemicals are based on both laboratory animal studies and human epidemiological research; in most cases, the epidemiological studies are relatively new and the literature is just beginning to develop. Among the chemicals being studied for potential effects on childhood neurological development are organophosphate pesticides, polybrominated diphenyl ether flame retardants (PBDEs), phthalates, bisphenol A (BPA), polycyclic aromatic hydrocarbons (PAHs), arsenic, and perchlorate. Exposure to all of these chemicals is widespread in the United States for both children and adults. [64]

Organophosphate pesticides can interfere with the proper function of the nervous system when exposure is sufficiently high. [65] Many children may have low capacity to detoxify organophosphate pesticides through age 7 years. [66] In addition, recent studies have reported an association between prenatal organophosphate exposure and childhood ADHD in a U.S. community with relatively high exposures to organophosphate pesticides, [67] as well as with exposures found within the general U.S. population. [68] Other recent studies have described associations between prenatal organophosphate pesticide exposures and a variety of neurodevelopmental deficits in childhood, including reduced IQ, perceptual reasoning, and memory. [69-71]

Studies of certain PBDEs have found adverse effects on behavior, learning, and memory in laboratory animals. [72-74] A recent epidemiological study in New York City reported significant associations between children's prenatal exposure to PBDEs and reduced performance on IQ tests and other tests of neurological development in 6-year-old children. [75] Another study in the Netherlands reported significant associations between children's prenatal exposure to PBDEs and reduced performance on some neurodevelopmental tests in 5- and 6-year-old children, while associations with improved performance were observed for other tests. [76]

Two studies of a group of New York City children ages 4 to 9 years reported associations between prenatal exposure to certain phthalates and behavioral deficits, including effects on attention, conduct, and social behaviors. [77,78] Some of the behavioral deficits observed in these studies are similar to those commonly displayed in children with ADHD and conduct disorder. Studies conducted in South Korea of children ages 8 to 11 years reported that children with higher levels of certain phthalate metabolites in their urine were more inattentive and hyperactive, displayed more symptoms of ADHD, and had lower IQ compared with those who had lower levels. [79,80] The exposure levels in these studies are comparable to typical exposures in the U.S. population.

In 2008, the NTP concluded that there is "some concern" for effects of early-life (including prenatal) BPA exposure on brain development and behavior, based on findings of animal studies conducted at relatively low doses. [81] An epidemiological study conducted in Ohio reported an association between prenatal exposure to BPA and effects on children's behavior (increased hyperactivity and aggression) at age 2 years. [82] Another study of prenatal BPA exposure in New York City reported no association between prenatal BPA exposure and social behavior deficits in testing conducted at ages 7 to 9 years. [78]

A series of recent studies conducted in New York City has reported that children of women who were exposed to increased levels of polycyclic aromatic hydrocarbons (PAHs, produced when gasoline and other materials are burned) during pregnancy are more likely to have experienced adverse effects on neurological development (for example, reduced IQ and behavioral problems). [83,84]

Early-life exposure to arsenic has been associated with measures of reduced cognitive function, including lower scores on tests that measure neurobehavioral and intellectual development, in four studies conducted in Asia; however there are some inconsistencies in the findings of these studies. [85] These findings are from countries where arsenic levels in drinking water are generally much higher than in the United States due to high levels of naturally occurring arsenic in groundwater. [86]

Perchlorate is a naturally occurring and man-made chemical that has been found in drinking water [87] and foods [88,89] in the United States. Exposure to elevated levels of perchlorate inhibits iodide uptake into the thyroid gland, thus possibly disrupting the function of the thyroid and potentially leading to a reduction in the production of thyroid hormone. [90,91] Moderate deficits in maternal thyroid hormone levels during early pregnancy have been linked to reduced childhood IQ scores and other neurodevelopmental effects. [92-94]

Interactions of environmental contaminants and other environmental factors may combine to increase the risk of neurodevelopmental disorders. For example, exposure to lead may have stronger effects on neurodevelopment among children with lower socioeconomic status. [21,95]

A child's brain and nervous system are vulnerable to adverse impacts from pollutants because they go through a long developmental process beginning shortly after conception and continuing through adolescence. [96,97] This complex developmental process requires the precise coordination of cell growth and movement, and may be disrupted by even short-term exposures to environmental contaminants if they occur at critical stages of development. This disruption can lead to neurodevelopmental deficits that may have an effect on the child's achievements and behavior even when they do not result in a diagnosable disorder.

1.1 ATTENTION-DEFICIT/HYPERACTIVITY DISORDER (ADHD)

Attention-deficit/hyperactivity disorder (ADHD) is a disruptive behavior disorder characterized by symptoms of inattention and/or hyperactivity-impulsivity, occurring in several settings and more frequently and severely than is typical for other individuals in the same stage of development. [98] ADHD can make family and peer relationships difficult, diminish academic performance, and reduce vocational achievement.

As the medical profession has developed a greater understanding of ADHD through the years, the name of this condition has changed. The

American Psychiatric Association adopted the name "attention deficit disorder" in the early 1980s and revised it to "attention deficit/ hyperactivity disorder" in 1987. [99] Many children with ADHD have a mix of inattention and hyperactivity/impulsivity behaviors, while some may display primarily hyperactive behavior traits, and others display primarily inattentive traits. It is possible for an individual's primary symptoms of ADHD to change over time. [20] Children with ADHD frequently have other disorders, with parents reporting that about half of children with ADHD have a learning disability and about one in four have a conduct disorder. [2,100]

Other disorders, including anxiety disorders, depression, and learning disabilities, can be expressed with signs and symptoms that resemble those of ADHD. A diagnosis of ADHD requires a certain amount of judgment on the part of a doctor, similar to diagnosis of other mental disorders. Despite the variability among children diagnosed with the disorder and the challenges involved in diagnosis, ADHD has good clinical validity, meaning that impaired children share similarities, exhibit symptoms, respond to treatment, and are recognized with general consistency across clinicians. [20]

A great deal of research on ADHD has focused on aspects of brain functioning that are related to the behaviors associated with ADHD. Although this research is not definitive, it has found that children with ADHD generally have trouble with certain skills involved in problem-solving (referred to collectively as executive function). These skills include working memory (keeping information in mind while briefly doing something else), planning (organizing a sequence of activities to complete a task), response inhibition (suppressing immediate responses when they are inappropriate), and cognitive flexibility (changing an approach when a situation changes). Children with ADHD also generally have problems in maintaining sustained attention to a task (referred to as vigilance), and/or maintaining readiness to respond to new information (referred to as alertness). [20,101,102]

While uncertainties remain, findings to date indicate that ADHD is caused by combinations of genetic and environmental factors. [20,103-106] Much of the research on environmental factors has focused on the fetal environment. Maternal smoking during pregnancy has been associated with increased risk of ADHD in the child in numerous studies, however, this continues to be an active area of research as scientists consider whether other factors related to smoking (e.g., genetic factors, maternal mental health, stress, alcohol use, and low birth weight) may be responsible for associations attributed to smoking. [17,19,107] Findings regarding ADHD and maternal consumption of alcohol during pregnancy are considered more limited and inconsistent. [19,20] Preterm birth and low birth weight have also been found to increase the likelihood that a child will have ADHD. [16,18,20] Psychosocial adversity (representing factors such as low socioeconomic status and in-home conflict) in childhood may also play a role in ADHD. [108]

The potential role of environmental contaminants in contributing to ADHD, either alone or in conjunction with certain genetic susceptibilities or other environmental factors, is becoming better understood as a growing number of studies look explicitly at the relationship between ADHD and exposures to environmental contaminants.

Among environmental contaminants known or suspected to be developmental neurotoxicants, lead has the most extensive evidence of a potential contribution to ADHD. A number of recent epidemiological studies (all published since 2006, with data gathered beginning in 1999 or more recently) conducted in the United States and Asia have reported relationships between increased levels of lead in a child's blood and increased likelihood of ADHD. [55,109-115] In most of these studies, blood lead levels were comparable to levels observed currently in the United States. The potential contribution of childhood lead exposure to the risk of ADHD may be amplified in children of women who smoked cigarettes during pregnancy. [110] In addition, several studies have reported relationships between blood lead levels and the aspects of brain functioning that are most affected in children with ADHD, including sustained attention, alertness, and problem-solving skills (executive functions, specifically cognitive flexibility, working memory, planning, and response inhibition). [22,44,55,116-119] Similar results have been observed in laboratory animal studies. [55,96,120-122] The NTP has concluded that childhood lead exposure is "associated with increased diagnosis of attention-related behavioral problems." [22]

Although no studies evaluating a potential association between PCBs and ADHD itself have been published, a study in Massachusetts reported a relationship between levels of PCBs measured in cord blood and increased ADHD-like behaviors observed by teachers in children at ages 7 to 11 years. PCB levels in this study were generally lower than those measured in other epidemiological studies of PCBs and childhood neurological development. [40] Other research findings also suggest that PCBs may play a role in contributing to ADHD. Several studies in U.S. and European populations, most having elevated exposure to PCBs through the diet, have found generally consistent associations with aspects of brain function that are most affected in children with ADHD, including alertness and problem-solving skills (executive functions, specifically response inhibition, working memory, cognitive flexibility, and planning). [54,55] Studies in laboratory animals have similar findings regarding the mental functions affected by PCB exposure. [55,96]

Studies of other environmental chemicals reporting associations with ADHD or related outcomes have been published in recent years, but findings tend to be much more limited than for lead and PCBs. Findings for phthalates and organophosphate pesticides were noted above. In addition, three studies have reported associations between ADHD or impulsivity and concentrations of certain perfluorinated chemicals measured in the blood of children. [123-125] Studies of mercury have produced generally mixed findings of associations with ADHD or related symptoms and mental functions. [29,111,118,126-128]

1.2 LEARNING DISABILITY

Learning disability (or learning disorder) is a general term for a neurological disorder that affects the way in which a child's brain can receive, process, retain, and respond to information. A child with a learning disability may have trouble learning and using certain skills, including reading, writing, listening, speaking, reasoning, and doing math, although learning disabilities vary from child to child. Children with learning disabilities usually have average or above-average intelligence, but there are differences in the way their brains process information. [129]

As with many other neurodevelopmental disorders, the causes of learning disabilities are not well understood. Often learning disabilities run in the family, suggesting that heredity may play a role in their development. Problems during pregnancy and birth, such as drug or alcohol use during pregnancy, low birth weight, lack of oxygen, or premature or prolonged labor, may also lead to learning disabilities. [130]

As is the case with other neurodevelopmental outcomes, there are generally many more studies of lead exposure that are relevant to learning disabilities than for other environmental contaminants. Several studies have found associations between lead exposure and learning disabilities or reduced classroom performance that are independent of IQ. [119,120,131-133] Exposures to lead have been associated with impaired memory and difficulties or impairments in rule learning, following directions, planning, verbal abilities, speech processing, and classroom performance in children. [22,119,131,134-137] Other findings that may indicate contributions from environmental contaminants to learning disabilities include a study that found associations of both maternal smoking during pregnancy and childhood exposure to environmental tobacco smoke with parent report of a child with a learning disability diagnosis; [138] associations of prenatal mercury exposure with dysfunctions in children's language abilities and memory, [29,30] and associations of prenatal PCB exposure with poorer concentration and memory deficits compared with unexposed children. [39,45]

1.3 AUTISM SPECTRUM DISORDERS

Autism spectrum disorders (ASDs) are a group of developmental disabilities defined by significant social, communication, and behavioral impairments. The term "spectrum disorders" refers to the fact that although people with ASDs share some common symptoms, ASDs affect different people in different ways, with some experiencing very mild symptoms and others experiencing severe symptoms. ASDs encompass autistic disorder and the generally less severe forms, Asperger's syndrome and pervasive developmental disorder-not otherwise specified (PDD-NOS). Children with ASDs may lack interest in other people, have trouble showing or talking about feelings, and avoid or resist physical contact. A range of communication problems are seen in children with ASDs: some speak very well, while many children with an ASD do not speak at all. Another hallmark characteristic of ASDs is the demonstration of restrictive or repetitive interests or behaviors, such as lining up toys, flapping hands, rocking his or her body, or spinning in circles. [139]

To date, no single risk factor sufficient to cause ASD has been identified; rather each case is likely to be caused by the combination of multiple genetic and environmental risk factors. [140-142] Several ASD research findings and hypotheses may imply an important role for environmental contaminants. First, there has been a sharp upward trend in reported prevalence that cannot be fully explained by factors such as younger ages at diagnosis, migration patterns, changes in diagnostic criteria, inclusion of milder cases, or increased parental age. [8,9,143-146] Also, the neurological signaling systems that are impaired in children with ASDs can be affected by certain environmental chemicals. For example, several pesticides are known to interfere with acetylcholine (Ach) and γ-aminobutyric acid (GABA) neurotransmission, chemical messenger systems that have been altered in certain subsets of autistic individuals. [147] Some studies have reported associations between certain pharmaceuticals taken by pregnant women and increased incidence of autism, which may suggest that there are biological pathways by which other chemical exposures during pregnancy could increase the risk of autism. [148]

Furthermore, some of the identified genetic risk factors for autism are de novo mutations, meaning that the genetic defect is not present in either of the parents' genes, yet can be found in the genes of the child when a new genetic mutation forms in a parent's germ cells (egg or sperm), potentially from exposure to contaminants. [140,142,149,150] Many environmental contaminants have been identified as agents capable of causing mutations in DNA, by leading to oxidative DNA damage and by inhibiting the body's normal ability to repair DNA damage. [151] Some children with autism have been shown to display markers of increased oxidative stress, which may strengthen this line of reasoning. [152-154] Many studies have linked increasing paternal and maternal age with increased risk of ASDs. [144,146,155-157] The role of parental age in increased autism risk might be explained by evidence that shows advanced parental age can contribute significantly to the frequency of de novo mutations in a parent's germ cells. [151,158,159] Advanced parental age signifies a longer period

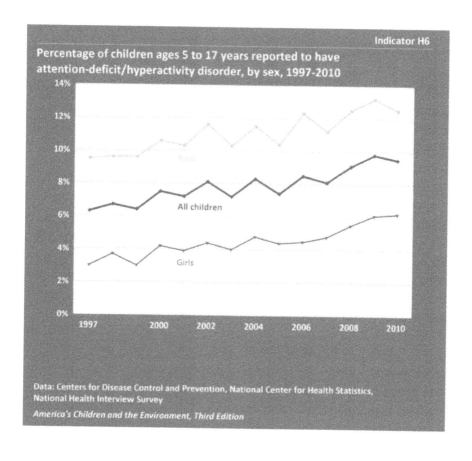

FIGURE 1: Data for this indicator are obtained from an ongoing annual survey conducted by the National Center for Health Statistics. Survey data are representative of the U.S. civilian noninstitutionalized population. A parent or other knowledgeable adult in each sampled household is asked questions regarding the child's health status, including if they have ever been told the child has Attention Deficit/Hyperactivity Disorder (ADHD).

- From 1997 to 2010, the proportion of children ages 5 to 17 years reported to have ever been diagnosed with attention-deficit/hyperactivity disorder (ADHD) increased from 6.3% to 9.5%. The increasing trend was statistically significant for children overall, and for both boys and girls considered separately.
- For the years 2007–2010, the percentage of boys reported to have ADHD (12.4%) was higher than the rate for girls (5.7%). This difference was statistically significant. (See Table H6a.)
- In 2007–2010, 11.6% of children of "All Other Races," 10.7% of White non-Hispanic children,
- 10.2% of Black non-Hispanic children, 4.8% of Hispanic children, and 1.7% of Asian non-Hispanic children were reported to have ADHD. (See Table H6b.) These differences were statistically significant, after accounting for the influence of other demographic differences (i.e., differences in age, sex, and family income), with two exceptions: there was no statistically significant difference between children of "All Other Races" and White non-Hispanic children, or between children of "All Other Races" and Black non-Hispanic children.
- In 2007–2010, 11.3% of children from families living below the poverty level were reported to have ADHD compared with 8.6% of children from families living at or above the poverty level. This difference was statistically significant. (See Table H6b.)

of time when environmental exposures may act on germ cells and cause DNA damage and de novo mutations. Finally, a recent study concluded that the role of genetic factors in ASDs has been overestimated, and that environmental factors play a greater role than genetic factors in contributing to autism. [141] This study did not evaluate the role of any particular environmental factors, and in this context "environmental factors" are defined broadly to include any influence that is not genetic.

Studies, limited in number and often limited in research design, have examined the possible role that certain environmental contaminants may play in the development of ASDs. A number of these studies have focused on mercury exposures. Earlier studies reported higher levels of mercury in the blood, baby teeth, and urine of children with ASDs compared with control children; [160-162] however, another more recent study reported

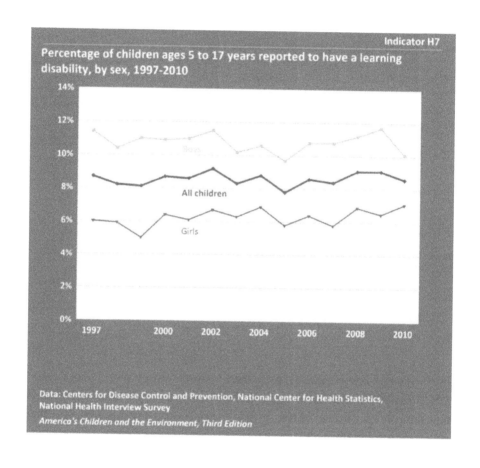

FIGURE 2: Data for this indicator are obtained from an ongoing annual survey conducted by the National Center for Health Statistics. Survey data are representative of the U.S. civilian noninstitutionalized population. A parent or other knowledgeable adult in each sampled household is asked questions regarding the child's health status, including if they have ever been told the child has a learning disability.

- In 2010, 8.6% of children ages 5 to 17 years had ever been diagnosed with a learning disability. There was little change in this percentage between 1997 and 2010.
- For the years 2007–2010, the percentage of boys reported to have a learning disability (10.9%) was higher than for girls (6.6%). This difference was statistically significant. (See Table H7a.)
- The reported prevalence of learning disability varies by race and ethnicity. The highest percentages of learning disability are reported for children of "All Other Races" (11.2%), Black non-Hispanic children (10.2%), and White non-Hispanic children (9.3%). By comparison, 7.2% of Hispanic children are reported to have a learning disability, and Asian non-Hispanic children have the lowest prevalence of learning disability, at 2.7%. (See Table H7b.)
- The prevalence of learning disability reported for Hispanic children and for Asian non-Hispanic children were lower than for the remaining race/ethnicity groups, and these differences were statistically significant. The difference in prevalence between Hispanic and Asian non-Hispanic children was also statistically significant.
- For the years 2007–2010, the percentage of children reported to have a learning disability was higher for children living below the poverty level (12.6%) compared with those living at or above the poverty level (7.9%), a statistically significant difference. (See Table H7b.)

no difference in the blood mercury levels of children with autism and typically developing children. [163] Proximity to industrial and power plant sources of environmental mercury was reported to be associated with increased autism prevalence in a study conducted in Texas. [164]

Thimerosal is a mercury-containing preservative that is used in some vaccines to prevent contamination and growth of harmful bacteria in vaccine vials. Since 2001, thimerosal has not been used in routinely administered childhood vaccines, with the exception of some influenza vaccines. [165] The Institute of Medicine has rejected the hypothesis of a causal relationship between thimerosal-containing vaccines and autism. [166]

Some studies have also considered air pollutants as possible contributors to autism. A study conducted in the San Francisco Bay Area reported an association between the amount of certain airborne pollutants at a child's place of birth (mercury, cadmium, nickel, trichloroethylene, and vinyl chloride) and the risk for autism, but a similar study in North Carolina and West Virginia did not find such a relationship. [167,168] Another study in California reported that mothers who lived near a freeway at the time of delivery were more likely to have children diagnosed with autism, suggesting that exposure to traffic-related air pollutants may play a role in contributing to ASDs. [169]

Finally, a study in Sweden reported an increased risk of ASDs in children born to families living in homes with polyvinyl chloride (PVC) flooring, which is a source of certain phthalates in indoor environments. [170]

1.4 INTELLECTUAL DISABILITY (MENTAL RETARDATION)

The most commonly used definitions of intellectual disability (also referred to as mental retardation) emphasize subaverage intellectual functioning before the age of 18, usually defined as an IQ less than 70 and impairments in life skills such as communication, self-care, home living, and social or interpersonal skills. Different severity categories, ranging from mild to severe retardation, are defined on the basis of IQ scores. [171,172] "Intellectual disability" is used as the preferred term for this condition in the disabilities sector, but the term "mental retardation" continues to be used in the contexts of law and public policy when designating eligibility for state and federal programs. [171]

Researchers have identified some causes of intellectual disability, including genetic disorders, traumatic injuries, and prenatal events such as maternal infection or exposure to alcohol. [172,173] However, the causes of intellectual disability are unknown in 30–50% of all cases. [173] The causes are more frequently identified for cases of severe retardation (IQ less than 50), whereas the cause of mild retardation (IQ between 50 and 70) is unknown in more than 75% of cases. [174,175] Exposures to environmental contaminants could be a contributing factor to the cases of mild retardation where the cause is unknown. Exposure to high levels of lead and mercury have been associated with intellectual disability.23, [176-178] Furthermore, lead, mercury, and PCBs all have been found to have adverse effects on intelligence and cognitive functioning in children, [22,26,43,52,179] and recent studies have reported associations of a number of other environmental contaminants with childhood IQ deficits, including organophosphate pesticides, [69-71] PBDEs, [75] phthalates, [79] and PAHs. [83,180] Exposure to environmental contaminants that reduce IQ has the potential to increase the proportion of the population with IQ less than 70, thus increasing the incidence of intellectual disability in an exposed population. [181-183]

1.5 INDICATORS IN THIS SECTION

The four indicators that follow provide the best nationally representative data available on the prevalence of neurodevelopmental disorders among U.S. children over time. The indicators present the number of children ages 5 to 17 years reported to have ever been diagnosed with ADHD (Indicator H6), learning disabilities (Indicator H7), autism (Indicator H8), and intellectual disability (Indicator H9). These four conditions are examples of neurodevelopmental disorders that may be influenced by exposures to environmental contaminants. Intellectual disability and learning disabilities are disorders in which a child's cognitive or intellectual development is affected, and ADHD is a disorder in which a child's behavioral development is affected. Autism spectrum disorders are disorders in which a child's behavior, communication, and social skills are affected.

- Indicator H6: Percentage of children ages 5 to 17 years reported to have attentiondeficit/hyperactivity disorder, by sex, 1997–2010
- Indicator H7: Percentage of children ages 5 to 17 years reported to have a learning disability, by sex, 1997–2010
- Indicator H8: Percentage of children ages 5 to 17 years reported to have autism, 1997–2010
- Indicator H9: Percentage of children ages 5 to 17 years reported to have intellectual disability (mental retardation), 1997–2010

About the Indicators: Indicators H6, H7, H8, and H9 present information about the number of children who are reported to have ever been diagnosed with four different neurodevelopmental disorders: attention-deficit/hyperactivity disorder (ADHD), learning disabilities, autism, and intellectual disability. The data come from a national survey that collects health information from a representative sample of the population each year. The four indicators show how the prevalence of children's neurode-

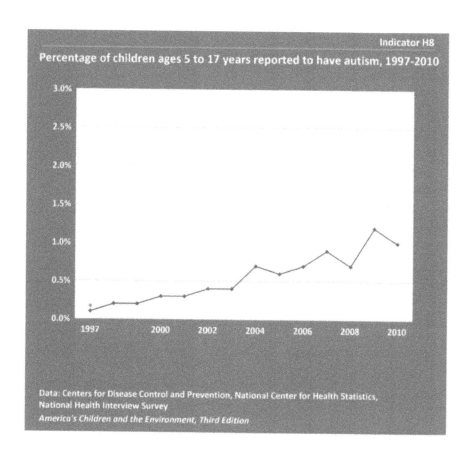

FIGURE 3: Data for this indicator are obtained from an ongoing annual survey conducted by the National Center for Health Statistics. Survey data are representative of the U.S. civilian noninstitutionalized population. A parent or other knowledgeable adult in each sampled household is asked questions regarding the child's health status, including if they have ever been told the child has autism.

- The percentage of children ages 5 to 17 years reported to have ever been diagnosed with autism rose from 0.1% in 1997 to 1.0% in 2010.This increasing trend was statistically significant.
- For the years 2007–2010, the rate of reported autism was more than three times higher in boys than in girls, 1.5% and 0.4%, respectively. This difference was statistically significant. (See Table H8a.)
- The reported prevalence of autism varies by race/ethnicity. The highest prevalence of autism is for children of "All Other Races" (1.7%) and White non-Hispanic children (1.1%). Autism prevalence was lower among Asian non-Hispanic children (0.8%), Black non-Hispanic children (0.7%), and Hispanic children (0.6%). (See Table H8b.)
- The prevalence of autism for both White non-Hispanic children and children of "All Other Races" was statistically significantly different from the prevalence for both Black non-Hispanic children and Hispanic children.
- For the years 2007–2010, the prevalence of autism was similar for children living below the poverty level and those living at or above the poverty level. (See Table H8b.)

velopmental disorders has changed over time, and, when possible, how the prevalence differs between boys and girls.

1.6 NATIONAL HEALTH INTERVIEW SURVEY

The National Health Interview Survey (NHIS) provides nationally representative data on the prevalence of ADHD, learning disabilities, autism, and intellectual disability (mental retardation) in the United States each year. NHIS is a large-scale household interview survey of a representative sample of the civilian noninstitutionalized U.S. population, conducted by the National Center for Health Statistics (NCHS). The interviews are conducted in person at the participants' homes. From 1997–2005, interviews

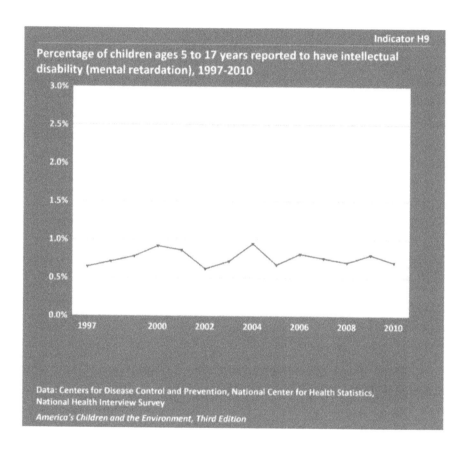

FIGURE 4: Data for this indicator are obtained from an ongoing annual survey conducted by the National Center for Health Statistics. Survey data are representative of the U.S. civilian noninstitutionalized population. A parent or other knowledgeable adult in each sampled household is asked questions regarding the child's health status, including if they have ever been told the child has mental retardation.

- In 2010, 0.7% of children ages 5 to 17 years were reported to have ever been diagnosed with intellectual disability (mental retardation). There was little change in this percentage between 1997 and 2010.
- In 2007–2010, the percentage of boys reported to have intellectual disability (0.9%) was higher than for girls (0.6%). This difference was statistically significant. (See Table H9a.)
- In 2007–2010, there was little difference by race/ethnicity in the reported prevalence of intellectual disability. (See Table H9b.)
- In 2007–2010, 1.2% of children from families with incomes below the poverty level were reported to have intellectual disability, compared with 0.7% of children from families at or above the poverty level, a statistically significant difference. (See Table H9b.)

were conducted for approximately 12,000– 14,000 children annually. From 2006–2008, interviews were conducted for approximately 9,000– 10,000 children per year. In 2009 and 2010, interviews were conducted for approximately 11,000 children per year. The data are obtained by asking a parent or other knowledgeable household adult questions regarding the child's health status. NHIS asks "Has a doctor or health professional ever told you that <child's name> had Attention Deficit/Hyperactivity Disorder (ADHD) or Attention Deficit Disorder (ADD)? Autism? Mental Retardation?" Another question on the NHIS survey asks "Has a representative from a school or a health professional ever told you that <child's name> had a learning disability?"

1.7 DATA PRESENTED IN THE INDICATORS

The following indicators display the prevalence of ADHD, learning disabilities, autism, and intellectual disability among U.S. children, for the years 1997–2010. Diagnosing neurodevelopmental disorders in young children can be difficult: many affected children may not receive a diagnosis until they enter preschool or kindergarten. For this reason, the indicators here show children ages 5 to 17 years. Where data are sufficiently reliable, the indicators provide separate prevalence estimates for boys and girls.

Although the NHIS provides national-level data on the prevalence of neurodevelopmental disorders over a span of many years, NHIS data could underestimate the prevalence of neurodevelopmental disorders. Reasons for underestimation may include late identification of affected children and the exclusion of institutionalized children from the NHIS survey population. A diagnosis of a neurodevelopmental disorder depends not only on the presence of particular symptoms and behaviors in a child, but on concerns being raised by a parent or teacher about the child's behavior, as well as the child's access to a doctor and the accuracy of the doctor's diagnosis. Further, the NHIS relies on parents reporting that their child has been diagnosed with a neurodevelopmental disorder, and the accuracy of parental responses could be affected by cultural and other factors.

Long-term trends in these conditions are difficult to detect with certainty due to a lack of data to track prevalence over many years, as well as changes in awareness and diagnostic criteria, which could explain at least part of the observed increasing trends. [184-186] The NHIS questions also do not assess whether a child currently has a disorder; instead, they provide data on whether a child has ever been diagnosed with a disorder, regardless of their current status.

Survey responses for learning disabilities may be more uncertain than for the other three disorders presented. Whereas survey respondents are asked whether the child has been diagnosed with ADHD, autism, or intellectual disability (mental retardation) by a health professional, for learning disabilities an affirmative response may also include a school representative. It is possible that some parents may respond "yes" to the question regarding learning disabilities based on informal comments made at school, rather than a formal evaluation to determine whether the child has any specific learning disability; similarly, they may give a "yes" answer for children with diagnosed disorders that are not learning disabilities. For example, parents of children with intellectual disability might also respond "yes" to the learning disability question, thinking that any learning problems may apply, even though intellectual disability and learning disabilities are distinct conditions. [2]

Because autism is the only autism spectrum disorder (ASD) referred to in the survey, it is not clear how parents of children with other ASDs, i.e., Asperger's syndrome and PDD-NOS, may have responded. The estimates shown by Indicator H8 could represent underestimates of ASD prevalence if parents of children with Asperger's syndrome and PDD-NOS did not answer yes to the NHIS questions about autism.

In addition to the data shown in the indicator graphs, supplemental tables provide information regarding the prevalence of neurodevelopmental disorders for different age groups and prevalence by race/ethnicity, sex, and family income. These comparisons use the most current four years of data available. The data from four years are combined to increase the statistical reliability of the estimates for each race/ethnicity, sex, and family income group. The tables include prevalence estimates for the following race/ethnicity groups: White non-Hispanic, Black non-Hispanic, Asian non-Hispanic, Hispanic, and "All Other Races." The "All Others Races" category includes all other races not specified, together with those individuals who report more than one race. The limits of the sample design and sample size often prevent statistically reliable estimates for smaller race/ethnicity groups. The data are also tabulated for three income groups: all incomes, income below the poverty level, and greater than or equal to the poverty level.

Please see the Introduction to the Health section for discussion of statistical significance testing applied to these indicators.

1.8 OTHER ESTIMATES OF ADHD AND AUTISM PREVALENCE

In addition to NHIS, other NCHS studies provide data on prevalence of ADHD and ASDs among children. The National Survey of Children's Health (NSCH), conducted in 2003 by NCHS, found that 7.8% of children ages 4 to 17 years had ever been diagnosed with ADHD. The same survey, when conducted again in 2007, found that 9.5% of children ages 4 to 17 years had ever been diagnosed with ADHD. [7] Both estimates are somewhat higher than the ADHD prevalence estimates from the NHIS for those years. The 2007 NSCH also estimates that 7.2% of children ages 4 to 17 years currently have ADHD. The 2007 NSCH also provides information at the state level: North Carolina had the highest rate, with 15.6% of children ages 4 to 17 years having ever been diagnosed with ADHD; the rate was lowest in Nevada, at 5.6%. [7]

In 2002 and 2006, the Centers for Disease Control and Prevention performed thorough data gathering in selected areas to examine the prevalence of ASDs in eight-year-old children. The ASD prevalence estimate for 2002 was 0.66%, or 1 in 152 eight-year-old children, and the estimate for 2006 was 0.9%, or 1 in 110 eight-year-old children. [8,187] The 2007 NSCH also provides an estimate of 1.1% of children ages 3 to 17 years reported to have ASDs, or about 1 in 90. [188]

REFERENCES

1. Boyle, C.A., S. Boulet, L.A. Schieve, R.A. Cohen, S.J. Blumberg, M. Yeargin–Allsopp, S. Visser, and M.D. Kogan. 2011. Trends in the prevalence of developmental disabilities in US Children, 1997–2008. Pediatrics 127 (6):1034–42.
2. Pastor, P.N., and C.A. Reuben. 2008. Diagnosed attention deficit hyperactivity disorder and learning disability: United States, 2004– 2006. Vital and Health Statistics 10 (237).
3. Grandjean, P., and P.J. Landrigan. 2006. Developmental neurotoxicity of industrial chemicals. Lancet 368 (9553):2167–78.
4. Newschaffer, C.J., M.D. Falb, and J.G. Gurney. 2005. National autism prevalence trends from United States special education data. Pediatrics 115 (3):e277–82.
5. Prior, M. 2003. Is there an increase in the prevalence of autism spectrum disorders? Journal of Paediatrics and Child Health 39 (2):81–2.
6. Rutter, M. 2005. Incidence of autism spectrum disorders: changes over time and their meaning. Acta Paediatrica 94 (1):2–15.
7. Centers for Disease Control and Prevention. 2010. Increasing prevalence of parent–reported attention–deficit/hyperactivity disorder among children —— United States, 2003 and 2007. Morbidity and Mortality Weekly Report 59 (44):1439–43.
8. Centers for Disease Control and Prevention. 2009. Prevalence of autism spectrum disorders —— autism and developmental disabilities monitoring network, United States, 2006. Morbidity and Mortality Weekly Report 58 (SS 10):1–20.
9. Hertz–Picciotto, I., and L. Delwiche. 2009. The rise in autism and the role of age at diagnosis. Epidemiology 20 (1):84–90.
10. Newschaffer, C.J. 2006. Investigating diagnostic substitution and autism prevalence trends. Pediatrics 117 (4):1436–7.
11. Grupp–Phelan, J., J.S. Harman, and K.J. Kelleher. 2007. Trends in mental health and chronic condition visits by children presenting for care at U.S. emergency departments. Public Health Reports 122 (1):55–61.
12. Kelleher, K.J., T.K. McInerny, W.P. Gardner, G.E. Childs, and R.C. Wasserman. 2000. Increasing identification of psychosocial problems: 1979–1996. Pediatrics 105 (6):1313–21.

13. U.S. Department of Education. 2007. 27th Annual (2005) Report to Congress on the Implementation of the Individuals with Disabilities Education Act, Vol. 1. Washington, DC.

14. Aarnoudse–Moens, C.S.H., N. Weisglas–Kuperus, J.B. van Goudoever, and J. Oosterlaan. 2009. Meta–analysis of neurobehavioral outcomes in very preterm and/or very low birth weight children. Pediatrics 124 (2):717–728.

15. Banerjee, T.D., F. Middleton, and S.V. Faraone. 2007. Environmental risk factors for attention–deficit hyperactivity disorder. Acta Pædiatrica 96 (9):1269–1274.

16. Bhutta, A.T., M.A. Cleves, P.H. Casey, M.M. Cradock, and K.J.S. Anand. 2002. Cognitive and behavioral outcomes of school–aged children who were born preterm. JAMA: The Journal of the American Medical Association 288 (6):728–737.

17. Herrmann, M., K. King, and M. Weitzman. 2008. Prenatal tobacco smoke and post-natal secondhand smoke exposure and child neurodevelopment. Current Opinion in Pediatrics 20 (2):184–190.

18. Institute of Medicine. 2007. Preterm Birth: Causes, Consequences, and Prevention. Edited by R. E. Behrman and A. S. Butler. Washington, DC: The National Academies Press.

19. Linnet, K.M., S. Dalsgaard, C. Obel, K. Wisborg, T.B. Henriksen, A. Rodriguez, A. Kotimaa, I. Moilanen, P.H. Thomsen, J. Olsen, et al. 2003. Maternal lifestyle factors in pregnancy risk of attention deficit hyperactivity disorder and associated behaviors: review of the current evidence. The American Journal of Psychiatry 160 (6):1028–40.

20. Nigg, J.T. 2006. What Causes ADHD? Understanding What Goes Wrong and Why. New York: The Guilford Press.

21. Weiss, B., and D.C. Bellinger. 2006. Social ecology of children's vulnerability to environmental pollutants. Environmental Health Perspectives 114 (10):1479–1485.

22. National Toxicology Program. 2012. NTP Monograph on Health Effects of Low–Level Lead. Research Triangle Park, NC: National Institute of Environmental Health Sciences, National Toxicology Program. http://ntp.niehs.nih.gov/go/36443.

23. U.S. Environmental Protection Agency. 1997. Mercury Study Report to Congress Volumes I to VII. Washington DC: U.S. Environmental Protection Agency Office of Air Quality Planning and Standards and Office of Research and Development. EPA–452/R–97–003. http://www.epa.gov/hg/report.htm.

24. Amin–Zaki, L., S. Elhassani, M.A. Majeed, T.W. Clarkson, R.A. Doherty, and M. Greenwood. 1974. Intra–uterine methylmercury poisoning in Iraq. Pediatrics 54 (5):587–95.

25. Harada, M. 1995. Minamata disease: methylmercury poisoning in Japan caused by environmental pollution. Critical Reviews in Toxicology 25 (1):1–24.

26. National Research Council. 2000. Toxicological Effects of Methylmercury. Washington, DC: National Academy Press.

27. Budtz–Jorgensen, E., P. Grandjean, and P. Weihe. 2007. Separation of risks and benefits of seafood intake. Environmental Health Perspectives 115 (3):323–7.

28. Crump, K.S., T. Kjellstrom, A.M. Shipp, A. Silvers, and A. Stewart. 1998. Influence of prenatal mercury exposure upon scholastic and psychological test performance: benchmark analysis of a New Zealand cohort. Risk Analysis 18 (6):701–13.

29. Debes, F., E. Budtz–Jorgensen, P. Weihe, R.F. White, and P. Grandjean. 2006. Impact of prenatal methylmercury exposure on neurobehavioral function at age 14 years. Neurotoxicology and Teratology 28 (5):536–47.

30. Grandjean, P., P. Weihe, R.F. White, F. Debes, S. Araki, K. Yokoyama, K. Murata, N. Sorensen, R. Dahl, and P.J. Jorgensen. 1997. Cognitive deficit in 7–year–old children with prenatal exposure to methylmercury. Neurotoxicology and Teratology 19 (6):417–28.

31. Kjellstrom, T., P. Kennedy, S. Wallis, and C. Mantell. 1986. Physical and mental development of children with prenatal exposure to mercury from fish. Stage 1: Preliminary tests at age 4. Sweden: Swedish National Environmental Protection Board.

32. Oken, E., and D.C. Bellinger. 2008. Fish consumption, methylmercury and child neurodevelopment. Current Opinion in Pediatrics 20 (2):178–83.

33. Myers, G.J., P.W. Davidson, C. Cox, C.F. Shamlaye, D. Palumbo, E. Cernichiari, J. Sloane–Reeves, G.E. Wilding, J. Kost, L.S. Huang, et al. 2003. Prenatal methylmercury exposure from ocean fish consumption in the Seychelles child development study. Lancet 361 (9370):1686–92.

34. Davidson, P.W., J.J. Strain, G.J. Myers, S.W. Thurston, M.P. Bonham, C.F. Shamlaye, A. Stokes–Riner, J.M. Wallace, P.J. Robson, E.M. Duffy, et al. 2008. Neurodevelopmental effects of maternal nutritional status and exposure to methylmercury from eating fish during pregnancy. Neurotoxicology 29 (5):767–75.

35. Lynch, M.L., L.S. Huang, C. Cox, J.J. Strain, G.J. Myers, M.P. Bonham, C.F. Shamlaye, A. Stokes–Riner, J.M. Wallace, E.M. Duffy, et al. 2011. Varying coefficient function models to explore interactions between maternal nutritional status and prenatal methylmercury toxicity in the Seychelles Child Development Nutrition Study. Environmental Research 111 (1):75–80.

36. Strain, J.J., P.W. Davidson, M.P. Bonham, E.M. Duffy, A. Stokes–Riner, S.W. Thurston, J.M. Wallace, P.J. Robson, C.F. Shamlaye, L.A. Georger, et al. 2008. Associations of maternal long–chain polyunsaturated fatty acids, methyl mercury, and infant development in the Seychelles Child Development Nutrition Study. Neurotoxicology 29 (5):776–782.

37. Lederman, S.A., R.L. Jones, K.L. Caldwell, V. Rauh, S.E. Sheets, D. Tang, S. Viswanathan, M. Becker, J.L. Stein, R.Y. Wang, et al. 2008. Relation between cord blood mercury levels and early child development in a World Trade Center cohort. Environmental Health Perspectives 116 (8):1085–91.

38. Oken, E., J.S. Radesky, R.O. Wright, D.C. Bellinger, C.J. Amarasiriwardena, K.P. Kleinman, H. Hu, and M.W. Gillman. 2008. Maternal fish intake during pregnancy, blood mercury levels, and child cognition at age 3 years in a US cohort. American Journal of Epidemiology 167 (10):1171–81.

39. Jacobson, J.L., and S.W. Jacobson. 2003. Prenatal exposure to polychlorinated biphenyls and attention at school age. Journal of Pediatrics 143 (6):780–8.

40. Sagiv, S.K., S.W. Thurston, D.C. Bellinger, P.E. Tolbert, L.M. Altshul, and S.A. Korrick. 2010. Prenatal organochlorine exposure and behaviors associated with attention deficit hyperactivity disorder in school–aged children. American Journal of Epidemiology 171 (5):593–601.

41. Stewart, P., S. Fitzgerald, J. Reihman, B. Gump, E. Lonky, T. Darvill, J. Pagano, and P. Hauser. 2003. Prenatal PCB exposure, the corpus callosum, and response inhibition. Environmental Health Perspectives 111 (13):1670–7.

42. Stewart, P., J. Reihman, B. Gump, E. Lonky, T. Darvill, and J. Pagano. 2005. Response inhibition at 8 and 9 1/2 years of age in children prenatally exposed to PCBs. Neurotoxicology and Teratology 27 (6):771–80.

43. Stewart, P.W., E. Lonky, J. Reihman, J. Pagano, B.B. Gump, and T. Darvill. 2008. The relationship between prenatal PCB exposure and intelligence (IQ) in 9–year–old children. Environmental Health Perspectives 116 (10):1416–22.

44. Stewart, P.W., D.M. Sargent, J. Reihman, B.B. Gump, E. Lonky, T. Darvill, H. Hicks, and J. Pagano. 2006. Response inhibition during Differential Reinforcement of Low Rates (DRL) schedules may be sensitive to low–level polychlorinated biphenyl, methylmercury, and lead exposure in children. Environmental Health Perspectives 114 (12):1923–9.

45. Vreugdenhil, H.J., P.G. Mulder, H.H. Emmen, and N. Weisglas–Kuperus. 2004. Effects of perinatal exposure to PCBs on neuropsychological functions in the Rotterdam cohort at 9 years of age. Neuropsychology 18 (1):185–93.

46. Darvill, T., E. Lonky, J. Reihman, P. Stewart, and J. Pagano. 2000. Prenatal exposure to PCBs and infant performance on the Fagan test of infant intelligence. Neurotoxicology 21 (6):1029–38.

47. Jacobson, J.L., and S.W. Jacobson. 1996. Intellectual impairment in children exposed to polychlorinated biphenyls in utero. New England Journal of Medicine 335 (11):783–9.

48. Jacobson, J.L., and S.W. Jacobson. 1997. Teratogen update: polychlorinated biphenyls. Teratology 55 (5):338–347.

49. Patandin, S., C.I. Lanting, P.G. Mulder, E.R. Boersma, P.J. Sauer, and N. Weisglas–Kuperus. 1999. Effects of environmental exposure to polychlorinated biphenyls and dioxins on cognitive abilities in Dutch children at 42 months of age. Journal of Pediatrics 134 (1):33–41.

50. Stewart, P., J. Reihman, E. Lonky, T. Darvill, and J. Pagano. 2000. Prenatal PCB exposure and neonatal behavioral assessment scale (NBAS) performance. Neurotoxicology and Teratology 22 (1):21–9.

51. Walkowiak, J., J.A. Wiener, A. Fastabend, B. Heinzow, U. Kramer, E. Schmidt, H.J. Steingruber, S. Wundram, and G. Winneke. 2001. Environmental exposure to polychlorinated biphenyls and quality of the home environment: effects on psychodevelopment in early childhood. Lancet 358 (9293):1602–7.

52. Schantz, S.L., J.J. Widholm, and D.C. Rice. 2003. Effects of PCB exposure on neuropsychological function in children. Environmental Health Perspectives 111 (3):357–576.

53. Jacobson, J.L., S.W. Jacobson, and H.E. Humphrey. 1990. Effects of exposure to PCBs and related compounds on growth and activity in children. Neurotoxicology and Teratology 12 (4):319–26.

54. Boucher, O., G. Muckle, and C.H. Bastien. 2009. Prenatal exposure to polychlorinated biphenyls: a neuropsychologic analysis. Environmental Health Perspectives 117 (1):7–16.

55. Eubig, P.A., A. Aguiar, and S.L. Schantz. 2010. Lead and PCBs as risk factors for attention deficit/hyperactivity disorder. Environmental Health Perspectives 118 (12):1654–1667.

56. Ribas–Fito, N., M. Sala, M. Kogevinas, and J. Sunyer. 2001. Polychlorinated biphenyls (PCBs) and neurological development in children: a systematic review. Journal of Epidemiology and Community Health 55 (8):537–46.

57. Schantz, S.L., J.C. Gardiner, D.M. Gasior, R.J. McCaffrey, A.M. Sweeney, and H.E.B. Humphrey. 2004. Much Ado About Something: The Weight of Evidence for PCB Effects on Neuropsychological Function. Psychology in the Schools 41 (6):669–679.

58. Wigle, D.T., T.E. Arbuckle, M.C. Turner, A. Berube, Q. Yang, S. Liu, and D. Krewski. 2008. Epidemiologic evidence of relationships between reproductive and child health outcomes and environmental chemical contaminants. Journal of Toxicology and Environmental Health Part B Critical Reviews 11 (5–6):373–517.

59. Agency for Toxic Substances and Disease Registry (ATSDR). 2000. Toxicological Profile for Polychlorinated Biphenyls (PCBs). Atlanta, GA: U.S. Department of Health and Human Services, Public Health Service. http://www.atsdr.cdc.gov/toxprofiles/tp.asp?id=142&tid=26.

60. Chen, Y.C., Y.L. Guo, C.C. Hsu, and W.J. Rogan. 1992. Cognitive development of Yu–Cheng ("oil disease") children prenatally exposed to heat–degraded PCBs. Journal of the American Medical Association 268 (22):3213–8.

61. Chen, Y.C., M.L. Yu, W.J. Rogan, B.C. Gladen, and C.C. Hsu. 1994. A 6–year follow–up of behavior and activity disorders in the Taiwan Yucheng children. American Journal of Public Health 84 (3):415–21.

62. Lai, T.J., X. Liu, Y.L. Guo, N.W. Guo, M.L. Yu, C.C. Hsu, and W.J. Rogan. 2002. A cohort study of behavioral problems and intelligence in children with high prenatal polychlorinated biphenyl exposure. Archives of General Psychiatry 59 (11):1061–6.

63. Rogan, W.J., B.C. Gladen, K.L. Hung, S.L. Koong, L.Y. Shih, J.S. Taylor, Y.C. Wu, D. Yang, N.B. Ragan, and C.C. Hsu. 1988. Congenital poisoning by polychlorinated biphenyls and their contaminants in Taiwan. Science 241 (4863):334–6.

64. Centers for Disease Control and Prevention. 2009. Fourth National Report on Human Exposure to Environmental Chemicals. Atlanta, GA: CDC. http://www.cdc.gov/exposurereport/.

65. Eskenazi, B., A. Bradman, and R. Castorina. 1999. Exposures of children to organophosphate pesticides and their potential adverse health effects. Environmental Health Perspectives 107 (Suppl. 3):409–19.

66. Huen, K., Harley, K., Brooks, J., Hubbard, A., Bradman, A., Eskenazi, B., Holland, N. 2009. Developmental changes in PON1 enzyme activity in young children and effects of PON1 polymorphisms. Environmental Health Perspectives 117 (10):1632–8.

67. Marks, A.R., K. Harley, A. Bradman, K. Kogut, D.B. Barr, C. Johnson, N. Calderon, and B. Eskenazi. 2010. Organophosphate pesticide exposure and attention in young Mexican–American children: the CHAMACOS study. Environmental Health Perspectives 118 (12):1768–74.

68. Bouchard, M.F., D.C. Bellinger, R.O. Wright, and M.G. Weisskopf. 2010. Attention–Deficit/Hyperactivity Disorder and urinary metabolites of organophosphate pesticides. Pediatrics 125 (6):e1270–e1277.

69. Bouchard, M.F., J. Chevrier, K.G. Harley, K. Kogut, M. Vedar, N. Calderon, C. Trujillo, C. Johnson, A. Bradman, D.B. Barr, et al. 2011. Prenatal exposure to organophosphate pesticides and IQ in 7–year old children. Environmental Health Perspectives doi:10.1289/ehp.1003185.

70. Engel, S.M., J. Wetmur, J. Chen, C. Zhu, D.B. Barr, R.L. Canfield, and M.S. Wolff. 2011. Prenatal exposure to organophosphates, paraoxonase 1, and cognitive development in childhood. Environmental Health Perspectives doi: 10.1289/ehp.1003183.

71. Rauh, V., S. Arunajadai, M. Horton, F. Perera, L. Hoepner, D.B. Barr, and R. Whyatt. 2011. 7–Year neurodevelopmental scores and prenatal exposure to chlorpyrifos, a common agricultural pesticide. Environmental Health Perspectives doi: 10.1289/ehp.1003160.

72. Costa, L.G., G. Giordano, S. Tagliaferri, A. Caglieri, and A. Mutti. 2008. Polybrominated diphenyl ether (PBDE) flame retardants: environmental contamination, human body burden and potential adverse health effects. Acta Biomed 79 (3):172–83.

73. Gee, J.R., and V.C. Moser. 2008. Acute postnatal exposure to brominated diphenylether 47 delays neuromotor ontogeny and alters motor activity in mice. Neurotoxicology and Teratology 30 (2):79–87.

74. Rice, D.C., E.A. Reeve, A. Herlihy, R.T. Zoeller, W.D. Thompson, and V.P. Markowski. 2007. Developmental delays and locomotor activity in the C57BL6/J mouse following neonatal exposure to the fully–brominated PBDE, decabromodiphenyl ether. Neurotoxicology and Teratology 29 (4):511–20.

75. Herbstman, J.B., A. Sjodin, M. Kurzon, S.A. Lederman, R.S. Jones, V. Rauh, L.L. Needham, D. Tang, M. Niedzwiecki, R.Y. Wang, et al. 2010. Prenatal exposure to PBDEs and neurodevelopment. Environmental Health Perspectives 118 (5):712–9.

76. Roze, E., L. Meijer, A. Bakker, K.N. Van Braeckel, P.J. Sauer, and A.F. Bos. 2009. Prenatal exposure to organohalogens, including brominated flame retardants, influences motor, cognitive, and behavioral performance at school age. Environmental Health Perspectives 117 (12):1953–8.

77. Engel, S.M., A. Miodovnik, R.L. Canfield, C. Zhu, M.J. Silva, A.M. Calafat, and M.S. Wolff. 2010. Prenatal phthalate exposure is associated with childhood behavior and executive functioning. Environmental Health Perspectives 118 (4):565–71.

78. Miodovnik, A., S.M. Engel, C. Zhu, X. Ye, L.V. Soorya, M.J. Silva, A.M. Calafat, and M.S. Wolff. 2011. Endocrine disruptors and childhood social impairment. Neurotoxicology 32 (2):261–267.

79. Cho, S.–C., S.–Y. Bhang, Y.–C. Hong, M.–S. Shin, B.–N. Kim, J.–W. Kim, H.–J. Yoo, I.H. Cho, and H.–W. Kim. 2010. Relationship between environmental phthalate exposure and the intelligence of school–age children. Environmental Health Perspectives 118 (7):1027–1032.

80. Kim, B.N., S.C. Cho, Y. Kim, M.S. Shin, H.J. Yoo, J.W. Kim, Y.H. Yang, H.W. Kim, S.Y. Bhang, and Y.C. Hong. 2009. Phthalates exposure and attention–deficit/hyperactivity disorder in school–age children. Biological Psychiatry 66 (10):958–63.

81. National Toxicology Program. 2008. NTP–CERHR Monograph on the Potential Human Reproductive and Developmental Effects of Bisphenol A. Research Triangle Park, NC: National Institute of Environmental Health Sciences, National Toxicology Program. http://ntp.niehs.nih.gov/ntp/ohat/bisphenol/bisphenol.pdf.

82. Braun, J.M., K. Yolton, K.N. Dietrich, R. Hornung, X. Ye, A.M. Calafat, and B.P. Lanphear. 2009. Prenatal bisphenol A exposure and early childhood behavior. Environmental Health Perspectives 117 (12):1945–1952.

83. Perera, F.P., Z. Li, R. Whyatt, L. Hoepner, S. Wang, D. Camann, and V. Rauh. 2009. Prenatal airborne polycyclic aromatic hydrocarbon exposure and child IQ at age 5 years. Pediatrics 124 (2):e195–202.

84. Perera, F.P., S. Wang, J. Vishnevetsky, B. Zhang, K.J. Cole, D. Tang, V. Rauh, and D.H. Phillips. 2011. PAH/Aromatic DNA Adducts in Cord Blood and Behavior Scores in New York City Children. Environmental Health Perspectives doi:10.1289/ehp.1002705.

85. Smith, A.H., and C.M. Steinmaus. 2009. Health effects of arsenic and chromium in drinking water: recent human findings. Annual Review of Public Health 30:107–22.

86. Sambu, S., and R. Wilson. 2008. Arsenic in food and water—a brief history. Toxicology and Industrial Health 24 (4):217–26.

87. U.S. Environmental Protection Agency. 2011. Perchlorate Retrieved February 11, 2011 from http://www.epa.gov/safewater/contaminants/unregulated/perchlorate.html.

88. Kirk, A.B., P.K. Martinelango, K. Tian, A. Dutta, E.E. Smith, and P.K. Dasgupta. 2005. Perchlorate and iodide in dairy and breast milk. Environmental Science & Technology 39 (7):2011–7.

89. Sanchez, C.A., L.M. Barraj, B.C. Blount, C.G. Scrafford, L. Valentin–Blasini, K.M. Smith, and R.I. Krieger. 2009. Perchlorate exposure from food crops produced in the lower Colorado River region. Journal of Exposure Science & Environmental Epidemiology 19 (4):359–68.

90. Greer, M.A., G. Goodman, R.C. Pleus, and S.E. Greer. 2002. Health effects assessment for environmental perchlorate contamination: the dose response for inhibition of thyroidal radioiodine uptake in humans. Environmental Health Perspectives 110 (9):927–37.

91. National Research Council. 2005. Health Implications of Perchlorate Ingestion. Washington, DC: National Academies Press. http://www.nap.edu/catalog.php?record_id=11202.

92. Haddow, J.E., G.E. Palomaki, W.C. Allan, J.R. Williams, G.J. Knight, J. Gagnon, C.E. O'Heir, M.L. Mitchell, R.J. Hermos, S.E. Waisbren, et al. 1999. Maternal thyroid deficiency during pregnancy and subsequent neuropsychological development of the child. New England Journal of Medicine 341 (8):549–55.

93. Miller, M.D., K.M. Crofton, D.C. Rice, and R.T. Zoeller. 2009. Thyroid–disrupting chemicals: interpreting upstream biomarkers of adverse outcomes. Environmental Health Perspectives 117 (7):1033–41.

94. Morreale de Escobar, G., M.J. Obregon, and F. Escobar del Rey. 2000. Is neuropsychological development related to maternal hypothyroidism or to maternal hypothyroxinemia? The Journal of Clinical Endocrinology and Metabolism 85 (11):3975–87.

95. Bellinger, D.C. 2008. Lead neurotoxicity and socioeconomic status: conceptual and analytical issues. Neurotoxicology 29 (5):828–32.

96. Rice, D.C. 2000. Parallels between attention deficit hyperactivity disorder and behavioral deficits produced by neurotoxic exposure in monkeys. Environmental Health Perspectives 108 (Suppl. 3):405–408.

97. Rodier, P.M. 1995. Developing brain as a target of toxicity. Environmental Health Perspectives 103 Suppl. 6:73–6.
98. American Psychiatric Association. 2000. Diagnostic and Statistical Manual of Mental Disorders, Fourth Edition Text Revision. Washington D.C.: American Psychiatric Association.
99. American Psychiatric Association. 1987. Diagnostic and Statistical Manual of Mental Disorders, Third Edition Text Revision (DSM–III–R). Washington, D.C.
100. Larson, K., S.A. Russ, R.S. Kahn, and N. Halfon. 2011. Patterns of comorbidity, functioning, and service use for U.S. children with ADHD, 2007. Pediatrics 127 (3):462–470.
101. Aguiar, A., P.A. Eubig, and S.L. Schantz. 2010. Attention deficit/hyperactivity disorder: a focused overview for children's environmental health researchers. Environmental Health Perspectives 118 (12):1646–53.
102. Barkley, R.A. 2006. Attention–Deficit Hyperactivity Disorder: A Handbook for Diagnosis and Treatment, Third Edition. New York: The Guilford Press.
103. Biederman, J., and S.V. Faraone. 2005. Attention–deficit hyperactivity disorder. Lancet 366 (9481):237–48.
104. Faraone, S.V., and E. Mick. 2010. Molecular genetics of attention deficit hyperactivity disorder. Psychiatric Clinics of North America 33 (1):159–80.
105. Kieling, C., R.R. Goncalves, R. Tannock, and F.X. Castellanos. 2008. Neurobiology of attention deficit hyperactivity disorder. Child and Adolescent Psychiatric Clinics of North America 17 (2):285–307, viii.
106. Thapar, A., K. Langley, P. Asherson, and M. Gill. 2007. Gene–environment interplay in attention–deficit hyperactivity disorder and the importance of a developmental perspective. The British Journal of Psychiatry 190:1–3.
107. Langley, K., F. Rice, M.B. van den Bree, and A. Thapar. 2005. Maternal smoking during pregnancy as an environmental risk factor for attention deficit hyperactivity disorder behaviour. A review. Minerva Pediatrica 57 (6):359–71.
108. Nigg, J., M. Nikolas, and S.A. Burt. 2010. Measured gene–by–environment interaction in relation to attention–deficit/hyperactivity disorder. Journal of the American Academy of Child and Adolescent Psychiatry 49 (9):863–73.
109. Braun, J.M., R.S. Kahn, T. Froehlich, P. Auinger, and B.P. Lanphear. 2006. Exposures to environmental toxicants and attention deficit hyperactivity disorder in U.S. children. Environmental Health Perspectives 114 (12):1904–9.
110. Froehlich, T.E., B.P. Lanphear, P. Auinger, R. Hornung, J.N. Epstein, J. Braun, and R.S. Kahn. 2009. Association of tobacco and lead exposures with attention–deficit/hyperactivity disorder. Pediatrics 124 (6):e1054–63.
111. Ha, M., H.J. Kwon, M.H. Lim, Y.K. Jee, Y.C. Hong, J.H. Leem, J. Sakong, J.M. Bae, S.J. Hong, Y.M. Roh, et al. 2009. Low blood levels of lead and mercury and symptoms of attention deficit hyperactivity in children: a report of the children's health and environment research (CHEER). Neurotoxicology 30 (1):31–6.
112. Nigg, J.T., G.M. Knottnerus, M.M. Martel, M. Nikolas, K. Cavanagh, W. Karmaus, and M.D. Rappley. 2008. Low blood lead levels associated with clinically diagnosed attention–deficit/hyperactivity disorder and mediated by weak cognitive control. Biological Psychiatry 63 (3):325–31.

113. Nigg, J.T., M. Nikolas, G. Mark Knottnerus, K. Cavanagh, and K. Friderici. 2010. Confirmation and extension of association of blood lead with attention–deficit/hyperactivity disorder (ADHD) and ADHD symptom domains at population–typical exposure levels. The Journal of Child Psychology and Psychiatry 51 (1):58–65.

114. Roy, A., D. Bellinger, H. Hu, J. Schwartz, A.S. Ettinger, R.O. Wright, M. Bouchard, K. Palaniappan, and K. Balakrishnan. 2009. Lead exposure and behavior among young children in Chennai, India. Environmental Health Perspectives 117 (10):1607–11.

115. Wang, H.–L., X.–T. Chen, B. Yang, F.–L. Ma, S. Wang, M.–L. Tang, N.–G. Hao, and D.–Y. Ruan. 2008. Case–control study of blood lead levels and attention–deficit hyperactivity disorder in Chinese children Environmental Health Perspectives 116 (10):1401–1406.

116. Canfield, R.L., M.H. Gendle, and D.A. Cory–Slechta. 2004. Impaired neuropsychological functioning in lead–exposed children. Developmental Neuropsychology 26 (1):513–40.

117. Chiodo, L.M., S.W. Jacobson, and J.L. Jacobson. 2004. Neurodevelopmental effects of postnatal lead exposure at very low levels. Neurotoxicology and Teratology 26 (3):359–71.

118. Nicolescu, R., C. Petcu, A. Cordeanu, K. Fabritius, M. Schlumpf, R. Krebs, U. Kramer, and G. Winneke. 2010. Environmental exposure to lead, but not other neurotoxic metals, relates to core elements of ADHD in Romanian children: performance and questionnaire data. Environmental Research 110 (5):476–83.

119. Surkan, P.J., A. Zhang, F. Trachtenberg, D.B. Daniel, S. McKinlay, and D.C. Bellinger. 2007. Neuropsychological function in children with blood lead levels <10 microg/dL. Neurotoxicology 28 (6):1170–7.

120. Rice, D.C. 1996. Behavioral effects of lead: commonalities between experimental and epidemiologic data. Environmental Health Perspectives 104 (Suppl. 2):337–51.

121. Rossi–George, A., M.B. Virgolini, D. Weston, M. Thiruchelvam, and D.A. Cory–Slechta. 2011. Interactions of lifetime lead exposure and stress: behavioral, neurochemical and HPA axis effects. Neurotoxicology 32 (1):83–99.

122. Virgolini, M.B., A. Rossi–George, R. Lisek, D.D. Weston, M. Thiruchelvam, and D.A. Cory–Slechta. 2008. CNS effects of developmental Pb exposure are enhanced by combined maternal and offspring stress. Neurotoxicology 29 (5):812–27.

123. Gump, B.B., Q. Wu, A.K. Dumas, and K. Kannan. 2011. Perfluorochemical (PFC) exposure in children: associations with impaired response inhibition. Environmental Science & Technology 45 (19):8151–9.

124. Hoffman, K., T.F. Webster, M.G. Weisskopf, J. Weinberg, and V.M. Vieira. 2010. Exposure to polyfluoroalkyl chemicals and attention deficit/hyperactivity disorder in U.S. children 12–15 years of age. Environmental Health Perspectives 118 (12):1762–7.

125. Stein, C.R., and D.A. Savitz. 2011. Serum perfluorinated compound concentration and attention deficit/hyperactivity disorder in children aged 5 to 18 years. Environmental Health Perspectives 119 (10):1466–71.

126. Cheuk, D.K., and V. Wong. 2006. Attention–deficit hyperactivity disorder and blood mercury level: a case–control study in Chinese children. Neuropediatrics 37 (4):234–40.

127. Julvez, J., F. Debes, P. Weihe, A. Choi, and P. Grandjean. 2010. Sensitivity of continuous performance test (CPT) at age 14 years to developmental methylmercury exposure. Neurotoxicology and Teratology 32 (6):627–632.

128. Plusquellec, P., G. Muckle, E. Dewailly, P. Ayotte, G. Begin, C. Desrosiers, C. Despres, D. Saint–Amour, and K. Poitras. 2010. The relation of environmental contaminants exposure to behavioral indicators in Inuit preschoolers in Arctic Quebec. Neurotoxicology 31 (1):17–25.

129. National Dissemination Center for Children with Disabilities. 2010. Disability Fact Sheet–No. 7: Learning Disabilities. Retrieved April 6, 2010 from http://www.nichcy. org/InformationResources/Documents/NICHCY%20PUBS/fs7.pdf.

130. National Center for Learning Disabilities. 2010. LD at a Glance. Retrieved April 6, 2010 from http://www.ncld.org/ld–basics/ldexplained/ basic–facts/learning–disabilities–at–a–glance.

131. Bellinger, D.C. 2008. Very low lead exposures and children's neurodevelopment. Current Opinion in Pediatrics 20 (2):172–177.

132. Marlowe, M., A. Cossairt, K. Welch, and J. Errera. 1984. Hair mineral content as a predictor of learning disabilities. Journal of Learning Disabilities 17 (7):418–21.

133. Pihl, R.O., and M. Parkes. 1977. Hair element content in learning disabled children. Science 198 (4313):204–6.

134. Leviton, A., D. Bellinger, E.N. Allred, M. Rabinowitz, H. Needleman, and S. Schoenbaum. 1993. Pre– and postnatal low–level lead exposure and children's dysfunction in school. Environmental Research 60 (1):30–43.

135. Lyngbye, T., O.N. Hansen, A. Trillingsgaard, I. Beese, and P. Grandjean. 1990. Learning disabilities in children: significance of lowlevel lead–exposure and confounding factors. Acta Paediatrica Scandinavica 79 (3):352–60.

136. Needleman, H.L., C. Gunnoe, A. Leviton, R. Reed, H. Peresie, C. Maher, and P. Barrett. 1979. Deficits in psychologic and classroom performance of children with elevated dentine lead levels. New England Journal of Medicine 300 (13):689–95.

137. Needleman, H.L., A. Schell, D.C. Bellinger, A. Leviton, and E.N. Allred. 1990. The long term effects of exposure to low doses of lead in childhood, an 11–year follow–up report. New England Journal of Medicine 322 (2):83–8.

138. Anderko, L., J. Braun, and P. Auinger. 2010. Contribution of tobacco smoke exposure to learning disabilities. Journal of Obstetric, Gynecologic, & Neonatal Nursing 39 (1):111–117.

139. Centers for Disease Control and Prevention. 2010. Autism Spectrum Disorders: Signs & Symptoms. Retrieved March 25, 2010 from http://www.cdc.gov/ncbddd/ autism/signs.html.

140. Beaudet, A.L. 2007. Autism: highly heritable but not inherited. Nature Medicine 13 (5):534–6.

141. Hallmayer, J., S. Cleveland, A. Torres, J. Phillips, B. Cohen, T. Torigoe, J. Miller, A. Fedele, J. Collins, K. Smith, et al. 2011. Genetic heritability and shared environmental factors among twin pairs with autism. Archives of General Psychiatry 68 (11):1095–102.

142. Levy, D., M. Ronemus, B. Yamrom, Y.–h. Lee, A. Leotta, J. Kendall, S. Marks, B. Lakshmi, D. Pai, K. Ye, et al. 2011. Rare de novo and transmitted copy–number variation in autistic spectrum disorders. Neuron 70 (5):886–897.

143. King, M., and P. Bearman. 2009. Diagnostic change and the increased prevalence of autism. International Journal of Epidemiology 38 (5):1224–1234.

144. King, M.D., C. Fountain, D. Dakhlallah, and P.S. Bearman. 2009. Estimated autism risk and older reproductive age. American Journal of Public Health 99 (9):1673–1679.

145. Liu, K.Y., M. King, and P.S. Bearman. 2010. Social influence and the autism epidemic. American Journal of Sociology 115 (5):1387–434.

146. Shelton, J.F., D.J. Tancredi, and I. Hertz–Picciotto. 2010. Independent and dependent contributions of advanced maternal and paternal ages to autism risk. Autism Research 3 (1):30–9.

147. Pessah, I.N., R.F. Seegal, P.J. Lein, J. LaSalle, B.K. Yee, J. Van De Water, and R.F. Berman. 2008. Immunologic and neurodevelopmental susceptibilities of autism. Neurotoxicology 29 (3):532–45.

148. Newschaffer, C.J., L.A. Croen, J. Daniels, E. Giarelli, J.K. Grether, S.E. Levy, D.S. Mandell, L.A. Miller, J. Pinto–Martin, J. Reaven, et al. 2007. The epidemiology of autism spectrum disorders. Annual Review of Public Health 28:235–58.

149. Sanders, S.J., A.G. Ercan–Sencicek, V. Hus, R. Luo, M.T. Murtha, D. Moreno–De–Luca, S.H. Chu, M.P. Moreau, A.R. Gupta, S.A. Thomson, et al. 2011. Multiple Recurrent De Novo CNVs, Including Duplications of the 7q11.23 Williams Syndrome Region, Are Strongly Associated with Autism. Neuron 70 (5):863–85.

150. Sebat, J., B. Lakshmi, D. Malhotra, J. Troge, C. Lese–Martin, T. Walsh, B. Yamrom, S. Yoon, A. Krasnitz, J. Kendall, et al. 2007. Strong association of de novo copy number mutations with autism. Science 316 (5823):445–9.

151. Kinney, D.K., D.H. Barch, B. Chayka, S. Napoleon, and K.M. Munir. 2010. Environmental risk factors for autism: do they help cause de novo genetic mutations that contribute to the disorder? Medical Hypotheses 74 (1):102–6.

152. James, S.J., P. Cutler, S. Melnyk, S. Jernigan, L. Janak, D.W. Gaylor, and J.A. Neubrander. 2004. Metabolic biomarkers of increased oxidative stress and impaired methylation capacity in children with autism. American Journal of Clinical Nutrition 80 (6):1611–7.

153. James, S.J., S. Melnyk, S. Jernigan, M.A. Cleves, C.H. Halsted, D.H. Wong, P. Cutler, K. Bock, M. Boris, J.J. Bradstreet, et al. 2006. Metabolic endophenotype and related genotypes are associated with oxidative stress in children with autism. American Journal of Medical Genetics Part B: Neuropsychiatric Genetics 141B (8):947–56.

154. Deth, R., C. Muratore, J. Benzecry, V.A. Power–Charnitsky, and M. Waly. 2008. How environmental and genetic factors combine to cause autism: A redox/methylation hypothesis. Neurotoxicology 29 (1):190–201.

155. Croen, L.A., D.V. Najjar, B. Fireman, and J.K. Grether. 2007. Maternal and paternal age and risk of autism spectrum disorders. Archives of Pediatric & Adolescent Medicine 161 (4):334–40.

156. Grether, J.K., M.C. Anderson, L.A. Croen, D. Smith, and G.C. Windham. 2009. Risk of autism and increasing maternal and paternal age in a large North American population. American Journal of Epidemiology 170 (9):1118–26.

157. Lauritsen, M.B., C.B. Pedersen, and P.B. Mortensen. 2005. Effects of familial risk factors and place of birth on the risk of autism: a nationwide register–based study. Journal of Child Psychology and Psychiatry 46 (9):963–71.

158. Chandley, A.C. 1991. On the parental origin of de novo mutation in man. Journal of Medical Genetics 28 (4):217–23.

159. Crow, J.F. 2000. The origins, patterns and implications of human spontaneous mutation. Nature Reviews Genetics 1 (1):40–7.

160. Adams, J.B., J. Romdalvik, V.M. Ramanujam, and M.S. Legator. 2007. Mercury, lead, and zinc in baby teeth of children with autism versus controls. Journal of Toxicology and Environmental Health A 70 (12):1046–51.

161. Bradstreet, J., D.A. Geier, J.J. Kartzinel, J.B. Adams, and M.R. Feier. 2003. A case–control study of mercury burden in children with autistic spectrum disorders. Journal of American Physicians and Surgeons 8 (3).

162. Desoto, M.C., and R.T. Hitlan. 2007. Blood levels of mercury are related to diagnosis of autism: a reanalysis of an important data set. Journal of Child Neurology 22 (11):1308–11.

163. Hertz–Picciotto, I., P.G. Green, L. Delwiche, R. Hansen, C. Walker, and I.N. Pessah. 2010. Blood mercury concentrations in CHARGE Study children with and without autism. Environmental Health Perspectives 118 (1):161–6.

164. Palmer, R.F., S. Blanchard, and R. Wood. 2009. Proximity to point sources of environmental mercury release as a predictor of autism prevalence. Health Place 15 (1):18–24.

165. Centers for Disease Control and Prevention. Mercury and Thimerosal: Vaccine Safety. CDC. Retrieved October 12, 2010 from http://www.cdc.gov/vaccinesafety/Concerns/thimerosal/index.html.

166. Institute of Medicine. 2004. Immunization Safety Review: Vaccines and Autism. Washington, DC: National Academies Press. http://www.nap.edu/catalog.php?record_id=10997.

167. Kalkbrenner, A.E., J.L. Daniels, J.–C. Chen, C. Poole, M. Emch, and J. Morrissey. 2010. Perinatal Exposure to Hazardous Air Pollutants and Autism Spectrum Disorders at Age 8. Epidemiology 21 (5):631–41.

168. Windham, G.C., L. Zhang, R. Gunier, L.A. Croen, and J.K. Grether. 2006. Autism spectrum disorders in relation to distribution of hazardous air pollutants in the San Francisco Bay area. Environmental Health Perspectives 114 (9):1438–44.

169. Volk, H.E., I. Hertz–Picciotto, L. Delwiche, F. Lurmann, and R. McConnell. 2011. Residential Proximity to Freeways and Autism in the CHARGE Study. Environmental Health Perspectives 119 (6):873–7.

170. Larsson, M., B. Weiss, S. Janson, J. Sundell, and C.G. Bornehag. 2009. Associations between indoor environmental factors and parental–reported autistic spectrum disorders in children 6–8 years of age. Neurotoxicology 30 (5):822–31.

171. American Association of Intellectual and Developmental Disabilities. 2009. FAQ on Intellectual Disability. Retrieved March 23, 2009 from http://www.aamr.org/content_104.cfm?navID=22.

172. Schroeder, S.R. 2000. Mental retardation and developmental disabilities influenced by environmental neurotoxic insults. Environmental Health Perspectives 108 (Suppl. 3):395–9.

173. Daily, D.K., H.H. Ardinger, and G.E. Holmes. 2000. Identification and evaluation of mental retardation. American Family Physician 61 (4):1059–67, 1070.

174. Flint, J., and A.O. Wilkie. 1996. The genetics of mental retardation. British Medical Bulletin 52 (3):453–64.

175. Murphy, C., C. Boyle, D. Schendel, P. Decouflé, and M. Yeargin–Allsopp. 1998. Epidemiology of mental retardation in children. Mental Retardation and Developmental Disabilities Research Reviews 4 (1):6–13.

176. Bakir, F., H. Rustam, S. Tikriti, S.F. Al–Damluji, and H. Shihristani. 1980. Clinical and epidemiological aspects of methylmercury poisoning. Postgraduate Medical Journal 56 (651):1–10.

177. David, O., S. Hoffman, B. McGann, J. Sverd, and J. Clark. 1976. Low lead levels and mental retardation. Lancet 2 (8000):1376–9.

178. McDermott, S., J. Wu, B. Cai, A. Lawson, and C. Marjorie Aelion. 2011. Probability of intellectual disability is associated with soil concentrations of arsenic and lead. Chemosphere 84 (1):31–8.

179. U.S. Environmental Protection Agency. 2006. Air Quality Criteria for Lead (Final Report). Washington, DC: U.S. EPA, National Center for Environmental Assessment. EPA/600/R–05/144aF–bF. http://cfpub.epa.gov/ncea/isa/recordisplay.cfm?deid=158823.

180. Edwards, S.C., W. Jedrychowski, M. Butscher, D. Camann, A. Kieltyka, E. Mroz, E. Flak, Z. Li, S. Wang, V. Rauh, et al. 2010. Prenatal exposure to airborne polycyclic aromatic hydrocarbons and children's intelligence at age 5 in a prospective cohort study in Poland. Environmental Health Perspectives 118 (9):1326–31.

181. Fewtrell, L.J., A. Pruss–Ustun, P. Landrigan, and J.L. Ayuso–Mateos. 2004. Estimating the global burden of disease of mild mental retardation and cardiovascular diseases from environmental lead exposure. Environmental Research 94 (2):120–33.

182. U.S. Environmental Protection Agency. 1997. The Benefits and Costs of the Clean Air Act, 1970 to 1990. Washington, DC: U.S. EPA, Office of Air and Radiation. http://www.epa.gov/air/sect812/copy.html.

183. Weiss, B. 2000. Vulnerability of children and the developing brain to neurotoxic hazards. Environmental Health Perspectives 108 (Suppl. 3):375–81.

184. De Los Reyes, A., and A.E. Kazdin. 2005. Informant discrepancies in the assessment of childhood psychopathology: a critical review, theoretical framework, and recommendations for further study. Psychological Bulletin 131 (4):483–509.

185. Owens, P.L., K. Hoagwood, S.M. Horwitz, P.J. Leaf, J.M. Poduska, S.G. Kellam, and N.S. Ialongo. 2002. Barriers to children's mental health services. Journal of the American Academy of Child and Adolescent Psychiatry 41 (6):731–8.

186. U.S. Department of Health and Human Services. 1999. Mental Health: A Report of the Surgeon General—Executive Summary. Rockville, MD: U.S. DHS, Substance Abuse and Mental Health Services Administration, Center for Mental Health Services, National Institutes of Health, National Institute of Mental Health. http://www.surgeongeneral.gov/library/mentalhealth/pdfs/ExSummary–Final.pdf.

187. Centers for Disease Control and Prevention. 2007. Prevalence of autism spectrum disorders——autism and developmental disabilities monitoring network, 14 sites, United States, 2002. In: Surveillance Summaries. Morbidity and Mortality Weekly Report 56 (No. SS–1):12–28.

188. Kogan, M.D., S.J. Blumberg, L.A. Schieve, C.A. Boyle, J.M. Perrin, R.M. Ghandour, G.K. Singh, B.B. Strickland, E. Trevathan, and P.C. van Dyck. 2009. Prevalence of parent–reported diagnosis of autism spectrum disorder among children in the US, 2007. Pediatrics 124 (5):1395–403.

There is an appendix to this article that is not available in this version of the article. To view this additional information, please use the citation on the first page of this chapter.

CHAPTER 2

A STRATEGY FOR COMPARING THE CONTRIBUTIONS OF ENVIRONMENTAL CHEMICALS AND OTHER RISK FACTORS TO NEURODEVELOPMENT OF CHILDREN

DAVID C. BELLINGER

Assessments of the import of an association observed between an environmental chemical exposure and child neurodevelopment often focus solely on the magnitude of the effect size and its associated p-value (i.e., whether it is < 0.05). Effect size is expressed in various forms, as the difference between the mean scores of exposed and unexposed groups, the change in score per unit change in an exposure biomarker, or the change in risk (relative risk, odds ratio) associated with a particular value of the biomarker. Among the reasons cited to dismiss an effect size is that it is clinically unimportant (e.g., Kaufman 2001). This perspective fails to place the effect estimate in a public health context, however. Estimating the population burden attributable to a factor requires a metric that reflects not only the magnitude of the risk associated with the factor but also the frequency

Reproduced with permission from Environmental Health Perspectives. Bellinger DC. A Strategy for Comparing the Contributions of Environmental Chemicals and Other Risk Factors to Neurodevelopment of Children. Environmental Health Perspectives 120,4 (2012). doi: 10.1289/ehp.1104170.

with which the factor occurs in the population (Steenland and Armstrong 2006), a concept embodied in the environmentally attributable fraction model (Institute of Medicine 1981). Although a factor associated with a large impact would be a significant burden to a patient, it might not be a major contributor to population burden if it occurs rarely. Conversely, a factor associated with a modest but frequently occurring impact could contribute substantially to population burden.

The objective of this review was to describe a population-oriented approach to estimating risk factor burden as an alternative to the usual disease-oriented approach. This approach was then used to compare the population burdens associated with major medical, social, and chemical risks to child development.

2.1 METHODS

Several choices were required to apply the approach.

Risk factors. An effort was made to estimate the contributions to children's neurodevelopment of a wide range of medical conditions, including neurodevelopmental disorders, postnatal events, socioeconomic and psychosocial risks. The goal was not to provide an exhaustive accounting of all contributors, however, and the selection of risk factors was not based on a systematic review, but on the availability of data.

End point for comparison. In most studies, a battery of neurodevelopmental tests assessing many domains is administered. Full-Scale IQ (FSIQ) score is the end point most consistently reported across studies, however, and provides the best opportunity to conduct a comparative analysis. Among the instruments used to assess neurodevelopment in children, FSIQ tests tend to be the strongest psychometrically, and an extensive body of research demonstrates relationships between FSIQ and many important late outcomes (Neisser et al. 1996).

Evidence on which effect sizes are based. Given the typical heterogeneity of the effect sizes derived from individual epidemiologic studies, basing the calculation on the effect size from a single study, particularly one of the first reported (Ioannidis 2005), would be an invitation to controversy. An effect estimate derived from a meta-analysis or pooled analysis, conducted by subject matter experts applying a transparent protocol for study inclusion and weighting, reflects the weight of evidence available on a risk factor. Therefore, preference was given to effect estimates based on a meta-analysis or pooled analysis that provided evidence supporting a statistically significant association between a risk factor and FSIQ. In some cases, when such an analysis was not available, a single study was used, preferably one that was population based and with a large sample size. However, this was done in recognition that the effect size would likely differ, to an uncertain extent, if based on an analysis that integrated the findings of multiple studies.

Population to which to generalize findings. A population of 25.5 million 0- to 5-year-old children in the United States was assumed (Federal Interagency Forum on Child and Family Statistics 2011).

Method used to estimate FSIQ loss. For a categorical risk factor (i.e., one that a child either has or does not), the published prevalence of the factor in 0- to 5-year-old children was multiplied by the difference between the FSIQ scores of children with and without the risk factor (i.e., the effect size) to estimate the total FSIQ loss associated with it. If only an estimate of yearly incidence was available (e.g., the number of events per year among children 0–5 years of age), the incidence was multiplied by five (the number of yearly intervals in a population of 0- to 5-year-olds) to estimate the total number of children in the cohort who would be expected to have experienced the risk factor. When the prevalence/incidence among 0- to 5-year-olds was not available, it was estimated based on the prevalence/incidence for the closest age range for which it was available.

For risk factors represented by a continuous distribution, the numbers of 0- to 5-year-old children (or the age range closest to this) with values in specified intervals of the distribution were calculated (e.g., 25th–50th percentile; 90th–95th percentile). Based on the dose–effect relationship for the risk factor, slopes for the FSIQ loss per unit increase in the factor were calculated, either across the entire distribution or, in the case of a nonlinear relationship, over specific intervals of the exposure distribution. Within each interval, the slope was multiplied, first, by the midpoint value of the risk factor (or the distance between the midpoint value and the value below which no association has been found to exist between the risk factor and FSIQ) and, second, by the estimated number of children in the interval. The FSIQ losses of children within intervals were then summed to derive the total number of FSIQ points lost. (See Table 1 for an example.)

TABLE 1: Estimated numbers of FSIQ points lost from lead exposure for children in different intervals of the blood lead distribution.

Range of the BLL distribution (µg/dL)	Midpoint BLL (µg/dL)	FSIQ loss[a]	No. of children	No. of FSIQ points lost	
0 to 50th percentile (0–1.43)	0.72		0.37	12,750,000	4,717,500
50th to 75th percentile (1.43–2.10)	1.77		0.90	6,375,000	5,737,500
75th to 90th percentile (2.10–2.98)	2.54		1.30	3,825,000	4,972,500
90th to 95th percentile (2.98–3.80)	3.39		1.73	1,275,000	2,205,750
95th to 98th percentile (3.80–7.50)	5.65		2.88	765,000	2,203,200
> 98th percentile (> 7.50)	15		6.10	510,000	3,111,000

Abbreviation: BLL, blood lead level. [a]The FSIQ losses associated with blood lead intervals < 98th percentile were calculated by multiplying the midpoint BLL in an interval by −0.51 IQ points/µg/dL, the slope estimated for BLL < 10 µg/dL in the pooled analysis (Lanphear et al. 2005). The midpoint BLL of children with a BLL > 98th percentile was assumed to be 15, and the FSIQ loss was assumed to be 6.10 points (5.1 points lost up to a BLL of 10 µg/dL and an additional 1 point, which is one-half of the FSIQ loss estimated in the pooled analyses to be associated with an increase in BLL from 10 to 20 µg/dL).

The level of precision in the calculations reported here should not be overinterpreted. They are intended to provide only rough estimates of the FSIQ losses associated with different risk factors for purposes of comparison.

2.2 RESULTS

Medical conditions. Congenital heart disease. Karsdorp et al. (2007) conducted a meta-analysis in which estimates were derived for the FSIQ deficits associated with different forms of congenital heart disease, the most common structural birth defect. The scores of children with a ventricular or atrial septal defect were not impaired, but the scores of children with more complex lesions—such as tetralogy of Fallot (TOF), d-transposition of the great arteries (d-TGA), and hypoplastic left heart syndrome (HLHS)—were, with mean deficits of 2.55, 2.10, and 12.3 points, respectively. The incidence of TOF is 4 in 10,000 (Child 2004), or 10,200 cases in children 0–5 years of age in the United States. The incidence of d-TGA is 3 in 10,000 (Martins and Castela 2008), or 7,650 cases, and the incidence of HLHS is 2 in 10,000 (Barron et al. 2009), or 5,100 cases. Therefore, the estimated numbers of FSIQ points lost are 26,010 (TOF), 16,065 (d-TGA), and 62,730 (HLHS), totaling 104,805 points.

Preterm birth. Approximately 12.3% of U.S. children are born preterm (gestational age < 37 weeks) (Hamilton et al. 2010). In a meta-analysis of 15 studies (1,556 cases; 1,720 controls), Bhutta et al. (2002) calculated a mean FSIQ deficit among cases of 10.85 points, producing a total loss of 34,031,025 FSIQ points. The severity of preterm birth likely influences the magnitude of the deficit, but separate estimates for specific intervals of gestational age were not available. The estimate of 10.85 points is based on studies published between 1988 and 2001, and it is possible that the deficit among contemporary samples of children born preterm has been reduced by improvements in neonatal intensive care practices. In some cohorts born after 2000, FSIQ at age 5 years is approximately the expected mean of 100, even among infants born at 28 weeks of gestation and with birth weights of approximately 1,000 g (Lind et al. 2011).

Type 1 diabetes. The prevalence of type 1 diabetes in U.S. children is approximately 1 in 500 (~ 51,000 children). In a meta-analysis of 19 studies (1,393 cases; 751 controls), Gaudieri et al. (2008) estimated standardized effect sizes of –0.35 and –0.28 for two constructs, crystallized intelligence (i.e., ability to apply skills, knowledge, and experience) and fluid intelligence (i.e., ability to think logically to solve novel problems), respectively, in children with early-onset disease (diagnosis at < 7 years of age) compared with controls. The mean of these two, as a proxy for FSIQ, is –0.315, corresponding to 4.73 points. Among children with late-onset disease, the effect sizes for crystallized and fluid intelligence were –0.20 and –0.14, respectively, or a mean effect size of –0.17, corresponding to

2.55 points. If half of the cases are assumed to be early onset and half late onset, the total FSIQ loss is estimated to be 185,640 points.

Acute lymphocytic leukemia. The most common malignancy in children, acute lymphocytic leukemia, occurs with an annual incidence of 10 in 100,000, primarily in 2- to 5-year-olds, resulting in a total of 12,750 cases among children < 5 years of age in the United States. In a meta-analysis involving 28 studies of children treated with cranial radiation, intrathecal chemotherapy, or both, the average weighted standardized effect size for FSIQ was –0.71, corresponding to 10.65 points (Campbell et al. 2007). Therefore, the estimated FSIQ loss is 135,788 points.

Brain tumors. Brain tumors are the most common solid tumor diagnosis in children and the second leading cause of death by disease. The annual incidence is 2.35 in 100,000 children (Mulhern and Butler 2004), representing 599 cases yearly among U.S. children. In a meta-analysis of 32 studies involving 1,096 children, Robinson et al. (2010) reported a weighted standardized effect size of –0.83 for FSIQ, corresponding to a loss of 12.45 points. Therefore, the total FSIQ loss is 37,288 points. Significant heterogeneity of the effect sizes across studies was noted, most likely reflecting cohort differences in tumor subtype (e.g., medulloblastoma vs. astrocytoma) or differences in treatment protocols. Because of data limitations, however, tumor-specific estimates could not be made.

Duchenne muscular dystrophy. Duchenne muscular dystrophy is the most common form of muscular dystrophy, occurring in 2.9 in 10,000 male births (therefore, approximately 1.5 in 10,000 total births [Centers for Disease Control and Prevention (CDC) 2009a]. This corresponds to 3,825 cases in U.S. children 0–5 years of age. In a meta-analysis of 32 studies, which included 1,231 patients, Cotton et al. (2005) estimated a mean FSIQ of 82, representing a deficit of 18 points. Therefore, the total FSIQ loss is estimated to be 68,850 points.

Neurodevelopmental disorders. Autism spectrum disorders. The prevalence of autism spectrum disorders (ASDs) in the United States is approximately 1 in 110 (CDC 2009b), or 231,818 children in the 0- to 5-year age range. Although a meta-analysis of FSIQ scores of children with ASDs could not be found, Charman et al. (2011) conducted a population-based study in the United Kingdom that involved identifying each child in a population of 56,946 who had either a local diagnosis of an ASD or a

"Statement of Educational Needs." FSIQ was measured in the 156 children identified. The percentages of children in severity categories were as follows: 7.4% severe/profound (FSIQ < 35, or a loss of 65 points); 8.4% moderate (FSIQ 35–49, or an average loss of 58 points); 39.4% mild (FSIQ 50–69, or an average loss of 41 points); and 16.6% below average (FSIQ 70–84, or an average loss of 23 points). Another 25.4% were in the average range (85–114). Half of these children (12.7%) were assumed to have FSIQ scores between 85 and 99, with an average loss of 8 points. If these figures are applied to U.S. children, the estimated total FSIQ loss is 7,109,899 points.

Bipolar disorder. Based on the number of office visits that identify pediatric bipolar disorder as the reason (from the National Ambulatory Medical Care Survey of the National Center for Health Statistics, 1999–2003), Moreno et al. (2007) estimated the prevalence to be 6.67%. The weighted standardized effect size for FSIQ based on 10 studies included in a meta-analysis is –0.32, corresponding to a loss of 4.8 points (Joseph et al. 2008), producing an estimated total loss of 8,164,080 points.

Attention deficit hyperactivity disorder. Based on parent report (from the National Survey of Children's Health, United States, 2007), 7.2% of children 4–17 years of age have a current diagnosis of attention deficit hyperactivity disorder (ADHD) (CDC 2010a). In a meta-analysis that included 137 comparisons of FSIQ among children with ADHD and controls (Frazier et al. 2004), the weighted standardized effect size was –0.61 or 9.15 points, producing an estimated total loss of 16,799,400 points.

Postnatal events. Traumatic brain injury. The number of cases of traumatic brain injury (TBI) is estimated to be 475,000 annually among children 0–14 years of age, with the highest incidence among children 0–4 years of age (Langlois et al. 2005). An assumption that 40% of TBI events occur in children 0–5 years of age results in an estimate of ~ 950,000 cases in the United States. In a meta-analysis, Babikian and Asarnow (2009) provided estimates of the mean FSIQ deficits associated with TBI of differing severity, defined by Glasgow Coma Scale score (mild: 13–15; moderate: 9–12; severe: 3–8). Because recovery does occur, mostly in the 24 months after injury, the estimated FSIQ deficits present 24 months postinjury were used. The mean deficits associated with mild, moderate, and severe TBI were 4.47, 8.99, and 16.59 points, respectively. Narayan et al. (2002) reported that 80% of TBIs are mild, 10% moderate, and 10% severe. There-fore, the FSIQ loss associated with mild TBI is 3,397,200 points; moderate TBI, 854,050 points; and severe TBI, 1,576,050. The total estimated loss is therefore 5,827,300 points.

Socioeconomic, nutritional, and psychosocial risks. Nonorganic fail-ure to thrive. Some children fail to grow at the expected rate because of child abuse, neglect, parental mental disorder, and the like. Various criteria are used to identify cases, including weight below the 5th or 3rd percen-tile, a decrease of two major percentile lines on a growth chart, and < 80% expected weight. In a meta-analysis of studies in which cases were identi-fied from primary care settings, Corbett and Drewett (2004) reported a difference of 4.2 points in the FSIQ scores of cases (n = 502) and controls (n = 523). The various definitions used imply different prevalences, but if as many as 5% of children are assumed to be cases, the total estimated loss is 5,355,000 points.

Iron deficiency. In the National Health and Nutrition Examination Sur-vey (NHANES) 1999–2000, the prevalence of iron deficiency, defined as an abnormal value on two or more indicators (serum ferritin, transferring saturation, free erythrocyte protoporphyrin) was 7% in 1- to 2-year-olds and 5% in 3- to 5-year-olds (CDC 2002). In a meta-analysis of four sup-plementation trials (Sachdev et al. 2005), the weighted standardized effect size was 0.41, corresponding to an increase of 6.15 points in the FSIQ scores of iron-deficient children who received supplementation. Interpret-ing this value as an estimate of the loss among children who do not receive supplementation and assuming a prevalence of 6%, the estimated FSIQ loss in U.S. children from iron deficiency is 9,409,500 points.

Environmental chemical exposures. Methylmercury. Using NHANES 1999–2000 data, McDowell et al. (2004) reported the distribution of hair mercury levels in U.S. women of childbearing age (16–49 years). Levels for the 10th, 25th, 50th, 75th, 90th, and 95th percentiles were 0.04, 0.09, 0.19, 0.42, 1.11, and 1.73 µg/g, respectively. Axelrad et al. (2007) con-ducted a dose–response analysis that integrated the results of three major epidemiological studies (New Zealand, Faroe Islands, Seychelles Islands), identifying a regression coefficient of –0.18 child FSIQ points per micro-gram per gram increase in maternal hair during pregnancy. This coefficient was derived on the basis of maternal hair mercury levels considerably greater than those of U.S. women (means in the Seychelles Islands and Faroe Islands cohorts were 6.8 µg/g and 4.3 µg/g, respectively). To estimate FSIQ loss, it was assumed that the coefficient applies to hair mercury levels > 1.11 µg/g (90th percentile), approximately the value on which the methylmercury reference dose is based (Rice et al. 2003). A concentration of 1.73 µg/g (95th percentile) was assumed to be the midpoint hair mercury level of the 10% of U.S. women with a level > 1.11 µg/g. The estimated total FSIQ loss is therefore 284,580 points.

Some studies have reported adverse neurodevelopmental outcomes at maternal hair levels lower than those represented in the analyses by Axelrad et al. (e.g., Oken et al. 2008). If the slope of –0.18 FSIQ points per microgram per gram is assumed to hold over the full range of maternal hair mercury levels in U.S. women, the total loss would be 1,875,017 points.

Recent studies, as well as reanalyses of older studies, suggest that neurotoxicity of methylmercury is underestimated if account is not taken of the fact that fish consumption also provides exposure to beneficial nutrients (Budtz-Jorgensen et al. 2007; Lynch et al. 2011; Oken et al. 2008). Because this was not done in the analyses by Axelrad et al. (2007), the coefficient might underestimate the true slope and thus result in an underestimate of the total FSIQ loss.

Although NHANES data are nationally representative, concern has been expressed that the relatively small sample size (n = 1,726) resulted in inadequate sampling of subgroups at particular risk, such as the families of subsistence and sport fishermen (Knobeloch et al. 2007) and certain ethnic groups in which fish is a particularly prominent part of the diet (Hightower et al. 2006) and among whom awareness of fish advisories is low (Knobeloch et al. 2005). If consumers of a diet high in fish are indeed underrepresented in NHANES, the FSIQ loss calculated on the basis of the distribution of hair mercury levels in that survey would be an underestimate. When exposure of women of childbearing age is concerned, it is also important to consider whether the body burden for a chemical increases with age (e.g., polychlorinated biphenyls and, to a lesser extent, methylmercury). If burden is positively associated with age, risk will be overestimated unless age-specific natality rates are taken into account (Axelrad and Cohen 2011).

Organophosphate pesticides. In NHANES 1999–2004, the 5th, 10th, 25th, 50th, 75th, 90th, and 95th percentiles of the distribution of total urinary dialkyl phosphate (DAP) metabolites in pregnant women were 7.3, 9.3, 27.0, 65.0, 151.7, 237.2, and 483.5 nmol/L, respectively (CDC 2011b). A meta-analysis that provides the dose–effect relationship between total DAP metabolites and children's FSIQ is not available, but Bouchard et al. (2011) and Engel et al. (2011) both reported on the association between total urinary DAP metabolites in pregnant women and childhood FSIQ. In the cohort studied by Engel et al. (2007), the median total urinary DAP metabolite concentration was 82 nmol/L (interquartile range of 35–195). In the cohort studied by Bouchard et al. (2011), the range was roughly 50–500 nmol/L. The ranges observed in these studies are therefore reasonable approximations of the upper half of the distribution of urinary DAP concentrations of U.S. pregnant women. Bouchard et al. (2011) reported that a 10-fold increase in total urinary DAP was associated with a loss of 5.6 FSIQ points [95% confidence interval (CI): –9.0, –2.2; n = 297], whereas Engel et al. (2011) reported that a 10-fold increase was associated with a loss of 1.39 points (95% CI: –4.5, 1.77; n = 140). Weighting the effect estimates by sample size produces an expected loss of 4.25 FSIQ points for a 10-fold increase in urinary DAP over this range, or a slope of –0.01 point/nmol/L. The studies do not provide information about the dose–effect relationship < 50 nmol/L, so this slope was applied only to the 50% of U.S. children with DAP levels > 65.0 nmol/L (the median). The studies also do not provide information about the relationship > 500 nmol/L, so the FSIQ loss for the 5% of U.S. children with a level > 483.5 nmol/L was assumed to be 4.25 points. Combining the slope and the distribution of total urinary DAP levels produces a total estimated loss of 16,899,488 points. If levels < 50th percentile are associated with FSIQ loss, the total would be greater.

Lead. In NHANES 2005–2006, the 50th, 75th, 90th, 95th, and 98th percentiles of the blood lead distribution for U.S. children 1–5 years of age were 1.43, 2.10, 2.98, and 3.80 µg/dL, respectively (CDC 2011a). The 98th percentile was not reported, but in NHANES 2003–2004, it was 10.0 µg/dL (CDC 2009c). Based on the percentage declines observed between NHANES 2003–3004 and 2005–2006 in the 90th and 95th percentiles (23.6% and 25.5%, respectively), I estimated that the 98th percentile in NHANES 2005–2006 was 7.5 µg/dL. Estimates of the dose–effect relationship relating blood lead level to FSIQ in children were taken from the pooled analysis of Lanphear et al. (2005). This analysis, involving > 1,300 children who participated in seven international prospective studies, identified a supralinear relationship over the range of 2.4–30 µg/dL. The best fits over narrower ranges were linear, however. An increase in blood lead level from 2.4 to 10 µg/dL was associated with a decrement of 3.9 FSIQ points (i.e., a slope of –0.51 points/µg/dL). This slope was also assumed to apply to blood lead levels between 0 and 2.4 µg/dL, as recent risk assessments have concluded that it is not possible to identify a blood lead level below which no adverse impact can be discerned [European Food Safety Authority 2010; Joint FAO/WHO (Food and Agriculture Organization/ World Health Organization) Expert Committee on Food Additives 2010]. In the pooled analysis, an increase in blood lead from 10 to 20 µg/dL was associated with an additional decrement of 1.9 FSIQ points. A blood lead level of 15 µg/dL was assumed for the 2% of children with a blood lead level above the 98th percentile and an average loss of 6.1 points (5.1 points for the range of 0–10 µg/dL plus one additional point for the increase > 10 µg/dL). For children with blood lead levels < 10 µg/dL, the midpoint blood lead level for each interval was multiplied by –0.51 and the product then multiplied by the number of children in the interval. For children with levels > 10 µg/dL, the assumed midpoint of 15 µg/dL was multiplied by 6.1 points. The total estimated FSIQ loss is therefore 22,947,450 points (Table 1). An uncertainty analysis was conducted using the lower and upper bounds of the 95% CIs for the slopes estimated in the pooled analysis. Assuming the lower and upper bounds yields an estimated total FSIQ loss of 14,185,905 and 31,277,154 points, respectively.

2.3 DISCUSSION

Based on the estimated number of FSIQ points lost, the population burdens associated with environmental chemical exposures of children are surprisingly large—in some cases larger than those estimated for major medical conditions and events (Table 2). This is attributable not so much to the magnitude of the effect sizes associated with chemicals, but to the prevalence of exposures associated with adverse impacts. For example, in the case of lead, because of the absence of a threshold, every child contributes at least a little to population morbidity, and the cumulative impact is substantial, even if the lower bound of the CI for the effect size is used. Furthermore, most of the total morbidity is contributed by children with blood lead levels < 10 µg/dL rather than by children with levels > 10 µg/dL, the current CDC level of concern (Table 1). This illustrates the principle, applied in evaluating the impart of radiation exposure, that "it is the total dose falling on the whole population which determines the burden of health effects" (Rose 1991), and that "a large number of people at a small risk may give rise to more cases of disease than the small number who are at a high risk" (Rose 1985). This led Rose (1981) to argue in favor of supplementing individually based interventions, which target those at high risk, with population-based interventions designed to shift the population distribution of a health index in the direction of lower risk.

TABLE 2: Estimated FSIQ point losses associated with different risk factors in a population of 25.5 million children.

Risk factor	Total no. of FSIQ points lost
Medical conditions	
Congenital heart disease	104,805
Preterm birth	34,031,025
Type 1 diabetes	185,640
Acute lymphocytic leukemia	135,788
Brain tumors	37,288
Duchenne muscular dystrophy	68,850
Neurodevelopmental disorders	
ASDs	7,109,899
Pediatric bipolar disorder	8,164,080
ADHD	16,799,400
Postnatal traumatic brain injury	5,827,300
Socioeconomic, nutritional, psychosocial factors	
Nonorganic failure to thrive	5,355,000
Iron deficiency	9,409,500
Environmental chemical exposures	
Methylmercury	284,580
Organophosphate pesticides	16,899,488
Lead	22,947,450

Another illustration of the important distinction between individual and population risk is provided by the epidemiology of Down syndrome. As individuals, older women are at substantially greater risk than younger women of delivering a child with Down syndrome, as the relative risk associated with a maternal age > 44 years is approximately 50 compared with women < 30 years. The birth rate among younger women is so much higher, however, that 50% of children with Down syndrome are born to women < 30 years of age. Despite its large relative risk, maternal age has a modest attributable fraction, and much of the population burden is contributed by women who, individually, are at low risk. Although a factor that increases the odds ratio of a serious disease by 10-fold is clearly important for an affected individual, if it only increases the number of cases from 0.1 in 1,000,000 to 1 in 1,000,000, its import for population health is modest.

The notion that individuals with values on a health index that are not sufficiently extreme to meet diagnostic criteria may contribute substantially to population burden has been widely discussed in the context of chronic disease epidemiology. Applying categorical disease labels to individuals is necessary for clinical management and resource allocation. However, for many diseases that are defined using cutoff values of continuously distributed measurements (e.g., hypertension, diabetes, depression), the important question, as Rose (1993) noted, is not whether an individual "has" the disease but "how much of it" one has. Quoting Pickering, Rose (1993) lamented that "medicine in its present state can count up to two but not beyond," tending to regard disease and health as nonoverlapping states. Goldberg (2000) observed that in insisting on categorical diagnoses, "rather than carving nature at the joints, we appear to be merely drawing lines in the fog."

The strategies used to estimate the population health burden associated with chemicals have generally reflected a disease-oriented approach rather than a population-oriented approach. It is frequently noted that a modest shift in the mean IQ score in a population will be accompanied by a substantial increase in the percentage of individuals with extremely low scores. For example, Needleman et al. (1982) showed that the median verbal IQ scores of children with high and low dentine lead levels differed by only 5 or 6 points, but scores < 80 were three times more frequent in the high-lead group. This difference is surely important, but the cumulative frequency distributions of the two groups differed throughout the entire range and, in fact, never intersected. Focusing solely on the difference between the distributions in the extreme left tail fails to acknowledge that the differences over the rest of the range of verbal IQ scores are also germane to population burden.

A disease-oriented approach underlies the protocol used by the WHO to estimate the global burden of disease, in that it is only health states associated with an *International Classification of Diseases* (ICD) code that contribute to burden (WHO 2009). Fewtrell et al. (2003) used this protocol to estimate the burden attributable to lead. With regard to neurodevelopment, it was only children whose FSIQ score would be expected to be reduced to ≤ 70 (ICD category: mild mental retardation) as a result of lead exposure who contributed to the burden estimate. That a substantial fraction of the overall FSIQ loss in the calculations reported in this review is contributed by children with blood lead levels at the lower end of the exposure distribution, among whom few would be expected to meet criteria for mild mental retardation, indicates that a disease-oriented approach likely underestimates the contribution of lead to neurodevelopmental morbidity.

The population approach advocated here is consistent with the strategy economists use to assign monetary value to changes in FSIQ, which does not focus solely on the extreme low tail of the distribution. In estimating the economic benefits of reducing children's lead exposure, Grosse et al. (2002) estimated that each FSIQ point lost reduces future work productivity by 1.76–2.38%, regardless of an individual's initial FSIQ, a monetary loss placed by Gould (2009) at $17,815 in discounted lifetime earnings.

The important risk factors for FSIQ loss likely vary across cultural and regional settings. Although the intellectual burden associated with undernutrition, infectious diseases, and parasitic diseases is far greater among children in developing than in developed countries (Walker et al. 2007), exposures to environmental chemicals are also greater. In 2000, < 10% of children worldwide had a blood lead level > 20 µg/dL, but 99% of them lived in developing countries (Fewtrell et al. 2003), where tragic episodes of mass fatalities continue to occur (CDC 2010b).

The approach described in this review can be used to carry out a range-finding analysis of newly identified exposures and to prioritize research needs. For example, concern has been raised about the neurodevelopmental effects of children's exposures to bisphenol A (Braun and Hauser 2011), polybrominated diphenyl ethers (Herbstman et al. 2010), and phthalates (Engel et al. 2010), but meta-analyses of these exposures have not been published. Keeping in mind that the effect estimates reported in initial studies of a risk factor tend to be larger than those reported in later studies (Ioannidis 2005), one can nevertheless estimate the total FSIQ loss using the limited data available to get a preliminary sense of how important an exposure might be on a population basis.

Finally, the approach can be helpful in evaluating the impact of interventions to reduce population exposures. Applying it to the blood lead level data collected in NHANES II (1976–1980) (Mahaffey et al. 1982) yields an estimated FSIQ loss of 119,990,842 points for that cohort of children, suggesting that measures taken in recent decades to reduce blood lead levels of children have produced a substantial reduction in neurodevelopmental morbidity. The approach could also be used to compare the anticipated benefits of alternative regulatory initiatives based on the expected impact of an initiative on a biomarker distribution.

2.4 LIMITATIONS

Use of FSIQ as the basis for calculations. FSIQ was chosen as the end point for comparing risk factors, but this might not be the outcome that captures the most important impact of a risk factor. For example, among children with a TBI, deficits in visual-perceptual function are more prominent than deficits in FSIQ (Babikian and Asarnow 2009), and verbal memory and executive function are typically more impaired than FSIQ in children with bipolar disorder (Joseph et al. 2008). Because FSIQ averages performance over multiple domains, it is a poor metric for expressing the impact of a risk factor that selectively impairs certain domains, as has been suggested for methylmercury (Grandjean et al. 2006). Some risk factors, such as environmental tobacco smoke, might have their greatest impact on a child's risk of behavioral disorders such as ADHD (Froehlich et al. 2009; Lindberg et al. 2010). Therefore, for other end points, the relative importance of risk factors might differ from what was observed for FSIQ.

In some studies, the FSIQ scores of children with a risk factor were compared with the scores of children in the standardization sample of the test used, whereas in others it was compared with the scores of a control group. Each strategy has advantages. Use of a control group can provide better control for confounding when studying a risk factor that tends to occur more often in particular subgroups of children (e.g., sickle cell disease). However, if the control group differs from the exposed group on important predictors of neurodevelopment and if adjustment for such factors is inadequate, the effect size derived could over- or underestimate the true value, depending on the circumstances.

Data used to support the calculations. The calculations carried out for different risk factors varied in terms of the quantity of data available (i.e., the number of studies, the number of children contributing data), resulting in differences in the weight and strength of the evidence that a risk factor is causally related to children's FSIQ. For some risk factors, such as fetal alcohol syndrome/alcohol-related neurodevelopmental disabilities and environmental tobacco smoke, a published meta-analysis could not be found.. For other risk factors, the available meta-analyses involved ecologic comparisons not suitable for calculating FSIQ loss. For fluorosis (Tang et al. 2008) and arsenicosis (Dong and Su 2009), for example, meta-analyses reported only the mean FSIQ deficits of children in areas with endemic disease compared with control areas.

Although relying on a meta-analysis reduces the problems associated with selecting a single study as the basis for calculations, such an analysis might not be accurate if it included studies that suffer from biases. Here I relied on the subject-matter experts who conducted the analyses to select the data on which to base the effect estimates. In some analyses, the effect estimates reported showed significant heterogeneity. This might reflect the presence of effect modification by characteristics that varied across studies (Bellinger 2009) or to methodological factors such as differences in the amount of exposure measurement error, which usually biases estimation toward the null (Grandjean et al. 2004). It could also be attributable to the presence of residual confounding in some of the studies included. Historically, confounding has been of prime importance, and the focus of most contention, in studies of environmental chemical exposures, because of the frequent regulatory and economic implications of the causal inferences drawn. Equivalent attention might not be paid to such issues in studies of other risk factors and, to the extent that confounders have not been identified and adjusted for in the individual studies, the overall effect estimates derived in meta-analyses might be inaccurate.

For iron deficiency, the results of intervention trials provided the effect estimate. Even if studies suggest that supplementation improves cognitive outcomes, the effect size might underestimate the FSIQ loss if supplementation does not fully reverse the impact of iron deficiency. In a meta-analysis of Chinese studies, the FSIQ deficit of children living in iodine-deficient areas was 12.45 points compared with children from iodine-sufficient areas (Qian et al. 2005). Children from iodine-deficient areas in which women received iodine supplementation during pregnancy recovered only 8.7 points, however. Prospective observational studies that do not involve supplementation would provide purer estimates of the impact of nutrient deficiencies, although ethical considerations might prevent such studies

For some risk factors (e.g., iron deficiency, methylmercury), the effect estimates were derived from studies conducted on non-U.S. samples. Important regional differences in the distributions of potential effect modifiers could reduce the appropriateness of extrapolating the effect estimates to U.S. children. For example, the impact of a micronutrient deficiency might be greater among children with comorbid health conditions, and the effect estimate derived on the basis of such a sample would overestimate the impact of the deficiency among children who lack the comorbidities. Also, the effect estimates derived in some meta-analyses (e.g., of methylmercury) were derived on the basis of exposures that differ substantially from those of U.S. children, potentially compromising their usefulness.

Conceptual issues. Some risk factors for which calculations were made are likely to lie on the same causal pathway as other risk factors. For example, because increased exposure to air pollutants has been associated with preterm birth, some portion of the burden calculated for preterm birth might represent an indirect effect of such exposures (Llop et al. 2010). In some cases, it might be possible to disentangle the contributions of different risk factors. For instance, Braun et al. (2006) estimated that one in five ADHD cases can be attributed to children with a blood lead level > 2 μg/dL. The WHO Global Burden of Disease methodology addresses this general problem by establishing disease "envelopes" (WHO 2009). For example, the total number of known deaths from hepatocellular carcinoma establishes an upper bound for the number of cases that can be attributed to its various causes (e.g., hepatitis B, hepatitis C, alcoholism, aflatoxin exposure). If the number of deaths attributed to all causes exceeds this total, double counting has likely occurred. Because FSIQ loss is not a reported disease, however, such bounding cannot be used to constrain the calculations.

Finally, it is likely that risk factors interact with one another to influence FSIQ of children. For example, not only do children living in poverty tend to experience greater exposures to environmental chemicals than do children living in advantaged circumstances (Elliott et al. 2004), but increasing evidence also suggests that material hardship, increased stress, and lack of enrichment opportunities exacerbate chemical neurotoxicity (Weiss and Bellinger 2006). Because of limitations in the available data, the impact of such interactions could not be estimated.

2.5 CONCLUSION

Any effort to compare the neurodevelopmental burden associated with different risk factors is limited by the data available and the assumptions required. It was possible to estimate the total loss of FSIQ points in the population of 0- to 5-year-old U.S. children for a variety of risk factors, including three environmental chemicals: methylmercury, organophosphate pesticides, and lead. Despite the limitations of the approach, it appears that when population impact is considered, the contributions of chemicals to FSIQ loss in children are substantial, in some cases exceeding those of other recognized risk factors for neurodevelopmental impairment in children. The primary reason for this is the relative ubiquity of exposure. As a community, we have not effectively communicated this point to risk assessors and other decision makers, despite the fact that a risk assessment that focuses solely on individual risk and fails to consider the problem in a public health context is potentially misleading.

REFERENCES

1. Axelrad DA, Bellinger DC, Ryan LM, Woodruff TJ. Dose–response relationship of prenatal mercury exposure and IQ: an integrated analysis of epidemiologic data. Environ Health Perspect. 2007;115:609–615.

2. Axelrad DA, Cohen J. Calculating summary statistics for population chemical biomonitoring in women of childbearing age with adjustment for age-specific natality. Environ Res. 2011;111:149–155.

3. Babikian T, Asarnow R. Neurocognitive outcomes and recovery after pediatric TBI: meta-analytic review of the literature. Neuropsychology. 2009;23:283–296.

4. Barron DJ, Kilby MD, Davies B, Wright JG, Jones TJ, Brown WJ. 2009. Hypoplastic left heart syndrome. Lancet 374 (9689551–564.564

5. Bellinger DC. Interpreting epidemiologic studies of developmental neurotoxicity: conceptual and analytic issues. Neurotoxicol Teratol. 2009;31:267–274.

6. Bhutta AT, Cleves MA, Casey PH, Cradock MM, Anand KJS. Cognitive and behavioral outcomes of school-aged children who were born preterm. JAMA. 2002;288:728–737.

7. Bouchard MF, Chevrier J, Harley KG, Kogut K, Vedar M, Calderon N, et al. Prenatal exposure to organophosphate pesticides and IQ in 7-year-old children. Environ Health Perspect. 2011;119:1189–1195.

8. Braun JM, Hauser R. Bisphenol A and children's health. Curr Opin Pediatr. 2011;23:233–239.

9. Braun JM, Kahn RS, Froehlich T, Auinger P, Lanphear BP. Exposures to environmental toxicants and attention deficit hyperactivity disorder in U.S. children. Environ Health Perspect. 2006;114:1904–1909.

10. Budtz-Jorgensen E, Grandjean P, Weihe P. Separation of risks and benefits of seafood intake. Environ Health Perspect. 2007;115:323–327.

11. Campbell LK, Scaduto M, Sharp W, Dufton L, Van Slyke D, Whitlock JA, et al. A meta-analysis of the neurocognitive sequelae of treatment for childhood acute lymphocytic leukemia. Pediatr Blood Cancer. 2007;49:65–73.

12. CDC (Centers for Disease Control and Prevention) Iron deficiency–United States, 1999–2000. MMWR Morb Mortal Wkly Rep. 2002;51(40):897–899.

13. CDC (Centers for Disease Control and Prevention) Prevalence of Duchenne/Becker muscular dystrophy among males aged 5–24 years — four states, 2007. MMWR Morb Mortal Wkly Rep. 2009a;58(4):1119–1222.

14. CDC (Centers for Disease Control and Prevention) Prevalence of autism spectrum disorders—autism and developmental disabilities monitoring network, United States, 2006. MMWR Morb Mortal Wkly Rep. 2009b;58(5510):1–20.

15. CDC (Centers for Disease Control and Prevention) Atlanta, GA: U.S. Department of Health and Human Services, Centers for Disease Control and Prevention; 2009c. Fourth National Report on Human Exposure to Environmental Chemicals.

16. CDC (Centers for Disease Control and Prevention) Increasing prevalence of parent-reported attention-deficit/hyperactivity disorder among children: United States, 2003–2007. MMWR Morb Mortal Wkly Rep. 2010a;59(44):1439–1443.

17. CDC (Centers for Disease Control and Prevention) Notes from the field: outbreak of acute lead poisoning among children aged < 5 years–Zamfara, Nigeria. MMWR Morb Mortal Wkly Rep. 2010b;59:846.

18. CDC (Centers for Disease Control and Prevention) Fourth National Report on Human Exposure to Environmental Chemicals, Updated Tables, February 2011. 2011a. Available: http://www.cdc.gov/exposurereport/pdf/updated_Tables.pdf [accessed 8 December 2011]

19. CDC (Centers for Disease Control and Prevention) Questionnaires, Datasets, and Related Documentation. 2011b. Available: http://www.cdc.gov/nchs/nhanes/nhanes_questionnaires.htm [accessed 8 December 2011]

20. Charman T, Pickles A, Simonoff E, Chandler S, Loucas T, Baird G. IQ in children with autism spectrum disorders: data from the Special Needs and Autism project (SNAP). Psychol Med. 2011;41:619–627.

21. Child JS. Fallot's tetralogy and pregnancy: prognostication and prophesy. J Am Coll Cardiol. 2004;44:181–183.

22. Corbett SS, Drewett RF. To what extent is failure to thrive in infancy associated with poorer cognitive development? A review and meta-analysis. J Child Psychol Psychiatry. 2004;45:641–654.

23. Cotton SM, Voudouris NJ, Greenwood KM. Association between intellectual functioning and age in children and young adults with Duchenne muscular dystrophy: further results from a meta-analysis. Dev Med Child Neurol. 2005;47:257–265.

24. Dong J, Su S-Y. The association between arsenic and children's intelligence: a meta-analysis. Biol Trace Elem Res. 2009;129:88–93.

25. Elliott MR, Wang Y, Lowe RA, Kleindorfer PR. Environmental justice: frequency and severity of US chemical industry accidents and the socioeconomic status of surrounding communities. J Epidemiol Community Health. 2004;58:24–30.

26. Engel SM, Berkowitz GS, Barr DB, Teitelbaum SL, Siskind J, Meisel SJ, et al. Prenatal organophosphate metabolites and organochlorine levels and performance on the Brazelton Neonatal Behavioral Assessment Scale in a multiethnic pregnancy cohort. Am J Epidemiol. 2007;165:1397–1404.

27. Engel SM, Miodovnik A, Canfield RL, Zhu C, Silva MJ, Calafat AM, et al. Prenatal phthalate exposure is associated with childhood behavior and executive functioning. Environ Health Perspect. 2010;118:565–571.

28. Engel SM, Wetmur J, Chen J, Zhu C, Barr DB, Canfield RL, et al. Prenatal exposure to organophosphates, paraoxonase 1, and cognitive development in childhood. Environ Health Perspect. 2011;119:1182–1188.

29. European Food Safety Authority 2010. Scientific opinion on lead in food. EFSA J 81570; doi:[Online 20 April 2010]10.2903/j.efsa.2010.1570 [Cross Ref]

30. Federal Interagency Forum on Child and Family Statistics. America's Children: Key National Indicators of Well-Being, 2011. 2011. Available: http://www.childstats.gov/americaschildren/tables/pop1.asp [accessed 8 December 2011]

31. Fewtrell L, Kaufmann R, Ustin-Pruss A. Geneva: World Health Organization; 2003. Lead. Assessing The Environmental Burden of Disease at National and Local Levels. Environmental Burden of Disease Series, No. 2.

32. Frazier TW, Demaree HA, Youngstrom EA. Meta-analysis of intellectual and neuropsychological test performance in attention-deficit/hyperactivity disorder. Neuropsychology. 2004;18:543–555.

33. Froehlich TE, Lanphear BP, Auinger P, Hornung R, Epstein JN, Braun J, et al. Association of tobacco and lead exposure with attention-deficit/hyperactivity disorder. Pediatrics. 2009;124:e1054–e1063.

34. Gaudieri PA, Chen R, Greer TF, Holmes CS. Cognitive function in children with type 1 diabetes. A meta-analysis. Diabetes Care. 2008;31:1892–1897.

35. Goldberg D. Plato versus Aristotle: categorical and dimensional models for common mental disorders. Compr Psychiatry. 2000;41:8–13.

36. Gould E. Childhood lead poisoning: conservative estimates of the social and economic benefits of lead hazard control. Environ Health Perspect. 2009;117:1162–1167.

37. Grandjean P, Budtz-Jorgensen E, Keiding N, Weihe P. Underestimation of risk due to exposure misclassification. Int J Occup Environ Health. 2004;17:131–136.

38. Grandjean P, Cordier S, Kjellstrom T. In: Human Developmental Neurotoxicology (Bellinger DC, ed). New York:Taylor & Francis Group, 25–42; 2006. Developmental neurotoxicity associated with dietary exposure to methylmercury from seafood and freshwater fish.

39. Grosse SD, Matte TD, Schwartz J, Jackson RJ. Economic gains resulting from the reduction in children's exposure to lead in the United States. Environ Health Perspect. 2002;110:563–569.

40. Hamilton BE, Martin JA, Ventura SJ. Births: preliminary data for 2008. Natl Vital Stat Rep. 2010;58(16) Available: http://www.cdc.gov/nchs/data/nvsr/nvsr58/nvsr58_16.pdf[accessed 21 February 2012]

41. Herbstman JB, Sjodin A, Kurzon M, Lederman SA, Jones RS, Rauh V, et al. Prenatal exposure to PBDEs and neurodevelopment. Environ Health Perspect. 2010;118:712–719.

42. Hightower JM, O'Hare A, Hernandez GT. Blood mercury reporting in NHANES: identifying Asian, Pacific Islander, Native American, and multiracial groups. Environ Health Perspect. 2006;114:173–175.

43. Institute of Medicine. Washington, DC: National Academy Press; 1981. Costs of Environment-Related Health Effects: A Plan for Continuing Study.

44. Ioannidis JP. 2005. Why most published research findings are false. PLoS Med 2e124; doi:[Online 30 August 2005]10.1371/journal.pmed.0020124 [Cross Ref]

45. Joint FAO/WHO Expert Committee on Food Additives. Report of 73rd Meeting: Summary and Conclusions. 2010. Available: http://whqlibdoc.who.int/trs/WHO_TRS_960_eng.pdf [accessed 22 February 2012]

46. Joseph MF, Frazier TW, Youngstrom EA, Soares JC. A quantitative and qualitative review of neurocognitive performance in pediatric bipolar disorder. J Child Adolesc Psychopharmacol. 2008;18:595–605.

47. Karsdorp PA, Everaerd W, Kindt M, Mulder BJM. Psychological and cognitive functioning in children and adolescents with congenital heart disease: a meta-analysis. J Pediatr Psychol. 2007;32:527–541.

48. Kaufman AS. How dangerous are low (not moderate or high) doses of lead for children's intellectual development? Arch Clin Neuropsychol. 2001;16:403–431.

49. Knobeloch L, Anderson HA, Imm P, Peters D, Smith A. Fish consumption, advisory awareness, and hair mercury levels among women of childbearing age. Environ Res. 2005;97:220–227.

50. Knobeloch L, Gliori G, Anderson H. Assessment of methylmercury exposure in Wisconsin. Environ Res. 2007;103:205–210.

51. Langlois JA, Rutland-Brown W, Thomas KE. The incidence of traumatic brain injury among children in the United States: differences by race. J Head Trauma Rehabil. 2005;20:229–238.

52. Lanphear BP, Hornung R, Khoury J, Yolton K, Baghurst P, Bellinger DC, et al. Low-level environmental lead exposure and children's intellectual function: an international pooled analysis. Environ Health Perspect. 2005;113:894–899.

53. Lind A, Korkman M, Lehtonen L, Lapinleimu H, Parkkola R, Matomaki J, et al. Cognitive and neuropsychological outcomes at 5 years of age in preterm children born in the 2000s. Dev Med Child Neurol. 2011;23:256–262.

54. Lindberg F, Cnattingins S, D'Onofrio B, Altman D, Lambe M, Hultman C, et al. Maternal smoking during pregnancy and intellectual performance in young adult Swedish male offspring. Paediatr Perinat Epidemiol. 2010;24:79–87.

55. Llop S, Ballester F, Estarlich M, Esplugues A, Rebagliato M, Iniguez C. Preterm birth and exposure to air pollutants during pregnancy. Environ Res. 2010;110:778–785.

56. Lynch ML, Huang LS, Cox C, Strain JJ, Myers GJ, Bonham MP, et al. Varying coefficient models to explore interactions between maternal nutritional status and prenatal methylmercury toxicity in the Seychelles Child Development Study. Environ Res. 2011;111:75–80.

57. Mahaffey KR, Annest JL, Roberts J, Murphy RS. National estimates of blood lead levels: United States, 1976–1980. Association with selected demographic and socioeconomic factors. N Engl J Med. 1982;307(10):573–579.

58. Martins P, Castela E. Transposition of the great arteries. Orphanet J Rare Dis. 2008;3:27.

59. McDowell MA, Dillon CF, Osterloh J, Bolger PM, Pellizarri E, Fernando R, et al. Hair mercury levels in U.S. children and women of childbearing age: reference range data from NHANES 1999–2000. Environ Health Perspect. 2004;112:1165–1171.

60. Moreno C, Laje G, Blanco C, Jiang H, Schmidt AB, Olfson M. National trends in the outpatient diagnosis and treatment of bipolar disorder in youth. Arch Gen Psychiatry. 2007;64:1032–1039.

61. Mulhern RK, Butler RW. Neurocognitive sequelae of childhood cancers and their treatment. Pediatr Rehab. 2004;7:1–14.

62. Narayan R, Michel ME, Ansell B, Baethmann A, Biegon A, Bracken MB, et al. Clinical trials in head injury. J Neurotrauma. 2002;19:503–557.

63. Needleman HL, Leviton A, Bellinger D. Lead-associated intellectual deficit. N Engl J Med. 1982;306:367. [Letter]

64. Neisser U, Boodoo G, Bouchard TJ, Boykin AW, Brody N, Ceci SJ, et al. Intelligence: knowns and unknowns. Am Psychol. 1996;51:77–101.

65. Oken E, Radesky J, Wright RO, Bellinger DC, Amarasiriwardena C, Kleinman KP, et al. Maternal fish intake during pregnancy, blood mercury levels, and child cognition at age 3 years in a US cohort. Am J Epidemiol. 2008;167:1171–1178.

66. Oken E, Wright RO, Kleinman KP, Bellinger D., Amarasiriwardena CJ, Hu H, et al. Maternal fish consumption, hair mercury, and infant cognition in a U.S. cohort. Environ Health Perspect. 2005;113:1376–1380.

67. Qian M, Wang D, Watkins WE, Gebski V, Yan YQ, Li M, et al. The effects of iodine on intelligence in children: a meta-analysis of studies conducted in China. Asia Pac J Clin Nutr. 2005;14:32–42.

68. Rice DC, Schoeny R, Mahaffey KR. Methods and rationale for derivation of a reference dose for methylmercury by the U.S. EPA. Risk Anal. 2003;23:107–115.

69. Robinson KE, Kuttesch JF, Champion JE, Andreotti CR, Hipp DW, Bettis A, et al. A quantitative meta-analysis of neurocognitive sequelae in survivors of pediatric brain tumors. Pediatr Blood Cancer. 2010;55:525–531.

70. Rose G. Strategy of prevention: lessons from cardiovascular disease. BMJ. 1981;282:1847–1851.

71. Rose G. Sick individuals and sick populations. Int J Epidemiol. 1985;14:32–38.

72. Rose G. Environmental health: problems and prospects. J R Coll Physicians Lond. 1991;5:48–52.

73. Rose G. Mental disorder and the strategies of prevention. Psychol Med. 1993;23:553–555.

74. Sachdev HPS, Gera T, Nestel P. Effect of iron supplementation on mental and motor development in children: systematic review of randomised controlled trials. Public Health Nutr. 2005;8:117–132.

75. Steenland K, Armstrong B. An overview of methods for calculating the burden of disease due to specific risk factors. Epidemiology. 2006;17:512–519.

76. Tang Q-Q, Du J, Ma H-H, Jiang S-J, Zhou Z-J. Fluoride and children's intelligence: a meta-analysis. Biol Trace Elem Res. 2008;126:115–120.

77. Walker SP, Wachs TD, Gardner JM, Lozoff B, Wasserman GA, Pollitt E, et al. Child development: risk factors for adverse outcomes in developing countries. Lancet. 2007;369:145–157.

78. Weiss B, Bellinger DC. Social ecology of children's vulnerability to environmental pollutants. Environ Health Perspect. 2006;114:1479–1485.

79. WHO (World Health Organization) Geneva: World Health Organization; 2009. GBD Study Operations Manual, January 2009.

CHAPTER 3

DECODING NEURODEVELOPMENT: FINDINGS ON ENVIRONMENTAL EXPOSURES AND SYNAPTIC PLASTICITY

ANGELA SPIVEY

What makes one person different from the next? In large part it's that our individual brains are wired a bit differently; each neuron in each person's brain has a different set of synapses connecting to a different set of neurons. When we're born, most of the major functional subregions of the brain and their interconnections are in place, but various experiences and environmental exposures affect which synaptic connections become stronger and which become weaker. Different areas of the brain have this synaptic plasticity—or ability to grow stronger or weaker connections—at different time periods, and the timing of these "critical periods" is tightly regulated.

The field of neurobiology is humming with new findings on the intricate workings that orchestrate this process, too many to describe in one story. But of special interest are key discoveries by investigators at the National Institute of Environmental Health Sciences (NIEHS) about some

Reproduced with permission from Environmental Health Perspectives. Spivey A. Decoding Neurodevelopment: Findings on Environmental Exposures and Synaptic Plasticity. Environmental Health Perspectives 120 (2012); http://dx.doi.org/10.1289/ehp.120-a70 .

of the basic mechanisms involved in synaptic plasticity, and work by other investigators that explores the hypothesis that environmental toxicants that disrupt synaptic plasticity at critical periods play a role in disorders that have roots in early brain development, such as autism spectrum disorders (ASDs), attention deficit/hyperactivity disorder, and schizophrenia. [1,2]

3.1 THE CONSPIRACY AGAINST PLASTICITY IN CA2

All areas of the brain were once thought equally capable of rewiring them-selves in response to environmental input, but Serena Dudek, principal investigator of the NIEHS Synaptic and Developmental Plasticity Group, has revealed that one region of the brain has what she and colleagues have termed a "conspiracy against plasticity," with the neurons there exhibiting a remarkable stability in synaptic strength in response to electrical stimula-tion. [3] This region, CA2, is part of the hippocampus, an important center of learning and memory. The other regions of the hippocampus, CA1 and CA3, have been heavily studied, but CA2 had been largely ignored; it was long considered simply a transition area between the other regions. [3,4]

Dudek began studying CA2 because she wanted to figure out exactly how critical periods for phenomena such as ocular dominance are con-trolled. Ocular dominance refers to the preference of the brain for input from one eye over the other, and development of ocular dominance pro-vides a simple example of synaptic plasticity at work in everyday life. When a baby is born with a cataract or other condition in only one eye, the problem ideally should be corrected before 2 years of age and no later than age 8. [5] That's because the longer the brain receives information from only one eye, the weaker its connections to the inactive eye will become, until that eye is wired out of the circuit, even if the physical condition itself is later corrected. [6] But if an adult loses vision in one eye for a time, the consequences are not so dire; the connections to receive information from both eyes are already formed, and the opportunity for that part of the brain to rewire itself has closed.

In rodent models Dudek noticed that a particular gene, *TREK-1*, was highly expressed in a layer of the adult visual cortex that wasn't particu-larly plastic, and that its expression appeared to increase as the animal aged and the critical period for plasticity in that region closed. [7] "This gene was one of several that might have been predicted to prevent plasticity, and so we were surprised to see that it showed up in this area of the hippocampus, CA2. [8] As we studied CA2, it turned out that the area was a lot different [from CA1 and CA3]," Dudek says.

THE BASICS OF NEURAL ACTIVITY

Neurons are polarized brain cells: that is, the outside of the cell membrane is positively charged, while the inside is negatively charged. On each neuron a large antenna-like tree of dendrites receives synapses from many other neurons, and a single axon branches to contact many other neurons. Neurons communicate with each other using chemical signals that they release at synapses, where the axon terminals contact another neuron's dendrites.

Some chemicals alter the activity of ion channels, while others alter neuronal metabolism. When enough excitatory synapses are activated simultaneously, the neuron conducts a regenerative electrical wave of depolarization along its axon. This electrical wave is known as an "action potential," sometimes referred to as the "firing" of a neuron. When the depolarization arrives at the axon terminals, or synapses, the resulting calcium entry triggers the release of vesicles containing chemical messengers called neurotransmitters, and the process begins again.

Synaptic plasticity is the ability of the synapses to strengthen or weaken their connections. A simple way to think of strengthening a synapse is the insertion of postsynaptic receptors. When the number of receptors is increased, neurotransmitters can have more effect. When postsynaptic receptors are removed, neurotransmitters make less of an impact per transmission.

Veer

In their studies of CA2, Dudek and colleagues used the patch-clamp technique to measure the response of neurons in slices of rodent hippocampus to electrical stimulation; these responses include either the firing of "action potentials" or else the smaller electrical activity of synapses [see "The Basics of Neural Activity," this page]. Repeated high-frequency electrical stimulation to other regions of the hippocampus typically causes a long-lasting boost in the strength of synapse; this is called long-term potentiation. But stimulating slices from CA2 yielded no such increase. [3]

"Up until we discovered this five years ago, I would have thought that the cellular profile of all the pyramidal [primary excitatory] cells in the cerebral cortex was similar enough that their synaptic plasticity would be very similar. But we're finding that that is clearly not the case," Dudek says. Neuroscientists are excited about her findings in CA2 because they open up new opportunities for delving into the workings of plasticity, especially for better understanding the factors that reduce or prevent it.

3.2 BIDIRECTIONAL ACTIVITY

In earlier work, when Dudek was a PhD student, she conducted the first studies demonstrating that synaptic plasticity goes in both directions. Many neuroscientists had shown that long-term potentiation occurs, but no one had shown that the opposite—long-term depression—also could be induced. Dudek and colleagues demonstrated that a repeated stimulation of synapses at frequencies lower than those required to induce long-term potentiation would result in prolonged synaptic weakening in hippocampal slices. [9]

Later, Dudek collaborated with John Hepler, a professor of pharmacology at Emory University, to find that *RGS14*, a gene highly enriched in CA2, keeps plasticity turned off. When Hepler knocked out *RGS14* in rodents, the animals learned faster, especially in spatial activities, and Dudek showed that plasticity had been turned back on in CA2. [10] It may seem odd that the brain has a "Homer Simpson gene," as *RGS14* has been nicknamed, that keeps the brain from learning. But Hepler suggests that such mechanisms may be vital for processing the world in a way that enables normal function.

"Think about everything that you encounter every day: You forget the vast majority of it, and that's a good thing—you have to filter out what's important and what's not important," Hepler says. "You could also think about *RGS14* and CA2 as important devices for filtering which memories are important to retain and which are not."

Most recently, Dudek and colleagues have found that CA2 is probably the "caffeine center" of the brain. In both brain slices and live animals, they demonstrated that a dose of caffeine equivalent to about 2 cups of coffee for a human almost doubled the transmissions of synapses in CA2 compared with those in controls. [11] At the same doses, caffeine had no effect on other areas of the hippocampus. Dudek thinks that CA2 gets such a jolt from caffeine because the region is rich in adenosine receptors. Adenosine is a neurotransmitter that normally inhibits synaptic transmission and plasticity; that is, it induces sleepiness. Caffeine is known to antagonize adenosine receptors.

3.3 THE HORMONE CONNECTION

Some of the signaling chemicals involved in plasticity are hormones. For instance, since the early twentieth century, it has been known that people deprived of iodine develop cognitive disabilities because the lack of iodine reduces production of thyroid hormone. [12] But many of the details of how thyroid hormone actually works in the brain are still largely unknown.

Researchers previously thought that thyroid hormone affected neurodevelopment mainly by regulating gene expression, a process that can take hours to produce effects. But in recent years, says David Armstrong, chief of the NIEHS Neurobiology Laboratory, it has become apparent that thyroid hormone also works via rapid events, such as binding to receptors that can regulate ion channel activity through cytoplasmic signaling mechanisms.

Armstrong and colleagues are finding out how thyroid hormone does its job in normal brain development. In a rat pituitary cell line, they showed that a nuclear receptor for thyroid hormone, TRβ, binds to phosphatidylinositol 3-kinase (PI3K), an enzyme that's essential for brain development and synaptic plasticity. [13] In unpublished work presented in

November 2011 at the Society for Neuroscience Annual Meeting, Armstrong's team showed exactly where TRβ binds to PI3K and that, when a mutation at this site prevents binding, rats' brains exhibited less plasticity, reduced synaptic response to an electrical stimulus, and reduced response to thyroid hormone. [14]

"If we change one tyrosine residue in the thyroid hormone receptor protein to a phenylalanine, which is a very conservative difference, then we see all these changes in the brain," Armstrong says. "So this must be an important mechanism for how thyroid hormone works."

Tracing these intricate basic mechanisms is the best route that Armstrong sees to the discovery of environmental toxicants that may disrupt brain development. Other approaches that involve exposing an animal to a suspected toxicant and observing behavioral changes that develop are too imprecise, in his view. "Especially for things like early learning disorders in humans, it's not so easy to map that [type of behavioral change] onto mouse behavior," he explains. "It's highly controversial what an autistic mouse would look like because they have a very different forebrain and cortex than we do and very different social behaviors."

Armstrong and other basic scientists therefore take the approach of nailing down the molecular mechanisms that underlie brain functions such as plasticity. Then they can develop high-throughput screens to identify toxicants that may perturb those mechanisms.

3.4 TOO MUCH EXCITEMENT?

How might a disruption in synaptic plasticity lead to developmental disorders such as ASDs? In order for senses such as vision to develop normally and become integrated into behavior, the brain changes in response to experience, says Michela Fagiolini, a neurobiologist at Harvard Medical School. Some evidence suggests that ASDs—a group of conditions of varying severity—begin in part with an underdeveloped ability to integrate visual information with auditory information when making out words. Other research has shown that autistic children process images of faces differently than nonautistic children. In one study, autistic children were more successful at recognizing facial expressions depicted with high spatial frequency; that is, their visual perception was more oriented to contrast and detail than that of nonautistic children, who focused on the overall composition of the faces. [15]

Normal plasticity requires a delicate balance between excitation and inhibition of synapses, according to Fagiolini. "We and others have shown that a balance between inhibition and excitation is actually critical for allowing the brain to become plastic and respond to the environment," she says. "This is different from what people thought in the past, when inhibition was thought to suppress plasticity. The new view is that you need a certain level of inhibition to allow the brain to sense and respond to the environment."

In one study, scientists genetically engineered mice to lack just 1 of 2 receptors for γ-aminobutyric acid (GABA), a neurotransmitter involved in inhibition of synaptic electrical excitement. [16] Without the proper inhibition, the visual cortex stayed in the immature state that normally occurs just before the onset of the critical period for ocular dominance. But enhancing GABA transmission with the drug benzodiazepine resulted in a normal-length critical period of plasticity, no matter the mouse's age.

Some scientists hypothesize that lack of inhibition of electrical activity in the brain caused by environmental toxicants may contribute to developmental disorders such as ASDs. For instance, Timothy syndrome, a very rare developmental disorder characterized by autism and cardiovascular irregularities, results from a mutation in the CaV1.2 voltage-gated calcium channel. [17] Voltage-gated ion channels open in response to electrical stimulation to allow entry of critical signaling ions including calcium, potassium, and sodium. Armstrong and colleagues found that this CaV1.2 mutation increases the duration of each channel opening by more than 10 times, and far more calcium enters the cells to the point it could become cytotoxic. [18]

Increased calcium entering through CaV1.2 channels also overstimulates any nearby ryanodine receptor calcium channels, which are thought to work with CaV1.2 to control synaptic plasticity as well as muscle coordination. [19,20] "Normally, ryanodine receptors are kept under tight control," says Isaac Pessah, chairman of the Department of Molecular Biosciences at the University of California, Davis. "For instance, in muscle cells such as those in the heart, ryanodine receptors' role is to contribute an intense signal only when they're called upon. When muscle contraction is needed, the receptors open briefly, release the calcium needed, then shut off quickly." But some polybrominated diphenyl ethers (PBDEs) and polychlorinated biphenyl ethers (PCBs), because of their structure, enhance the activity of ryanodine receptors. [19,21]

Pessah's group has shown that after exposure to PCBs, ryanodine receptors activate much more easily than usual, and they are, as Pessah says, "noisy." [19] "I call it 'chattering,'" he says. "That can be extremely confusing to cells." Pessah and colleague Pam Lein, also at UC Davis, have shown that some of the same PBDEs and PCBs that alter the activity of ryanodine receptors also affect activity-dependent growth of dendrites (the branches of neurons where synaptic receptors lie). [22]

"Activity-dependent growth is extremely important in neurodevelopment because not only does it develop the complexity needed to promote learning, it also is essential for 'coding' neural networks so that they're meaningful to the brain," Pessah says. He and Lein hypothesize that the effects of the environmental toxicants on neural development are mediated by their effects on ryanodine receptors in neurons, but that idea remains to be tested in animals.

3.5 WHAT DOES THIS MEAN FOR HUMANS?

More than 150 mutations in one type of ryanodine receptor (Ry1R1) have been well documented to heighten sensitivity to chemicals called halogenated alkanes, which are used as general anesthetics. A person may go his whole life unaware that he has such a mutation until he is given a halogenated anesthetic in the operating room, which could rapidly trigger a life-threatening response known as malignant hyperthermia. [23,24,25]

"We are convinced that this is an amazing demonstration of a gene-by-environment interaction in which the gene by itself is insufficient to cause an overt clinical phenotype, so you don't know that individuals are susceptible until they're subjected to an environmental stressor," Pessah says. He and other researchers are investigating the idea that ASDs and other developmental disorders similarly could begin with a small genetic variation that makes a person more susceptible to ryanodine receptor disruption.

Can human developmental disorders really be reduced to disruptions in synapses and chemicals? The idea may not be so farfetched. As Armstrong points out, until it was demonstrated a few years ago, scientists would not have predicted that intranasal administration of the hormone oxytocin, previously thought to be involved mostly in reproduction, could have a direct effect on complex human behavior such as trust. [26]

Because many of the mechanisms of neural plasticity are chemical processes, investigators predict that environmental chemicals are capable of disrupting them. However, although the molecules that regulate synaptic plasticity in mice and humans are almost identical, the cellular substrates of cognitive processes in the two species are quite different. So it remains to be seen what any of these findings mean for human neurodevelopment.

But even if basic work such as Dudek's and Armstrong's can pinpoint particular chemicals that disrupt plasticity in experiments at high concentrations, many steps will be required to determine the human health effects of environmentally relevant chemical exposures. "There won't ever be any one test that rules a chemical in or out as being neurotoxic," Armstrong says. "You have to test its toxicity at many levels."

REFERENCES

1. Hasan A, et al. Dysfunctional long-term potentiation-like plasticity in schizophrenia revealed by transcranial direct current stimulation. Behav Brain Res 224(1):15–22. 2011. http://dx.doi.org/10.1016/j.bbr.2011.05.017

2. Zhou R, et al. Abnormal synaptic plasticity in basolateral amygdala may account for hyperactivity and attention-deficit in male rat exposed perinatally to low-dose bisphenol-A. Neuropharmacology 60(5):789–798. 2011. http://dx.doi.org/10.1016/j. neuropharm.2011.01.031

3. Zhao M, et al. Synaptic plasticity (and the lack thereof) in hippocampal CA2 neurons. J Neurosci 27(44):12025–12032. 2007. http://dx.doi.org/10.1523/JNEURO-SCI.4094-07.2007

4. Jones MW, McHugh TJ. Updating hippocampal representations: CA2 joins the circuit. Trends Neurosci 34(10):526–535. 2011. http://dx.doi.org/10.1016/j. tins.2011.07.007

5. Mitchell DE, MacKinnon S. The present and potential impact of research on animal models for clinical treatment of stimulus deprivation amblyopia. Clin Exper Optom 85(1):5–18. 2002. http://dx.doi.org/10.1111/j.1444-0938.2002.tb03067.x

6. Banks MS, et al. Sensitive period for the development of human binocular vision. Science 190(4215):675–677. 1975. http://dx.doi.org/10.1126/science.1188363

7. Xu X, et al. mRNA expression of the lipid and mechano-gated 2P domain K+ channels during rat brain development. J Neurogenet 16(4):263–269. 2002. http://dx.doi.org/10.1080/01677060216294

8. Talley EM, et al. CNS distribution of members of the two-pore-domain (KCNK) potassium channel family. J Neurosci 21(19):7491–7505. 2001. http://www.ncbi.nlm.nih.gov/pubmed/11567039

9. Dudek SM, Bear MF. Homosynaptic long-term depression in area CA1 of hippocampus and effects of N-methyl-D-aspartate receptor blockade. Proc Natl Acad Sci USA 89(10):4363–4367. 1992. http://www.ncbi.nlm.nih.gov/pubmed/1350090/

10. Lee SE, et al. RGS14 is a natural suppressor of both synaptic plasticity in CA2 neurons and hippocampal-based learning and memory. Proc Natl Acad Sci USA 107(39):16994–16998. 2010. http://dx.doi.org/10.1073/pnas.1005362107

11. Simons SB, et al. Caffeine-induced synaptic potentiation in hippocampal CA2 neurons. Nature Neurosci 15(1):23–25. 2012. http://dx.doi.org/10.1038/nn.2962

12. Zimmerman MB. Research on iodine deficiency and goiter in the 19th and early 20th centuries. J Nutr 138(11):2060–2063. 2008. http://www.ncbi.nlm.nih.gov/pubmed/18936198

13. Storey NM, et al. Rapid signaling at the plasma membrane by a nuclear receptor for thyroid hormone. Proc Natl Acad Sci USA 103(13):5197–5201. 2006. http://dx.doi.org/10.1073/pnas.0600089103

14. Mizuno F, et al. Thyroid Hormone Signaling through Phosphatidylinositol 3-kinase Is Essential for Synaptic Plasticity in Mouse Hippocampal Pyramidal Neurons [abstract]. Presented at: Society for Neuroscience Annual Meeting, Washington, DC, 13 Nov 2011. Available: http://www.abstractsonline.com/Plan/ViewAbstract.aspx?sKey=5ba97878-21c1-44f4-b8a8-a36b5470b5fd&cKey=8239c459-cc37-4deb-9817-e503c5354aaf&mKey=%7B8334BE29-8911-4991-8C31-32B32DD5E6C8%7D [accessed 13 Jan 2012].

15. Vlamings PHJM, et al. 2010. Biol Psychiatr. Basic abnormalities in visual processing affect face processing at an early age in autism spectrum disorder. pp. 1107–1113. http://dx.doi.org/10.1016/j.biopsych.2010.06.024

16. Fagiolini M, Hensch TK. Inhibitory threshold for critical-period activation in primary visual cortex. Nature 404(6774):183–186. 2000. http://dx.doi.org/10.1038/35004582

17. Splawski I, et al. CaV1.2 calcium channel dysfunction causes a multisystem disorder including arrhythmia and autism. Cell 119(1):19–31. 2004. http://dx.doi.org/10.1016/j.cell.2004.09.011

18. Erxleben C, et al. Cyclosporin and Timothy syndrome increase mode 2 gating of CaV1.2 calcium channels through aberrant phosphorylation of S6 helices. Proc Natl Acad Sci USA 103(10):3932–3937. 2006. http://dx.doi.org/10.1073/pnas.0511322103

19. Pessah IN, et al. Minding the calcium store: ryanodine receptor activation as a convergent mechanism of PCB toxicity. Pharmacol Ther 125(2):260–285. 2010. http://dx.doi.org/10.1016/j.pharmthera.2009.10.009

20. Dai S, et al. Supramolecular assemblies and localized regulation of voltage-gated ion channels. Physiol Rev 89(2):411–452. 2009. http://dx.doi.org/10.1152/physrev.00029.2007

21. Kim KH, et al. Para- and ortho-substitutions are key determinants of polybrominated diphenyl ether activity toward ryanodine receptors and neurotoxicity. Environ Health Perspect 119(4):519–526. 2011. http://dx.doi.org/10.1289/ehp.1002728

22. Yang D, et al. Developmental exposure to polychlorinated biphenyls interferes with experience-dependent dendritic plasticity and ryanodine receptor expression in weanling rats. Environ Health Perspect 117(3):426–435. 2009. http://dx.doi.org/10.1289/ehp.11771

23. Zhou J, et al. 2010. Neuromuscular disorders and malignant hyperthermia. In: Miller's Anesthesia, 7th Edition (Miller RD, ed.). Philadelphia, PA:Churchill Livingstone:

24. Jurkat-Rott K, et al. Skeletal muscle channelopathies. J Neurol 249(11):1493–1502. 2002. http://dx.doi.org/10.1007/s00415-002-0871-5

25. Parness J, et al. The myotonias and susceptibility to malignant hyperthermia. Anesth Analg 109(4):)1054–1064. 2009. http://dx.doi.org/10.1213/ane.0b013e3181a7c8e5

26. Baumgartner T., et al. Oxytocin shapes the neural circuitry of trust and trust adaptation in humans. Neuron 58(4):639–650. 2008. http://dx.doi.org/10.1016/j.neuron.2008.04.009

CHAPTER 4

SEVEN-YEAR NEURODEVELOPMENTAL SCORES AND PRENATAL EXPOSURE TO CHLORPYRIFOS, A COMMON AGRICULTURAL PESTICIDE

IRGINIA RAUH, SRIKESH ARUNAJADAI, MEGAN HORTON, FREDERICA PERERA, LORI HOEPNER, DANA B. BARR, AND ROBIN WHYATT

Each year, thousands of new chemicals are released in the United States, with very little documentation about potential long-term human health risks (Landrigan et al. 2002). First registered in 1965 for agricultural and pest control purposes, chlorpyrifos (CPF; 0,0-diethyl-0-3,5,6-trichloro-2-pyridyl phosphorothioate) is a broad-spectrum, chlorinated organophosphate (OP) insecticide. Before regulatory action by the U.S. Environmental Protection Agency (EPA) to phase out residential use beginning in 2000, CPF applications were particularly heavy in urban areas, where the exposed populations included pregnant women (Berkowitz et al. 2003; Whyatt et al. 2002, 2003). In a sample of pregnant women in New York City (Perera et al. 2002) detectable levels of CPF were found in 99.7% of personal air samples, 100% of indoor air samples, and 64–70% of blood

Reproduced with permission from Environmental Health Perspectives. Rauh V, Arunajadai S, Horton M, Perera F, Hoepner L, Barr DB, and Whyatt R. Seven-Year Neurodevelopmental Scores and Prenatal Exposure to Chlorpyrifos, a Common Agricultural Pesticide. Environmental Health Perspectives **119**,8 (2011); doi:10.1289/ehp.1003160.

samples collected from umbilical cord plasma at delivery (Whyatt et al. 2002).

Early concerns about the possible neurotoxicity of OP insecticides for humans derived from rodent studies showing that prenatal and early post-natal exposures to CPF were associated with neurodevelopmental deficits, and these effects have been seen at exposure levels well below the threshold for systemic toxicity caused by cholinesterase inhibition in the brain (e.g., Slotkin and Seidler 2005). Evidence has accumulated over the past decade showing that noncholinergic mechanisms may play a role in the neurotoxic effects of CPF exposure in rodents, involving disruption of neural cell development, neurotransmitter systems (Aldridge et al. 2005; Slotkin 2004), and synaptic formation in different brain regions (Qiao et al. 2003). Such developmental disruptions have been associated with later functional impairments in learning, short-term working memory, and long-term reference memory (Levin et al. 2002).

In humans, OPs have been detected in amnionic fluid (Bradman et al. 2003) and are known to cross the placenta (Richardson 1995; Whyatt et al. 2005), posing a threat to the unborn child during a period of rapid brain development. Using urinary metabolites as the biomarker of exposure, several different birth cohort studies have reported that prenatal maternal nonspecific OP exposure was associated with abnormal neonatal reflexes (Engel et al. 2007; Young et al. 2005), mental deficits and pervasive development disorder at 2 years (Eskenazi et al. 2007), and attention problem behaviors and a composite attention-deficit/hyperactivity disorder indicator at 5 years of age (Marks et al. 2010).

Using a different biomarker of exposure (the parent compound of CPF in umbilical cord plasma), we have previously reported (in the same cohort as the present study) significant associations between prenatal exposure to CPF (> 6.17 pg/g) and reduced birth weight and birth length (Whyatt et al. 2004), increased risk of small size for gestational age (Rauh V, Whyatt R, Perera F, unpublished data), increased risk of mental and motor delay (< 80 points) and 3.5- to 6-point adjusted mean decrements on the 3-year Bayley Scales of Infant Development (Rauh et al. 2006), and evidence of increased problems related to attention, attention deficit hyperactivity disorder, and pervasive developmental disorder as measured by the Child Behavior Checklist at 2–3 years (Rauh et al. 2006). Taken together, these prospective cohort studies show a consistent pattern of early cognitive and behavioral deficits related to prenatal OP exposure, across both agricultural and urban populations, using different biomarkers of prenatal exposure.

We undertook the present study to identify the developmental consequences of prenatal exposure to CPF in a sample of New York City children at 7 years of age. Given the mechanisms proposed in the rodent literature, and early findings from prospective human studies involving nonspecific OP exposures, we hypothesized that prenatal exposure to CPF would be associated with neurodevelopmental deficits persisting into the early school years, when more refined neuropsychological tests are available to identify particular functional impairments.

4.1 MATERIALS AND METHODS

Participants and recruitment. The subjects for this report are participants in an ongoing prospective cohort study (Columbia Center for Children's Environmental Health) of inner-city mothers and their newborn infants (Perera et al. 2002). The cohort study was initiated in 1997 to evaluate the effects of prenatal exposures to ambient pollutants on birth outcomes and neurocognitive development in a cohort of mothers and newborns from low-income communities in New York City. Nonsmoking women (classified by self-report and validated by blood cotinine levels < 15 ng/mL), 18–35 years of age, who self-identified as African American or Dominican and who registered at New York Presbyterian Medical Center or Harlem Hospital prenatal clinics by the 20th week of pregnancy, were approached for consent. Eligible women were free of diabetes, hypertension, known HIV, and documented drug abuse and had resided in the area for at least 1 year. The study was approved by the Institutional Review Board of Columbia University. Informed consent was obtained from all participating mothers, and informed assent was obtained from all children as well, starting at 7 years of age.

Of 725 consenting women, 535 were active participants in the ongoing cohort study at the time of this report, and 265 of their children had reached the age of 7 years with complete data on the following: a) prenatal maternal interview data, b) biomarkers of prenatal CPF exposure level

from maternal and/or cord blood samples at delivery, c) postnatal covariates, and d) neurodevelopmental outcomes.

Maternal interview and assessment. A 45-min questionnaire was administered to each woman in her home by a trained bilingual interviewer
during the third trimester of pregnancy and annually thereafter. From the
interviews and medical records, the following sociodemographic and biomedical variables, among others, were available: race/ethnicity, infant sex,
household income, maternal age, maternal completed years of education
at child's age 7 years, birth weight, gestational age, and self-reported maternal exposure to environmental tobacco smoke (ETS) during pregnancy.

We measured maternal nonverbal intelligence by the Test of Nonverbal
Intelligence, 3rd edition (TONI-3) (Brown et al. 1997), a 15-min language-
free measure of general intelligence, administered when the child was 3
years of age. The quality of the care-taking environment was measured
by the Home Observation for Measurement of the Environment (HOME)
inventory when the child was 3 years of age (Caldwell and Bradley 1979)
to assess physical and interactive home characteristics. The mother report version of the Child Behavior Checklist for ages 6–18 years, a well-
validated measure of child behavior problems occurring in the preceding
2 months (Achenbach and Rescorla 2001), was administered at 7 years as
part of the larger cohort study.

Biological samples and pesticide exposure. A sample of umbilical cord
blood (30–60 mL) was collected at delivery, and a sample of maternal
blood (30–35 mL) was collected within 2 days postpartum by hospital
staff. Portions were sent to the Centers for Disease Control and Prevention
(Atlanta, GA) for analysis of CPF in plasma, as well as lead and cotinine, described in detail elsewhere (Perera et al. 2002; Whyatt et al. 2003).
Methods for the laboratory assay for CPF, including quality control, repro-
ducibility, and limits of detection (LODs), have also been previously published (Barr et al. 2002). In cases where the umbilical cord blood sample
was not collected (12% of subjects), mothers' values were substituted, using a formula previously derived from regression analyses (Whyatt et al.
2005). As previously reported, maternal and umbilical cord blood CPF
concentrations were similar (arithmetic means ± SDs of 3.9 ± 4.8 pg/g for
maternal blood and 3.7 ± 5.7 pg/g for cord blood) (Whyatt et al. 2005),
and CPF levels in paired maternal and umbilical cord plasma samples

were highly correlated (r = 0.76; p < 0.001, Spearman's rank), indicating that CPF was readily transferred from mother to fetus during pregnancy. Prenatal blood lead levels were available for a subset of children (n = 89). ETS exposure, measured by maternal self-report, was validated by cotinine levels in umbilical cord blood, as described in detail elsewhere (Rauh et al. 2004). We measured polycyclic aromatic hydrocarbon (PAH) exposure by personal air monitoring during the third trimester, using a previously described method, and excluding poor-quality samples (Perera et al. 2003). As previously described (Perera et al. 2003), we computed a composite log-transformed PAH variable from the eight correlated PAH air concentration measures (r-values ranging from 0.34 to 0.94; all p-values < 0.001 by Spearman's rank).

In the larger cohort study, > 40% of CPF exposure values for combined maternal and umbilical cord blood samples were below the LOD. Using a method suggested by Richardson and Ciampi (2003), we made a distributional assumption for the exposure variable (log-normal CPF), computed the expected value of the exposure (E) for all nondetects [E(X/X < LOD)], and assigned this value to all nondetects.

Measures of neurodevelopment. For the 7-year assessment, we selected the Wechsler Intelligence Scale for Children, 4th edition (WISC-IV), because of its revised structure based on the latest research in neurocognitive models of information processing (Wechsler 2003). The WISC-IV is sensitive to low-dose neurotoxic exposures, as demonstrated by studies of lead toxicity in 6- to 7.5-year-old children (Chiodo et al. 2004; Jusko et al. 2008; Rothenberg and Rothenberg 2005). The instrument measures four areas of mental functioning that are associated with, but distinct from, overall intelligence quotient (IQ) and is sensitive to cognitive deficits related to learning and working memory, which have been linked to CPF exposure in rodent studies (e.g., Levin et al. 2002). Each standardized scale has a mean of 100 and SD of 15. The Verbal Comprehension Index is a measure of verbal concept formation, a good predictor of school readiness (Hecht et al. 2000; Wechsler 2003); the Perceptual Reasoning Index measures nonverbal and fluid reasoning; the Working Memory Index assesses children's ability to memorize new information, hold it in short-term memory, concentrate, and manipulate information; the Processing Speed Index assesses ability to focus attention and quickly scan, discriminate, and sequentially order visual information; and the Full-Scale IQ score combines the four composite indices. The General Ability Index score is a summary score of general intelligence, similar to Full-Scale IQ, but excludes contributions from both Working Memory Index and Processing Speed Index (Wechsler 2003). WISC-IV scores may be influenced by socioeconomic background and/or child behavior problems particularly those related to anxiety (Wechsler 2003).

Data analysis. We conducted all analyses using the statistical program R (R Development Core Team 2010). We treated CPF exposure level (picograms per gram) as a continuous variable. We natural log (ln) transformed the WISC-IV Composite Index scores to stabilize the variance and to improve the linear model fit, based on regression diagnostics. Unadjusted correlation analyses were used to explore associations between CPF exposure and WISC-IV scores. We constructed smoothed cubic splines to explore the shape of the functional relationships between CPF exposure and each of the log-transformed WISC-IV indices. We compared the models in which CPF is entered as a single continuous outcome with those in which CPF is modeled using B-splines, using the Davidson–MacKinnon J-test for comparing nonnested models (Davidson and MacKinnon 1981).

Demographic, biomedical, and chemical exposure variables collected for the larger cohort study were available for possible inclusion in the present analysis. We used two different approaches for covariate selection and model fitting, for the purpose of determining the robustness of our results with respect to alternate methods. Covariates were initially selected based on prior literature and retained in the models if associated with either CPF exposure or the WISC-IV scales ($p < 0.10$ in univariate analyses). Multiple linear regression was used to test the effects of prenatal CPF exposure on each 7-year WISC-IV Index. We examined residuals for normality and homoscedasticity and detected no problems. In addition, we employed the least absolute shrinkage and selection operator (LASSO), a shrinkage with selection procedure that provides a more parsimonious approach to covariate selection and model fitting (Houwelingen 2001; Tibshirani 1996). This method minimizes the usual sum of squared errors, with a bound on the sum of the absolute values of the coefficients, thereby shrinking very unstable estimates toward zero, excluding redundant/irrelevant covariates, and avoiding overfitting (Zhao and Yu 2006). We used Sobel's indirect test to assess the influence of child behaviors on the estimates of CPF effect (MacKinnon et al. 2002; Sobel 1982). We used Sobel's indirect test to assess mediation (MacKinnon et al. 2002; Sobel 1982). Interaction terms including CPF and each additional covariate were tested in the models. Effect estimates, 95% confidence intervals (CIs), and p-values were calculated for all analytic procedures. Results were considered significant at $p < 0.05$.

4.2 RESULTS

The retention rate for the full cohort was 82% at the 7-year follow-up, with no significant sociodemographic differences between subjects retained in the study and those lost to follow-up (data not shown). Table 1 lists characteristics of the study sample with complete data on all variables (n = 265). Study families were predominantly low income, with 31% of mothers failing to complete high school by child's age 7 years, and 66% never married. The sample was largely full term (only 4% of children in the sample were < 37 weeks gestational age at delivery) and included very few low-birth-weight infants because a) we excluded high-risk pregnancies from the study cohort, and b) the timing of air monitoring in the third trimester of pregnancy eliminated early deliveries.

CPF exposure levels ranged from nondetectable to 63 pg/g. We imputed exposure levels in participants with nondetectable CPF (n = 115, 43%) according to assay-specific LOD values, with 93 subjects having LOD equal to 0.5 pg/g and 22 subjects having LOD equal to 1 pg/g.

Correlation analyses for exposures and cognitive outcomes. Unadjusted correlations between prenatal CPF exposure and log-transformed WISC-IV Composite Indices (Verbal Comprehension, Working Memory, Processing Speed, and Perceptual Reasoning), and Full-Scale IQ showed significant inverse associations between CPF exposure and a) Working Memory ($r = -0.21$, $p = < 0.0001$) and b) Full-Scale IQ ($r = -0.13$, $p = 0.02$). We observed a weak inverse correlation between CPF and Perceptual Reasoning ($r = -0.09$, $p = 0.09$), while associations of CPF with Verbal Comprehension ($r = -0.04$) and Processing Speed ($r = -0.01$) had p-values > 0.05.

TABLE 1: Demographic characteristics of the sample at 7-year follow-up (n = 265).

Characteristic	n (%) or mean ± SD (range)
Home quality[a]	40.23 ± 4.81 (23–52)
Income	
< $20,000	138 (52)
≥ $20,000	127 (48)
Maternal education[b]	
Years	12.22 ± 2.58 (1–20)
< High school degree	82 (31)
High school degree	183 (69)
Maternal IQ[c]	85.97 ± 13.46 (60–135)
Maternal race/ethnicity[d]	
Dominican	146 (55)
African American	119 (45)
Marital status	
Never married	175 (66)
Ever married	90 (34)
Child sex	
Male	117 (44)
Female	148 (56)
Gestational age (weeks)	39.3 ± 1.5 (30–43)
Birth weight (g)	3389.8 ± 493.5 (1,295–5,110)
Child age at testing (months)	85.97 ± 2.65 (74.90–101.5)
Prenatal chemical exposures	
ETS[e]	
Exposed	93 (35)
Not exposed	172 (65)
Cotinine (ng/mL)[f]	0.25 ± 0.92 (0.01–8.78)
Lead (μg/dL)[f]	1.09 ±.88 (0.15–7.45)
CPF (pg/g)[f]	3.17 ± 4.61 (0.09–32)
PAHs (ng/m³)[g]	3.37 ± 3.51 (0.50–36.5)

[a]As measured by the HOME inventory. [b]Completed years of education at child's age 7 years. [c]As measured by TONI-3. [d]Self-reported race/ethnicity (African American = 1; Dominican = 0). [e]Self-reported ever exposed to secondhand smoke in pregnancy (yes = 1; no = 2). [f]Measured in cord blood. [g]Measured by personal air sampling.

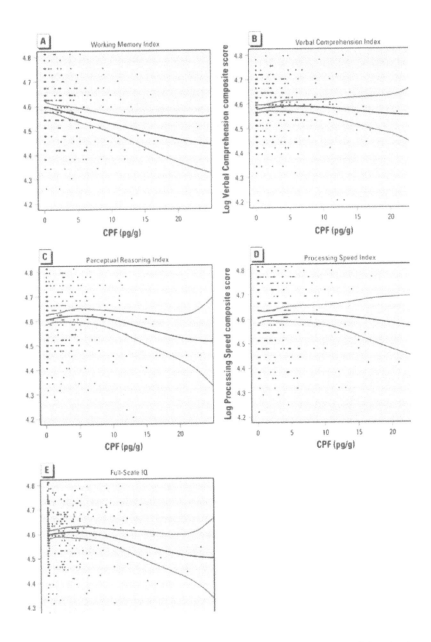

FIGURE 1: Smoothed cubic splines, superimposed over scatterplots, examining the shape of the associations between CPF exposure and (A) Working Memory Index, (B) Verbal Comprehension Index, (C) Perceptual Reasoning Index, (D) Processing Speed Index, and (E) Full-Scale IQ.

TABLE 2: Estimated associations between CPF (pg/g) and log-transformed Full-Scale IQ and each of four Composite Index scores from the WISC-IV from LASSO[a] and fully adjusted[b] linear regression models (n = 265).>

WISC-IV scale[c]	B-coefficient[c]	95% CI	p-Value
Full-Scale IQ			
LASSO	−0.003	−0.006 to 0.001	0.064
Fully adjusted	−0.003	−0.006 to 0.000	0.048
Working Memory Index			
LASSO	−0.006	−0.009 to −0.002	< 0.001
Fully adjusted	−0.006	−0.010 to −0.002	0.003
Verbal Comprehension Index			
LASSO	NAd	NA	NA
Fully adjusted	−0.002	−0.005 to 0.001	0.208
Perceptual Reasoning Index			
LASSO	NA	NA	NA
Fully adjusted	−0.002	−0.006 to 0.002	0.290
Processing Speed Index			
LASSO	NA	NA	NA
Fully adjusted	0.001	−0.004 to 0.005	0.728

NA, not assessed. [a]LASSO models were adjusted for maternal education, maternal IQ, and the HOME Inventory. [b]Fully adjusted models were adjusted for child sex, race/ethnicity, maternal IQ, maternal education income, child age at testing (months), ETS, and PAH. [c]All scales wereln transformed. [d]CPF was not retained in the final LASSO model.

Umbilical cord lead was not significantly correlated with CPF level (r = −0.08, p = 0.49) or WISC-IV scores (all p-values > 0.05) among the 89 children with lead data available. Lead was not significantly correlated with CPF level (r = −0.08, p = 0.49, as previously reported by Rauh et al. 2006) or with 7-year WISC-IV scores (all p-values > 0.05) among the 89 children with available data. To avoid excluding observations without lead data, we did not include lead as a covariate in regression models. ETS and (to a lesser extent) PAH were correlated with CPF (Spearman coefficients: 0.113, p = 0.01, and 0.07, p = 0.09, respectively) but were not significantly correlated (using the Mann–Whitney test for the dichotomous ETS variable) with any WISC-IV index (coefficients ranged from –0.02 to 0.03, and p-values ranged from 0.39 to 0.87). Birth weight was not significantly associated with any of the WISC-IV indices (all p-values > 0.05) and was not included in the final models.

Spline regression analysis. Examination of the smoothed cubic spline regression curves, superimposed over scatterplots, indicates subtle differences in shape of the functions (Figure 1). The log-transformed Working Memory Index and Full-Scale IQ appear to be approximately linear, whereas the other functions show some curvature across exposure levels, with sparse observations at the highest exposures. Using the Davidson–MacKinnon test for comparison of non-nested models (Davidson and MacKinnon 1981), we compared models in which CPF was entered as a single continuous outcome with those in which CPF was modeled using B-splines. We failed to reject the null hypothesis that the model with CPF as a continuous measure is adequate against the alternative that the model with CPF modeled using splines provided a better fit for each WISC-IV Index (p-values: Verbal Comprehension Index = 0.07, Perceptual Reasoning Index = 0.08, Processing Speed Index = 0.59, Working Memory Index = 0.40, and Full-Scale IQ = 0.08).

Estimation of linear models. Table 2 lists the estimated B-coefficients, 95% CIs, and p-values for the exposure variable and covariates for the best-fitting linear regression models predicting each WISC-IV outcome. Table 2 also includes the results of linear model selection using the LASSO technique, which eliminates covariates with unstable estimates and results in more parsimonious models. Because the LASSO method uses bootstrapping to obtain standard errors, the coefficient of any covariate may be shrunk to zero if that covariate is an unstable predictor—that is, if its significance depends on the particular subset of data used in the model. The two approaches yielded very similar estimates of CPF effect. Differences in estimates for the covariates in the two methods suggest that the contribution of some covariates to WISC-IV scores may be less stable. Results for both approaches show that, on average, a 1-pg/g increase in

CPF is associated with a decrease of −0.006 points in the log-transformed Working Memory score and a decrease of −0.003 points in the log-transformed Full-Scale IQ score. Because of the log transformation, estimated associations between CPF and actual Working Memory and Full-Scale IQ scores vary across the continuum of scores, such that the estimated deficit in the Working Memory score with a 1-pg/g increase in CPF ranges between 0.35 and 0.81 points, and the estimated decrease in Full-Scale IQ is between 0.20 and 0.40 points. The magnitude of these effects is more easily understood by calculating the neurodevelopmental deficit associated with an increase in CPF exposure equal to 1 SD (4.61 pg/g). On average, for each standard deviation increase in exposure, Full-Scale IQ declines by 1.4% and Working Memory declines by 2.8%. We found no significant interactions between CPF and any of the potential or final covariates, including the other chemical exposures measured during the prenatal period (ETS and PAH). Full model results for the linear regressions are provided in Supplemental Material, Table 1 (doi:10.1289/ehp.1003160), for the reader who is interested in the estimates of association between the covariates and outcomes for all of the WISC-IV index scales.

Sensitivity analysis of additional influences on Working Memory Index. To determine whether the observed CPF effect on the Working Memory Index was partially explained by its effect on general intelligence, we added the log-transformed General Ability Index, a general intelligence scale that does not include the Working Memory Index or Processing Speed Index, to the linear regression model. Although the estimate of the General Ability Index effect on Working Memory Index was significant (B-coefficient = 0.57; 95% CI, 0.44–0.70; $p < 0.001$), the estimate of the CPF effect remained unchanged (−0.006), and we found no evidence of interaction between CPF and General Ability Index ($p > 0.05$), suggesting that the Working Memory effect is targeted and does not depend upon level of general intelligence.

Because child performance on the Working Memory Index can be influenced by child behavior problems (Wechsler 2003), we conducted a supplementary analysis to rule out the possibility that the observed associations between CPF and the Working Memory Index might be affected by behavior problems, as measured by the clinically oriented diagnostic and statistical manual scales on the Child Behavior Checklist. We found no evidence of indirect "mediation" using Sobel's test, with p-values ranging from 0.31 to 0.99 (MacKinnon et al. 2002; Sobel 1982). Full model results are provided in Supplemental Material, Table 2 (doi:10.1289/ehp.1003160), for the reader who is interested in the estimates of association between child behavior problems and Working Memory Index.

Sensitivity analysis of the influence of LOD imputation. After obtaining all results, we recomputed all estimates of association between CPF and WISC-IV scores among subjects with detectable CPF levels only. Analysis with detects alone is known to give unbiased estimates of the parameters of interest (Little 1992). In the present sample, we observed no consistent differences in estimates when we excluded imputed CPF data (data not shown).

4.3 DISCUSSION

Results of this study showed that higher prenatal CPF exposure, as measured in umbilical cord blood plasma, was associated with decreases in cognitive functioning on two different WISC-IV indices, in a sample of urban minority children at 7 years of age. Specifically, for each SD increase in exposure (4.61 pg/g), Full-Scale IQ declined, on average, by 1.4% (0.94–1.8 points) and Working Memory Index scores declined by 2.8% (1.6–3.7 points). The dose–effect relationships between CPF exposure and log-transformed Working Memory Index and Full-Scale IQ scores are linear across the range of exposures in the study population, with no evidence for a threshold. Of the WISC-IV indices used as end points, the Working Memory Index was the most strongly associated with CPF exposure in this population.

Although no other epidemiologic studies have evaluated the neurotoxicity of prenatal CPF exposure on cognitive development at the time of school entry, several prior studies, using the present biomarker of exposure, have reported evidence of early cognitive and behavioral effects associated with a urinary biomarker of nonspecific OP exposure (Engel et al. 2007; Eskenazi et al. 2007; Young et al. 2005). Outcomes associated with exposure in these studies, as well as in our own earlier work (Rauh et al. 2006), have included attentional problems (e.g., Marks et al. 2010).

These prior findings are consistent with the present 7-year results, because working memory skills involve attentional processes. More important, problems in working memory may interfere with reading comprehension, learning, and academic achievement, although general intelligence remains in the normal range (Blair 2006). Working memory is less likely than full-scale IQ to be affected by socioeconomic or cultural conditions (Wechsler 2003), providing a useful, more targeted measure of possible neurotoxic effects on brain function.

Several different theories or models address how working memory operates in the human brain, but most agree that it involves a system of limited attention capacity, supplemented by more peripherally based storage systems (Baddeley and Logie 1999). Some theories emphasize the role of attentional control in working memory (e.g., Cowan 1999), whereas others stress a multicomponent model, including a control system of limited attentional capacity (the central executive control system), assisted by phonological and visuospatial storage systems (see review by Baddeley 2003). To date, most studies of the anatomical localization of working memory problems are based on clinical populations (individuals with specific brain lesions) (Vallar and Pagano 2002) and some neuroimaging studies in small numbers of normal subjects (Smith and Jonides 1997). More refined neuropsychological tests and neuroimaging studies are needed to determine whether CPF-related working memory deficits are primarily auditory (part of a phonological loop with implications for language acquisition) or primarily related to visuospatial short-term memory (reflecting nonverbal intelligence tasks).

Few human studies have focused on possible mechanisms underlying neurodevelopmental deficits associated with OP exposure, but there is evidence that certain genetic polymorphisms can affect CPF metabolism (e.g., Berkowitz et al. 2004). Such findings suggest that some populations may be more vulnerable and may exhibit adverse neurodevelopmental effects at much lower exposures than other populations (Berkowitz et al. 2004). Again, neuroimaging studies would be useful to determine if population differences in vulnerability to CPF are also reflected in population differences in brain abnormalities associated with exposure.

Although behavioral alterations observed in rodents may be imperfect analogues for humans, they have guided human studies by identifying specific deficits in locomotor activity, learning, and memory (e.g., Aldridge et al. 2005). In light of experimental evidence suggesting that CPF effects in rodents may be irreversible (Slotkin 2005), it will be important to determine how any neurocognitive deficits associated with prenatal CPF exposure might respond to treatment or early intervention. Here, we may benefit from studies of lead-exposed children that have demonstrated evidence of reversals in learning deficits as a result of environmental enrichment (Guilarte et al. 2003).

Some limitations of this study should be noted. Our sample consists of low-income, urban, minority children who may experience other unmeasured exposures or underlying health problems that could potentially confound or modify associations with pesticide exposure. Furthermore, in the absence of firm mechanistic evidence linking brain anomalies to more refined neuropsychological testing, the observed functional deficits at 7 years of age should be interpreted with caution. We cannot directly compare our findings with the results from the other epidemiological studies that have relied on urinary OP concentrations as the biomarker of exposure.

In June 2000, the U.S. EPA announced a phase-out of the sale of CPF for indoor residential use, with a complete ban effective 31 December 2001 (U.S. EPA 2000, 2002). After the ban, levels of CPF in personal and indoor air samples in our own cohort decreased by more than 65%, and plasma blood levels dropped by more than 80% (Whyatt et al. 2005), despite some lingering residential residues (Whyatt et al. 2007). From other parts of the country, there is evidence of continued low-dose exposures in children from food residues (Lu et al. 2006). Because agricultural use of CPF is still permitted in the United States, it is important that we continue to monitor the levels of exposure in potentially vulnerable populations, including pregnant women in agricultural communities, and evaluate the long-term neurodevelopmental implications of exposure to CPF and other OP insecticides.

REFERENCES

1. Achenbach TM, Rescorla LA. Burlington, VT: University of Vermont, Research Center for Children, Youth and Families; 2001. Manual for the ASEBA School-Age Forms and Profiles.

2. Aldridge JE, Meyer A, Seidler FJ, Slotkin TA. Alterations in central nervous system serotonergic and dopaminergic synaptic activity in adulthood after prenatal or neonatal chlorpyrifos exposure. Environ Health Perspect. 2005;113:1027–1031.

3. Baddeley A. Working memory: looking back and forward. Nat Rev Neurosci. 2003;4(10):829–839.

4. Baddeley AD, Logie RH. In: Models of Working Memory: Mechanisms of Active Maintenance AND Executive Control (Miyake A, Shah P, eds) New York:Cambridge University press, 28–61; 1999. Working memory: the multi-component model.

5. Barr DB, Barr JR, Maggio VL, Whitehead RD, Jr, Sadowski MA, Whyatt RM, et al. A multi-analyte method for the quantification of contemporary pesticides in human serum and plasma using high resolution mass spectrometry. J Chromatog B Anal Technol Biomed Life Sciences. 2002;778:99–111.

6. Berkowitz GS, Obel J, Deych E, Lapinski R, Godbold J, Liu Z, et al. Exposure to indoor pesticides during pregnancy in a multiethnic, urban cohort. Environ Health Perspect. 2003;111:79–84.

7. Berkowitz GC, Wetmur JG, Birman-Deych E, Obel J, Lapinski RH, Godbold JH, et al. In utero pesticide exposure, maternal paraoxonase activity, and head circumference. Environ Health Perspect. 2004;112:388–391.

8. Blair C. How similar are fluid cognition and general intelligence? A developmental neuroscience perspective on fluid cognition as an aspect of human cognitive ability. Behav Brain Science. 2006;29:109–125.

9. Bradman A, Barr DB, Claus Henn BG, Drumheller T, Curry C, Eskenazi B. Measurement of pesticides and other toxicants in amnionic fluid as a potential biomarker of prenatal exposure: a validation study. Environ Health Perspect. 2003;113:1802–1807.

10. Brown L, Sherbenou RJ, Johnson SK. Austin, TX: PRO-ED, Inc; 1997. Test of Nonverbal Intelligence: A Language-Free Measure of Cognitive Ability. 3rd ed.

11. Caldwell BM, Bradley RH. 1979. Home Observation for Measurement of the Environment. Little Rock:University of Arkansas Press.

12. Chiodo LM, Jacobson SW, Jacobson JL. Neurodevelopmental effects of postnatal lead exposure at very low levels. Neurotoxicol Teratol. 2004;26:359–371.

13. Cowan N. In: Models of Working Memory: Mechanisms of Active Maintenance and Executive Control (Miyake A, Shah P, eds). New York:Cambridge University Press, 62–101; 1999. An embedded-processes model of working memory.

14. Davidson R, MacKinnon J. Several tests for model specification in the presence of alternative hypotheses. Econometrica. 1981;49:781–793.

15. Engel SM, Berkowitz GS, Barr DB, Teitelbaum SL, Siskind J, Meisel SL, et al. Prenatal organophosphate metabolite and organochlorine levels and performance on the Brazelton Neonatal Behavioral Assessment Scale in a multiethnic pregnancy cohort. Am J Epidemiol. 2007;165:1397–1404.

16. Eskenazi B, Marks AR, Bradman A, Harley K, Barr DB, Johnson C, et al. Organophosphate pesticide exposure and neurodevelopment in young Mexican-American children. Environ Health Perspect. 2007;115:792–798.

17. Guilarte TR, Toscano CD, McGlothan JL, Weaver SA. Environmental enrichment reverses cognitive and molecular deficits induced by developmental lead exposure. Ann Neurol. 2003;53:50–56.

18. Hecht SA, Burgess SR, Torgesen RK, Wagner RK, Rashotte CA. Explaining social class differences in growth of reading skills from beginning kindergarten through fourth-grade: the role of phonological awareness, rate of access and print knowledge. Read Writ Interdisciplin J. 2000;12:99–127.

19. Houwelingen JC. Shrinkage and penalized likelihood as methods to improve predictive accuracy. Stat Neerl. 2001;55(1):17–34.

20. Jusko TA, Henderson CR, Lanphear BP, Cory-Slechta DA, Parsons PJ, Canfield RL. Blood lead concentrations < 10 µg/dL and child intelligence at 6 years of age. Environ Health Perspect. 2008;116:243–248.

21. Landrigan PJ, Schechter CB, Lipton JM, Fahs MC, Schwartz J. Environmental pollutants and disease in American children: estimates of morbidity, mortality, and costs for lead poisoning, asthma, cancer, and developmental disabilities. Environ Health Perspect. 2002;110:721–728.

22. Levin ED, Addy N, Baruah A, Elias A, Cannelle CN, Seidler FJ, et al. Prenatal chlorpyrifos exposure in rats causes persistent behavioral alternations. Neurotoxicol Teratol. 2002;24:733–741.

23. Little RJA. Regression with missing X's: a review. J Am Stat Assoc. 1992;87:1227–1237.

24. Lu C, Toepel K, Irish R, Fenske RA, Barr DB, Bravo R. Organic diets significantly lower children's dietary exposure to organophosphate pesticides. Environ Health Perspect. 2006;114:260–263.

25. MacKinnon DP, Lockwood CM, Hoffman JM, West SG, Sheets V. A comparison of methods to test mediation and other intervening variable effects. Psychol Methods. 2002;7:83–104.

26. Marks AR, Harley K, Bradman A, Kogut K, Barr DB, Johnson C, et al. Organophosphate pesticide exposure and attention in young Mexican-American children: the CHAMACOS Study. Environ Health Perspect. 2010;118:1768–1774.

27. Perera FP, Illman SM, Kinney PL, Whyatt RM, Kelvin EA, Shepard P, et al. The challenge of preventing environmentally related disease in young children: community-based research in New York City. Environ Health Perspect. 2002;110:197–204.

28. Perera FP, Rauh V, Tsai WY, Kinney P, Camann D, Barr D, et al. Effects of transplacental exposure to environmental pollutants on birth outcomes in a multiethnic population. Environ Health Perspect. 2003;111:201–205.

29. Qiao D, Seidler FJ, Tate CA, Cousins MM, Slotkin TA. Fetal chlorpyrifos exposure: adverse effects on brain cell development and cholinergic biomarkers emerge postnatally and continue into adolescence and adulthood. Environ Health Perspect. 2003;111:536–544.

30. R Development Core Team. Vienna: R Foundation for Statistical Computing; 2009. R: A Language and Environment for Statistical Computing.

31. Rauh VA, Garfinkel R, Perera FP, Andrews H, Barr D, Whitehead D, et al. 2006. Impact of prenatal chlorpyrifos exposure on neurodevelopment in the first three years of life among inner-city children. Pediatrics 118:e1845–e1859.

32. Rauh VA, Whyatt RM, Garfinkel R, Andrews H, Hoepner L, Reyes A, et al. Developmental effects of exposure to environmental tobacco smoke and material hardship among inner-city children. Neurotoxicol Teratol. 2004;26:373–385.

33. Richardson DB, Ciampi A. Effects of exposure measurement error when an exposure variable is constrained by a lower limit. Am J Epidemiol. 2003;57(4):355–363.

34. Richardson RJ. Assessment of the neurotoxic potential of chlorpyrifos relative to other organophosphorus compounds: a critical review of the literature. J Toxicol Environ Health. 1995;44:135–165.

35. Rothenberg SJ, Rothenberg JC. Testing the dose-response specification in epidemiology: public health and policy consequences for lead. Environ Health Perspect. 2005;113:1190–1195.

36. Slotkin TA. Cholinergic systems in brain development and disruption by neurotoxicants: nicotine, environmental tobacco smoke, organophosphates. Toxicol Appl Pharmacol. 2004;198:132–151.

37. Slotkin TA. In: Toxicity of Organophosphates and Carbamate Pesticides (Gupta RC, ed). San Diego:Academic Press, 293–314; 2005. Developmental neurotoxicity of organophosphates: a case study of chlorpyrifos.

38. Slotkin TA, Seidler FJ. The alterations in CNS serotonergic mechanisms caused by neonatal chlorpyrifos exposure are permanent. Dev Brain Res. 2005;158:115–119.

39. Smith EE, Jonides J. Working memory: a view from neuroimaging. Cogn Psychol. 1997;33:5–42.

40. Sobel ME. Asymptotic confidence intervals for indirect effects in structural equation models. Sociol Methodol. 1982;13:290–312.

41. Tibshirani R. Regression shrinkage and selection via the lasso. J R Stat Soc Series B Stat Methodol. 1996;58(1):267–288.

42. U.S. EPA (U.S. Environmental Protection Agency) Washington, DC: U.S. EPA; 2000. Chlorpyrifos Revised Risk Assessment and Agreement with Registrants.

43. U.S. EPA (U.S. Environmental Protection Agency) Washington, DC: U.S. EPA; 2002. Chlorpyrifos End-Use Products Cancellation Order.

44. Vallar G, Pagano C. Chichester, UK: Wiley, 249–270; 2002. Neuropsychological impairments of verbal short-term memory. In: Handbook of Memory Disorders (Baddeley AD, Kopelman MD, Wilson BA, eds)

45. Wechsler D. 2003. Wechsler Intelligence Scale for Children. 4th ed. San Antonio, TX:Psychological Corporation.

46. Whyatt RM, Barr DB, Camann DE, Kinney PL, Barr JR, Andrews HF, et al. Contemporary-use pesticides in personal air samples during pregnancy and blood samples at delivery among urban minority mothers and newborns. Environ Health Perspect. 2003;111:749–756.

47. Whyatt RM, Camann D, Perera FP, Rauh VA, Tang D, Kinney PL, et al. Biomarkers in assessing residential insecticide exposures during pregnancy and effects on fetal growth. Toxicol Appl Pharmacol. 2005;206:246–254.

48. Whyatt RM, Camann DE, Kinney PL, Reyes A, Ramirez J, Dietrich J, et al. 2002. Residential pesticide use during pregnancy among a cohort of urban minority women, Environ Health Perspect 110507–514.514

49. Whyatt RM, Garfinkel R, Hoepner LA, Holmes D, Borjas M, Perera FP, et al. 2007. Within and between home variability in indoor-air insecticide levels during pregnancy among an inner-city cohort from New York City, Environ Health Perspect 115383–390.390

50. Whyatt RM, Rauh VA, Barr DB, Camann DE, Andrews HF, Garfinkel R, et al. Prenatal insecticide exposure and birth weight and length among an urban minority cohort. Environ Health Perspect. 2004;112:1125–1132.
51. Young JG, Eskenazi B, Gladstone EA, Bradman A, Pedersen L, Johnson C, et al. Association between in utero organophosphate exposure and abnormal reflexes in neonates. Neurotoxicology. 2005;26:199–209.
52. Zhao P, Yu B. On model selection consistency of Lasso. J Machine Learn Res. 2006;7:2541–2563.

There are several supplemental files that are not available in this version of the article. To view this additional information, please use the citation on the first page of this chapter.

CHAPTER 5

FETAL AND NEONATAL ENDOCRINE DISRUPTORS

TOLGA ÜNÜVAR AND ATILLA BÜYÜKGEBIZ

5.1 INTRODUCTION

Endocrine disruptors (xenohormones) are exogenous substances or compounds that cause adverse health effects in the organism by disrupting the endocrine functions (1,2,3). Endocrine disruptions mostly occur on the basis of genetic predisposition. Natural or synthetic chemical endocrine disrupting substances that we are surrounded with and are exposed to in the modern world lead to clinical disorders by intervening with hormonal physiology (4). At first, endocrine disruptors were thought to act only via nuclear hormone receptors such as estrogen, androgen, progesterone, thyroid and retinoid receptors. However, recent studies have shown that the mechanism of action of endocrine disruptors is not that simple. Endocrine disruptors are thought to exert effects on endocrine and reproductive systems through nuclear receptors, non-nuclear steroid hormone receptors (membrane estrogen receptors), non-steroid receptors (neurotransmitter receptors such as serotonin, dopamine, norepinephrine receptors), orphan receptors (aryl hydrocarbon receptor), enzymatic path-

Fetal and Neonatal Endocrine Disruptors. Ünüvar T and Büyükgebiz A. © Journal of Clinical Research in Pediatric Endocrinology, *4,2 (2012). doi:10.4274/Jcrpe.569. Licensed under Creative Commons Attribution License.*

ways involving steroid biosynthesis and/or metabolism, and numerous other mechanisms (3). Endocrine disruptors are also known as endocrine modulators, hormone active agents, endocrine active agents, endocrine toxins or xenohormones (5,6). Molecules defined as endocrine disruptors constitute an extremely heterogeneous group and include synthetic chemicals used as industrial solvents/lubricants and their by-products (polychlorinated biphenyls, polybrominated biphenyls, dioxins), plastics (bisphenol A), plasticisers (phthalates), pesticides [methoxychlor, chlorphyrifos, dichlorodiphenyl-trichloroethane (DDT)], fungicides (vinclozolin) and pharmaceutical agents (diethylstilbestrol) (3). Natural chemicals found in human and animal food (phytoestrogens such as genistein, coumestrol) also act as endocrine disruptors (5,7) (Table 1). Different from adults, infants and children are not exposed only to chemical toxins in the environment but may also be exposed indirectly during their intrauterine life. Hundreds of toxic substances may affect the fetus via the placental cord and these substances may be excreted via the meconium. These include countless number of neuro-immune and endocrine toxic chemical components that may influence the critical steps of hormonal, neurological and immunological development. It has been demonstrated in animal and human studies that affected offsprings are not only born with congenital abnormalities but may also suffer from several health and behavioral problems throughout their lifespan (8). Measurement of endocrine disruptor levels in the umbilical cord blood of newborns is one of the several methods to determine intrauterine fetal exposure to chemical substances. In a study conducted in the US by the Environmental Working Group (EWG), 413 toxic substances were sought in the umbilical cord blood of 10 newborns, with positive results for 287 of these substances (Table 2). In the same study, many endocrine-disrupting chemical compounds including pharmaceutical agents, illegal drugs, heavy metals and pesticides were also detected in the meconium samples from the newborns. Children and especially newborns are more sensitive to environmental toxins compared to adults. Metabolic pathways in infants are immature, especially in the first months of life. Newborns differ from adults in their ability to metabolize, detoxify and eliminate many toxins. It has been demonstrated in various studies that newborns are affected from chemical toxins to a greater degree than adults (9). Although exposures have occurred during fetal life or during the neonatal period, the effect of these exposures may sometimes not be observed for many years. For these reasons, some of the states caused by endocrine disruptors are among examples of adult disease states of fetal origin (10). Owing to the fact that endocrine disruptors have low water solubility and high lipid solubility, they accumulate in fatty tissues. Thus, their long-term effects may be observed in later years.

TABLE 1: The most common chemicals found in the environment ([ref:5]5[/ref],[ref:7]7[/ref])

Category	Chemicals
Pesticides	
Herbicides	2,4-Dichlorophenoxyacetic acid, 2,4,5-Trichlorophenoxyacetic acid, Alacholor, Amitrole, Atrazine, Nitrophen, Trifluralin
Fungicides	Benomyl, Hexachlorobenzene, Iprodione, Mancozeb, Maneb, Metiram, Myclobutanil, Prokloraz, Procymidone, Triadimefon, Tributyltin, Vinclozolin, Zineb, Ziram
Insecticides	Carbaryl, Chlordane, Dicofol, Dieldrin, Dichlorodiphenyltrichloroethane and its metabolites, Endosulfan, Heptachlor, Epoxide, hexachloroyclohexane, Lindane, Metomil, Methoxychlor, Mirex, Oxychlodane, Parathion, Permetrine, Toxaphene, Trans-nonachlor
Nematocides	Aldicarb, Dibromochloropropane
Industrial compounds	Bisphenol A, Cadmium, Dioxins, Polybrominated biphenyls (PBBs), Polychlorinated biphenyls (PCBs), Pentachlorophenol, Pentanonylphenol, Phthalates, Ortho-chlorostyrene, Styrene dimers and trimers

5.1.1 EFFECTS OF ENDOCRINE DISRUPTORS ON GROWTH

Intrauterine exposure to endocrine disruptors has been associated with low birth weight, low height and low head circumference in the newborns. The main chemical compounds that affect growth in infancy are the chlorinated pesticide metabolites dichlorodiphenyldichloroethylene (DDE), organophosphate pesticides and polycyclic aromatic hydrocarbons (PAH). Growth retardation has been noted in a 5-year follow-up of children after prenatal exposure to dioxins polychlorinated dioxins and furans (PCDD/PCDFs) (11).

TABLE 2: Endocrine disruptors detected in umbilical cord blood ([ref:8]8[/ref])

Compound	Number of Screened Toxic Substances	Number of Positive Results	Source
Mercury	1	1	Dental filings, seafood
Polycyclic aromatic hydrocarbons (PAHs)	18	9	Combustion by-products in vehicle exhaust or smoking tobacco
Polybrominated dioxins and furans (PBDD/PBDFs)	12	7	Flame retardants
Polychlorinated dioxins and furans (PCDD/PCDFs)	17	11	By-products from plastic production, industrial bleaching, and incineration
Perfluorinated chemicals (PFCs)	12	9	Teflon®, carpet and fabric preservatives, food preserving stretch films
Chlorinated pesticides	28	21	Fish farms, fat-rich foods
Polybrominated diphenyl ethers (PBDEs)	46	32	Flame retardants
Polychlorinated napthalene	70	50	Wood preservatives, varnish, polish
Polychlorinated biphenyls (PCBs)	209	147	Machine oils and isolation materials

5.1.2 POLYCYCLIC AROMATIC HYDROCARBONS

These substances are found in combustion by-products associated with smoking, vehicle exhaust, factory chimneys, forest fires, and jet motors. It is well known that maternal smoking during pregnancy is associated with low birth weight (12). It has also been shown that air pollution in the cities is another source of PAH and that it is associated with low birth weight, reduced height and low head circumference in the newborn (13,14).

5.1.3 ORGANOPHOSPHATE PESTICIDES

It has been reported that intrauterine exposure to these substances is associated with height, weight and head circumference retardation in the newborns (15). Moreover, severe mental retardation, as well as abnormalities pertaining to the development of the brain, eyes, ears, teeth, heart, feet, breast and sexual organs (undescended testicles, microphallus, labial fusion) have been observed in affected infants at birth (16).

5.1.4 EFFECTS OF ENDOCRINE DISRUPTORS ON THE DEVELOPMENT OF THE IMMUNE SYSTEM

Some lead-containing endocrine-disrupting compounds have been shown to result in domination of T helper cells (TH2) in the fetal immune system, which in turn leads to an increased predisposition to asthma and allergies in newborns and infants (17). It has been shown that intrauterine exposure to dioxin leads to the development of autoimmunity in animals (18). Since most of the developmental activity in the immune system occurs in the first trimester of pregnancy, exposure to foreign substances during this period may have a greater impact. Depending on the time of impact, exposure to PAH may lead to imbalances in the immune system such as decrease in T cells, increase in B cells, and elevation in IgE levels (19). It has been found in animal studies that intrauterine exposure to polychlorinated biphenyls (PCBs) results in atrophy of the thymus. Respiratory tract infections have been noted to be more common and to show a tendency to recur more frequently in children exposed to PCB and DDE during the prenatal period as compared to children who are not affected (20,21). In addition to increased tendency for infections in infants affected by endocrine disruptors, immune response is also weakened. It was demonstrated in a Dutch study that insufficient amounts of antibodies were formed following measles-mumps-rubella vaccine in children exposed to PCB (21).

5.1.5 EFFECTS OF ENDOCRINE DISRUPTORS ON THE NERVOUS SYSTEM

As the blood-brain barrier has not yet completed its development during the fetal development of the nervous system, the fetus is more sensitive to all neurotoxins.

Mercury: High levels of mercury have been found in hair samples of infants born to women who have consumed high amounts of seafood during their pregnancy. These children may experience cognitive and behavioral disorders in later life (22).

Lead: Reduction in memory and problem-solving abilities have been noted in rats with prenatal lead exposure (23). Deficits in mental abilities have been reported in a 24-month follow-up of children with intrauterine exposure to high amounts of lead from maternal bone stores (24).

Polychlorinated biphenyls: Long-term neurological deficits and persistent behavioral problems have been reported in rats with neonatal PCB exposure. Also, intellectual functions have been found to be affected in infants whose mothers had consumed fish exposed to PCB during pregnancy (25). Reduction in comprehension and cognitive functions have been noted even in children born as late as six years after the incident in which their mothers were affected and these children were also observed to have significantly more behavioral and activity problems compared to the control group (26).

Organophosphate pesticides: Children with intrauterine exposure to organophosphate pesticides have been found to exhibit abnormal reflexes at the time of birth (27). These children were also noted to have poor short-term memory, slow response times as well as impaired mental development (28).

5.1.6 EFFECTS OF ENDOCRINE DISRUPTORS ON THE UROGENITAL SYSTEM

Sex steroids, and especially androgens are very important for normal intrauterine sexual development (29). Sexual differentiation of a male fetus is androgen-dependent (estrogen is also effective in a small degree). However, sexual differentiation of a female fetus is often independent of androgens and estrogens. Therefore, sexual development disorders related to endocrine disruptors, which excellently mimic estrogens and/or block androgens, lead to different clinical presentations in girls and boys (30) (Table 3).

TABLE 3: The potential effects of endocrine disruptors on the urogenital system

	Fetal/Neonatal	Prepubertal	Pubertal
Male	Intrauterine growth retardation	Premature pubarche	Small testicles and high FSH
	Undescended testicle		Precocious puberty
	Hypospadias		Delayed puberty
Female	Intrauterine growth retardation	Premature thelarche	Secondary central precocious puberty
		Peripheral precocious puberty	Polycystic ovary syndrome
		Premature pubarche	Delayed ovulatory cycles

FSH: follicle-stimulating hormone

5.1.7 THE MALE UROGENITAL SYSTEM

A weak association has been found between maternal serum concentrations of PCB, dichlorodiphenyltrichloroethane (DDT) and DDE (primary DDT metabolites) and occurrence of undescended testicles and hypospadias in infants born to these mothers (31,32). On the other hand, significant relationships between development of hypospadias or undescended testicle and consanguineous marriages or pesticide exposure have been reported (33). It has also been shown that 2,3,7,8-tetrachlorodibenzo-p-dioxin (TCDD) exposure of male rats during intrauterine and lactation periods leads to sexual differentiation in the brain and sexual behavior changes (34,35). Estrogen and testosterone levels in umbilical cord blood of newborns whose mothers were exposed to high levels of PCDD and PCDF were found to be lower compared to the control group (36). In a study conducted on Taiwanese boys exposed to intrauterine PCB and PCDF, a reduction in serum testosterone levels together with an increase in serum follicle-stimulating hormone (FSH) and estradiol levels during puberty were reported (37). It has been shown in experimental studies that phthalates have antiandrogenic and mild estrogenic effects and may cause ambiguous genitalia in male infants (38). The effects of certain specific endocrine disruptors on male urogenital system are presented in Table 4.

As the half-life of organochlorines is very long (years or even decades), intrauterine exposure should be suspected in children of prepubertal or pubertal ages admitted to hospital with genital abnormalities. Further studies are needed to clarify the effects of endocrine disruptors on the development of the male urogenital system (39).

TABLE 4: The effects of some specific endocrine disruptors on male urogenital system

Endocrine disruptors	Effects in animal model	Anticipated effects in humans	Possible mechanism of action
Vinclozolin	Hupospadias, undescended testicle		Epigenetic: Impaired DNA methylation in germ cells
DES	Hypospadias, undescended testicle, micropenis	Hypospadias, undescended testicle, micropensis, epididymal cyst	Increased estrogen receptor expression in the epididymis
			Reduction in IGFBP-3 level
DDT	Reduction in fertility	Undescended testicle	
DDE		Undescended testicle	
Phthalates	Reduction in anogential distance, undescended testicle, oligospermia	Reduction in anogenital distance and Leydig cell function, hypospadias	Reduction in testosterone synthesis
PCB	Reduced spermatogenesis, delayed puberty	Reduction in penis length, delayed sexual maturation, reduction in fertility, fetal testicular cancer	
BPA	Abnormal growth of prostate and urethra		Increased estrogen receptor expression in hypothalamus and androgen receptor expression in prostate

DES: diethylstilbestrol, DDT: dichlorodiphenyltrichloroethane, DDE: dichlorodiphenyl-dichloroethylene, PCB: polychlorinated biphenyl, BPA: bisphenol A, IGFBP-3: insulin-like growth factor-binding protein 3

5.1.8 THE FEMALE UROGENITAL SYSTEM

Dioxins: Although not classified as xenoestrogens, dioxins may lead to estrogenic or antiestrogenic effects depending on time of exposure, site (organ) of exposure and presence of estrogen. It has been demonstrated that tumor incidence is increased and latent period of tumor development is decreased in rats exposed to TCDD on the 15th day of gestation and to the chemical carcinogen dimethylbenzanthracene (DMBA) on the 50th day of gestation (40). There have also been studies reporting that fetal TCDD exposure increases breast cancer risk and leads to deterioration in breast tissue morphology (41). Kakeyama et al (42) reported that exposure to low-dose TCDD during the prenatal period led to early activation of the hypothalamic-pituitary-gonadal axis and precocious puberty in rats.

Bisphenol A: Bisphenol A (BPA), which is a xenoestrogen, is a chemical endocrine disruptor frequently encountered in every setting of daily life. While maternal exposure to BPA may indirectly affect the fetus, it may also affect the newborn directly through infant formulas, breast milk and preserved foods (43). In fact, high levels of BPA have been measured in human placental tissue as well as in maternal and fetal plasma at the time of birth (44). Urinary BPA levels measured in children and adolescents have been reported to be higher compared to adults (45). BPA has also been detected in the breast milk of lactating mothers. In the light of these findings, it can be suggested that human fetuses and newborns may readily be exposed to this chemical. Recent studies have reported that food is not the only source of BPA exposure and that parenteral applications may also be a source. BPA half-life in humans is much longer than expected (46). Morphological and developmental abnormalities were noted in the breast tissue of fetuses of mother rats exposed to BPA for 14 days starting from the 8th day of gestation. Mammary duct epithelial cell proliferation in these fetuses was found to be significantly greater compared to that in fetuses whose mothers were not exposed to BPA (47). It has also been observed that intraductal hyperplasias that are defined as preneoplastic lesions may appear in the 3rd postnatal month subsequent to this proliferation and increased ductal branching (48). In another study, 3-4-fold increase in precancerous lesions (intraductal proliferation) during puberty and adulthood has been shown to occur in rats as a result of fetal

BPA exposure (49). These results indicate that significant prenatal exposure to BPA leads to persistent changes in breast tissue structure and development, precancerous lesions and carcinoma in situ. Exposure to BPA and other chemicals with estrogen-like effects has been listed as one of the reasons for the increased incidence of breast cancer in modern societies in recent years.

TABLE 5: The effects of certain specific endocrine disruptors on female urogenital system

Endocrine disruptors	Effects in animal model	Anticipated effects in humans	Possible mechanism of action
Vinclozolin	Multisystem disorders , tumors		Epigenetic: Impaired DNA methylation in germ cells
DES	Predisposition to malignancies	Vaginal adenocarcinoma in infants of mothers who have used DES during pregnancy	Increased estrogen receptor expression in the epididymis Reduction in IGFBP 3 level
DDT/DDE	Early sexual development	Precocious puberty, increased risk for breast cancer	Neuroendocrine effects via aryl hydrocarbon and estrogen receptors
BPA	Mammary gland duct abnormalities, precocious puberty	Miscarriages	Inhibition of apoptotic activity in the breast tissue
PCB	Neuroendocrine effects, behavioral changes		Effects on estrogen and neurotransmitter receptors
Dioxins	Developmental abnormalities in the breast tissues		Aryl hydrocarbon receptor inhibition through cyclooxygenase 2
Phthalates		Premature thelarche	

DES: diethylstilbestrol, DDT: dichlorodiphenyltrichloroethane, DDE: dichlorodiphenyldichloroethylene, PCB: polychlorinated biphenyl, BPA: bisphenol A, IGFBP-3: insulin-like growth factor-binding protein 3

Polychlorinated compounds: Yang et al (50) reported that prenatal exposure to PCBs and PCDFs results in abnormal menstruations and very high FSH and estradiol levels in the follicular phase of the cycle in adolescent girls aged between 13 and 19 years. In a Chinese study, prenatal phthalate exposure (di-n-butyl phthalate (DBP) and di-2-ethylhexyl phthalate (DEHP) was shown to increase the risk of low birth weight (51).

Diethylstilbestrol: Epidemiological studies suggest that exposure to xenoestrogens, such as diethylstilbestrol (DES) and DDT, during the fetal period and during puberty increases the risk of developing cancer. In several studies, it has been reported that intrauterine DES exposure may cause cervical uterine and fallopian tube abnormalities, subfertility, infertility and ectopic pregnancies (52). The effects of certain specific endocrine disruptors on the female urogenital system are presented in Table 5. In newborns with intrauterine growth retardation and in those with sexual differentiation disorders such as hypospadias and undescended testicle, breast milk and maternal serum should be screened for endocrine disruptors and these biological samples should be preserved for further research. Research priority should be given to the identification of early markers and indicators of endocrine disruptors encountered in fetal life (39).

5.1.9 EFFECTS OF ENDOCRINE DISRUPTORS ON THYROID FUNCTION

PCBs: Although PCBs have been prohibited in many countries for years due to their very strongly lipophilic features, they can still be detected in human and animal tissue samples (5,53). PCB, especially their biologically active hydroxylated metabolites, has great structural similarity with thyroxine (T4). In animal studies, it has been shown that intrauterine PCB exposure has negative impact on thyroid hormone levels by leading to a decrease in total T4, free T4 (fT4) and total triiodothyronine (T3) and an increase in thyrotropin (TSH) level and that these effects are dose-dependent (54). There is strong evidence demonstrating reduced thyroid hormone levels in infants whose mothers experienced perinatal exposure to PCB or its hydroxylated metabolites (5,55,56,57). Antibodies against thyroid peroxidase and an increase in thyroid volume have also been noted in the follow-up of infants exposed to PCB (58,59). In another study, PCB levels measured in breast milk have been shown to correlate with low postpartum maternal thyroid hormone levels and high fetal TSH levels at postnatal 2nd-3rd months (54,60).

Dioxins: PCDDs and PCDFs are permanent and very toxic environmental pollutants that are formed as by-products from destruction of several chemical substances, including substances used in pesticide production and for bleaching of cellulose in paper production. These compounds initially diffuse into air, then into soil and then contaminate meat, fish, dairy products and breast milk. When pregnant rats were exposed to PCDD, in male offspring rats, the T4 levels were found to be decreased, while an increase was noted in TSH levels (61). Five-year follow-up revealed a positive correlation between serum thyroid hormone levels and PCDD/PCDF levels in children with prenatal exposure to dioxins (11).

Polybrominated diphenyl ethers: These substances are found in several materials used in daily life including plastic coating of electronic devices such as television and computer, in light bulbs, car spare parts, carpets and bedspreads, dye substances and synthetic textile products. Tetrabromobisphenol A (TBBPA) and polybrominated biphenyls are also classified within the same group as polybrominated diphenyl ethers (PBDE). TBBPA and PBDE show a closer structural similarity with thyroid hormone than PCB (53). Prenatal and postnatal thyroid hormone levels have been found to be low in rats with perinatal exposure to PBDE (62). Even low doses of PBDE have affected thyroid functions; T4 levels of offspring of pregnant rats exposed to PBDE have been found to be decreased at postnatal 3rd week (63).

Pesticides: DDT, hexachlorobenzene (HCB) and nonylphenol are the chemicals whose effects on thyroid functions have been investigated most frequently. Although these substances have been prohibited in many countries, they can be still detected in the environmental cycle as they are still being used in some countries and they have very long half-lives. Evidence regarding the disrupting effects of pesticides on thyroid hormones have been noted in numerous animal and toxicological studies (53).

Perfluorinated chemicals: Owing to their surface protecting features, perfluorinated chemicals (PFCs) are chemicals that are very frequently used in daily life. T4 levels have been found to be decreased in both pregnant rats and their offspring as a result of short- and long-term exposure to these substances (64,65). A transient increase in T4 and a decrease in TSH followed by a decrease in T4 and T3 have been noted following exposure to a single dose of PFC (66).

TABLE 6: Summary of effects of endocrine disruptors detected in umbilical cord blood and meconium samples (8)

Chemical compound	Sample source	Effects
Mercury	Merconium/Umbilical cord	Impairment of cognitive functions and alteration in mental status
Lead	Meconium	Neurological and immune system disorders
Polycyclic aromatic hydrocarbons (PAH)	Meconium/Umbilical cord	Allergy, asthma, and recurrent infections
Polybrominated dioxins and furans (PBDD/PBDFs)	Umbilical cord blood	Not studied
Polychlorinated dioxins and furans (PCDD/PCDFs)	Umbilical cord blood	Cognitive and behavioral problems, sex hormone disorders, growth retardation
Perfluorinated chemicals (PFC)	Umbilical cord blood	Thyroid hormone disorders
Chlorinated pesticides	Meconium/Umbilical cord	Recurrent infections, allergies, impairment of cognitive functions and decreased memory, obesity, attention deficit disorders
Polybrominated diphenyl ethers (PBDE)	Umbilical cord blood	Endocrine disorders in animal models
Polychlorinated naphthalene	Umbilical cord blood	Not studied
Polychlorinated biphenyls (PCBs)	Meconium/Umbilical cord	Recurrent infections, reduced respons to infection, inadequate immune response, reduction in intelligence quotient values, activity disorders, thyroid hormone disorders, sexual changes, hearing loss
Organophosphate pesticides	Meconium	Impairment of cognitive and mental functions

Phthalates: Phthalates are often impossible to avoid since they are widely present as additives in many plastic products and in several industrial and commercial products. They are found in soft plastic toys, floor coverings, home cleaning products, medical devices, blood bags, cosmetic products and air cleaners. As phthalates are water-soluble, they can reach the fetus via the amniotic fluid in pregnant mothers. Particularly newborns in contact with materials such as catheters and medical tubings in hospitals are exposed to phthalates and they may subsequently develop transient thyroid dysfunction. T3 and T4 levels have been found to be decreased in rats exposed to phthalates in a dose-dependent manner (67). Histopathological changes in the thyroid gland have been noted in some studies (68). Also, a negative correlation has been found between phthalate exposure and total T4 and fT4 levels in pregnant women (69).

BPA: BPA is a chemical that we are easily exposed to because it is found within the structure of many plastic products including food containers, plastic bottles, feeding bottles, and inner parts of cans. T4 levels have been found to be increased at postnatal 15 days in offspring of pregnant rats exposed to BPA (70). However, there have also been studies showing that BPA does not affect thyroid functions (71). Further studies are needed to evaluate the harmful effects of several groups of chemical disruptors on thyroid functions.

5.1.10 EFFECTS OF OTHER COMPOUNDS AS ENDOCRINE DISRUPTORS

In addition to those mentioned above, effects of other chemical compounds on the endocrine system have also been observed. Children with intrauterine exposure to HCB, a type of chlorine pesticide, were found to have a tendency for obesity when they reach 6 years of age, and they have been shown to have a 2.5-3-fold increased risk of being overweight compared to children not exposed to HCB, independent from diet type and daily activity (72). Testicular dysgenesis syndrome, a clinical entity which comprises testicular cancer, urogenital abnormalities and reduced semen quality, is thought to occur by contact of the fetal testis with endocrine disruptors during intrauterine development (73). Phytoestrogens are abundantly present in our daily food, and a 500 times greater estrogenic effect has been found in infants fed by soy-based formulas as compared to those fed by cow's milk-based formulas (74). Genistein, found in soy beans, is a weak estrogenic substance which may lead to several pathologies in the reproductive system and also in the thyroid gland through thyroid peroxidase inhibition (75). The effects of intrauterine exposure to endocrine disruptors, which can be detected in umbilical cord blood and meconium samples, are summarized in Table 6.

5.2 CONCLUSION

Endocrine disruptors are commonly found substances that we may encounter in every setting and condition in the modern world and it is virtually impossible to avoid the contact with these chemical compounds in our daily life. Epidemiological and toxicological studies that have been performed over the years and have provided scientific data for the protection of human health and wildlife have shown that nature as a whole is under risk due to these chemicals. These studies also provide evidence to inform local authorities about this threat and about preventive measures to be taken on the issue of endocrine disruptors, particularly with regard to pregnant women and children. These local measures should be considered as an initial step in prevention and global awareness studies should be performed in addition to local studies. Further animal and human studies are also needed to investigate the effects of intrauterine endocrine disruptor exposure on adult health.

REFERENCES

1. Wang MH, Baskin LS. Endocrine disruptors, genital development, and hypospadias. J Androl. 2008;29:499–505.
2. Lee MM. Endocrine Disrupters. A Current Review of Pediatric Endocrinology. 2007:109–118.
3. Phillips KP, Foster WG. Key developments in endocrine disrupter research and human health. J Toxicol Environ Health B Crit Rev. 2008;11:322–344.
4. Suk WA, Murray K, Avakian MD. Environmental hazards to children's health in the modern world. Mutat Res. 2003;544:235–242.
5. Abaci A, Demir K, Bober E, Buyukgebiz A. Endocrine disrupters - with special emphasis on sexual development. Pediatr Endocrinol Rev. 2009;6:464–475.
6. Foster WG, Agzarian J. Toward less confusing terminology in endocrine disruptor research. J Toxicol Environ Health B Crit Rev. 2008;11:152–161.
7. Whaley DA, Keyes D, Khorrami B. Incorporation of endocrine disruption into chemical hazard scoring for pollution prevention and current list of endocrine disrupting chemicals. Drug Chem Toxicol. 2001;24:359–420.

8. Crinnion WJ. Maternal levels of xenobiotics that affect fetal development and childhood health. Altern Med Rev. 2009;14:212–222.

9. Bruckner JV. Differences in sensitivity of children and adults to chemical toxicity: the NAS panel report. Regul Toxicol Pharmacol. 2000;31:280–285.

10. Barker DJ. The developmental origins of adult disease. Eur J Epidemiol. 2003;18:733–736.

11. Su PH, Chen JY, Chen JW, Wang SL. Growth and thyroid function in children with in utero exposure to dioxin: a 5-year follow-up study. Pediatr Res. 2010;67:205–210.

12. Leonardi-Bee J, Smyth A, Britton J, Coleman T. Environmental tobacco smoke and fetal health: systematic review and meta-analysis. Arch Dis Child Fetal Neonatal Ed. 2008;93:351–361.

13. Choi H, Jedrychowski W, Spengler J, Camann DE, Whyatt RM, Rauh V, et al. International studies of prenatal exposure to polycyclic aromatic hydrocarbons and fetal growth. Environ Health Perspect. 2006;114:1744–1750.

14. Choi H, Rauh V, Garfinkel R, Tu Y, Perera FP. Prenatal exposure to airborne polycyclic aromatic hydrocarbons and risk of intrauterine growth restriction. Environ Health Perspect. 2008;116:658–665.

15. Perera FP, Rauh V, Tsai WY, Kinney P, Camann D, Barr D, Bernert T, Garfinkel R, Tu YH, Diaz D, Dietrich J, Whyatt RM. Effects of transplacental exposure to environmental pollutants on birth outcomes in a multiethnic population. Environ Health Perspect. 2003;111:201–205.

16. Sherman JD. Chlorpyrifos (Dursban)-associated birth defects: report of four cases. Arch Environ Health. 1996;51:5–8.

17. Dietert RR, Zelikoff JT. Early-life environment, developmental immunotoxicology, and the risk of pediatric allergic disease including asthma. Birth Defects Res B Dev Reprod Toxicol. 2008;83:547–560.

18. Gogal RM, Holladay SD. Perinatal TCDD exposure and the adult onset of autoimmune disease. J Immunotoxicol. 2008;5:413–418.

19. Hertz-Picciotto I, Park HY, Dostal M, Kocan A, Trnovec T, Sram R. Prenatal exposures to persistent and non-persistent organic compounds and effects on immune system development. Basic Clin Pharmacol Toxicol. 2008;102:146–154.

20. Dallaire F, Dewailly E, Vezina C, Muckle G, Weber JP, Bruneau S, Ayotte P. Effect of prenatal exposure to polychlorinated biphenyls on incidence of acute respiratory infections in preschool Inuit children. Environ Health Perspect. 2006;114:1301–1305.

21. Weisglas-Kuperus N, Patandin S, Berbers GA, Sas TC, Mulder PG, Sauer PJ, Hooijkaas H. Immunologic effects of background exposure to polychlorinated biphenyls and dioxins in Dutch preschool children. Environ Health Perspect. 2000;108:1203–1207.

22. Davidson PW, Strain JJ, Myers GJ, Thurston SW, Bonham MP, Shamlaye CF, Stokes-Riner A, Wallace JM, Robson PJ, Duffy EM, Georger LA, Sloane-Reeves J, Cernichiari E, Canfield RL, Cox C, Huang LS, Janciuras J, Clarkson TW. Neurodevelopmental effects of maternal nutritional status and exposure to methylmercury from eating fish during pregnancy. Neurotoxicology. 2008;29:767–775.

23. Jett DA, Kuhlmann AC, Farmer SJ, Guilarte TR. Age-dependent effects of developmental lead exposure on performance in the Morris water maze. Pharmacol Biochem Behav. 1997;57:271–279.

24. Gomaa A, Hu H, Bellinger D, Schwartz J, Tsaih SW, Gonzalez-Cossio T, Schnaas L, Peterson K, Aro A, Hernandez-Avila M. Maternal bone lead as an independent risk factor for fetal neurotoxicity: a prospective study. Pediatrics. 2002;110:110–118.

25. Jacobson SW, Fein GG, Jacobson JL, Schwartz PM, Dowler JK. The effect of intrauterine PCB exposure on visual recognition memory. Child Dev. 1985;56:853–860..

26. Chen YC, Yu ML, Rogan WJ, Gladen BC, Hsu CC. A 6-year follow-up of behavior and activity disorders in the Taiwan Yu-cheng children. Am J Public Health. 1994;84:415–421.

27. Young JG, Eskenazi B, Gladstone EA, Bradman A, Pedersen L, Johnson C, Barr DB, Furlong CE, Holland NT. Association between in utero organophosphate pesticide exposure and abnormal reflexes in neonates. Neurotoxicology. 2005;26:199–209.

28. Jurewicz J, Hanke W. Prenatal and childhood exposure to pesticides and neurobehavioral development: review of epidemiological studies. Int J Occup Med Environ Health. 2008;21:121–132.

29. Norgil D, Main KM, Toppari J, Skakkebaek NE. Impact of exposure to endocrine disrupters in utero and in childhood on adult reproduction. Best Pract Res Clin Endocrinol Metab. 2002;16:289–309.

30. Toppari J, Kaleva M, Virtanen HE. Trends in the incidence of cryptorchidism and hypospadias, and methodological limitations of registry-based data. Hum Reprod Update. 2001;7:282–286.

31. Longnecker MP, Klebanoff MA, Brock JW, Zhou H, Gray KA, Needham LL, Wilcox AJ. Maternal serum level of 1,1-dichloro-2,2-bis(p-chlorophenyl)ethylene and risk of cryptorchidism, hypospadias, and polythelia among male offspring. Am J Epidemiol. 2002;155:313–322.

32. Bhatia R, Shiau R, Petreas M, Weintraub JM, Farhang L, Eskenazi B. Organochlorine pesticides and male genital anomalies in the child health and development studies. Environ Health Perspect. 2005;113:220–224.

33. Pierik FH, Burdorf A, Deddens JA, Juttmann RE, Weber RF. Maternal and paternal risk factors for cryptorchidism and hypospadias: a case-control study in newborn boys. Environ Health Perspect. 2004;112:1570–1576.

34. Kakeyama M, Sone H, Miyabara Y, Tohyama C. Perinatal exposure to 2,3,7,8-tetrachlorodibenzo-p-dioxin alters activity-dependent expression of BDNF mRNA in the neocortex and male rat sexual behavior in adulthood. Neurotoxicology. 2003;24:207–217.

35. Ikeda M, Mitsui T, Setani K, Tamura M, Kakeyama M, Sone H, Tohyama C, Tomita T. In utero and lactational exposure to 2,3,7,8-tetrachlorodibenzo-p-dioxin in rats disrupts brain sexual differentiation. Toxicol Appl Pharmacol. 2005;205:98–105.

36. Cao Y, Winneke G, Wilhelm M, Wittsiepe J, Lemm F, Furst P, Ranft U, Imohl M, Kraft M, Oesch-Bartlomowicz B, Kramer U. Environmental exposure to dioxins and polychlorinated biphenyls reduce levels of gonadal hormones in newborns: results from the Duisburg cohort study. Int J Hyg Environ Health. 2008;211:30–39.

37. Hsu PC, Lai TJ, Guo NW, Lambert GH, Leon Guo Y. Serum hormones in boys prenatally exposed to polychlorinated biphenyls and dibenzofurans. J Toxicol Environ Health A. 2005;68:1447–1456.

38. Gonc N. Endokrin Bozucular. Katkı Pediatri Dergisi. 2008;30:511–518.

39. Diamanti-Kandarakis E, Bourguignon JP, Giudice LC, Hauser R, Prins GS, Soto AM, Zoeller RT, Gore AC. Endocrine-disrupting chemicals: an Endocrine Society scientific statement. Endocr Rev. 2009;30:293–342.

40. Brown NM, Manzolillo PA, Zhang JX, Wang J, Lamartiniere CA. Prenatal TCDD and predisposition to mammary cancer in the rat. Carcinogenesis. 1998;19(9):1623–9.

41. Fenton SE. Endocrine-disrupting compounds and mammary gland development: early exposure and later life consequences. Endocrinology. 2006;147:18–24.

42. Kakeyama M, Sone H, Tohyama C. Perinatal exposure of female rats to 2,3,7,8-tetrachlorodibenzo-p-dioxin induces central precocious puberty in the offspring. J Endocrinol. 2008;197:351–358.

43. vom Saal FS, Akingbemi BT, Belcher SM, Birnbaum LS, Crain DA, Eriksen M, Farabollini F, Guillette LJ Jr, Hauser R, Heindel JJ, Ho SM, Hunt PA, Iguchi T, Jobling S, Kanno J, Keri RA, Knudsen KE, Laufer H, LeBlanc GA, Marcus M, McLachlan JA, Myers JP, Nadal A, Newbold RR, Olea N, Prins GS, Richter CA, Rubin BS, Sonnenschein C, Soto AM, Talsness CE, Vandenbergh JG, Vandenberg LN, Walser-Kuntz DR, Watson CS, Welshons WV, Wetherill Y, Zoeller RT. Chapel Hill bisphenol A expert panel consensus statement: integration of mechanisms, effects in animals and potential to impact human health at current levels of exposure. Reprod Toxicol. 2007;24:131–138.

44. Vandenberg LN, Hauser R, Marcus M, Olea N, Welshons WV. Human exposure to bisphenol A (BPA) Reprod Toxicol. 2007;24:139–177.

45. Calafat AM, Weuve J, Ye X, Jia LT, Hu H, Ringer S, Huttner K, Hauser R. Exposure to bisphenol A and other phenols in neonatal intensive care unit premature infants. Environ Health Perspect. 2009;117:639–644.

46. Calafat AM, Weuve J, Ye X, Jia LT, Hu H, Ringer S, Huttner K, Hauser R. Exposure to bisphenol A and other phenols in neonatal intensive care unit premature infants. Environ Health Perspect. 2009;117:639–644.

47. Stahlhut RW, Welshons WV, Swan SH. Bisphenol A data in NHANES suggest longer than expected half-life, substantial nonfood exposure, or both. Environ Health Perspect. 2009;117:784–789..

48. Vandenberg LN, Maffini MV, Wadia PR, Sonnenschein C, Rubin BS, Soto AM. Exposure to environmentally relevant doses of the xenoestrogen bisphenol-A alters development of the fetal mouse mammary gland. Endocrinology. 2007;148:116–127.

49. Vandenberg LN, Maffini MV, Schaeberle CM, Ucci AA, Sonnenschein C, Rubin BS, Soto AM. Perinatal exposure to the xenoestrogen bisphenol-A induces mammary intraductal hyperplasias in adult CD-1 mice. Reprod Toxicol. 2008;26:210–219.

50. Jenkins S, Raghuraman N, Eltoum I, Carpenter M, Russo J, Lamartiniere CA. Oral exposure to bisphenol a increases dimethylbenzanthracene-induced mammary cancer in rats. Environ Health Perspect. 2009;117:910–915.

51. Yang CY, Yu ML, Guo HR, Lai TJ, Hsu CC, Lambert G, Guo YL. The endocrine and reproductive function of the female Yucheng adolescents prenatally exposed to PCBs/PCDFs. Chemosphere. 2005;61:355–360.

52. Zhang Y, Lin L, Cao Y, Chen B, Zheng L, Ge RS. Phthalate levels and low birth weight: a nested case-control study of Chinese newborns. J Pediatr. 2009;155:500–544.

53. Newbold R. Cellular and molecular effects of developmental exposure to diethyl-stilbestrol: implications for other environmental estrogens. Environ Health Perspect. 1995;103:83–87.

54. Boas M, Main KM, Feldt-Rasmussen U. Environmental chemicals and thyroid function: an update. Curr Opin Endocrinol Diabetes Obes. 2009;16:385–391.

55. Chevrier J, Eskenazi B, Bradman A, Fenster L, Barr DB. Associations between prenatal exposure to polychlorinated biphenyls and neonatal thyroid-stimulating hormone levels in a Mexican-American population, Salinas Valley, California. Environ Health Perspect. 2007;115:1490–1496.

56. Meerts IA, Assink Y, Cenijn PH, Weijers BM, Bergman A, Koeman JH, Brouwer A. Placental transfer of a hydroxylated polychlorinated biphenyl and effects on fetal and maternal thyroid hormone homeostasis in the rat. Toxicol Sci. 2002;68:361–371.

57. Crofton KM, Kodavanti PR, rr-Yellin EC, Casey AC, Kehn LS. PCBs, thyroid hormones, and ototoxicity in rats: cross-fostering experiments demonstrate the impact of postnatal lactation exposure. Toxicol Sci. 2000;57:131–140.

58. Darnerud PO, Morse D, Klasson-Wehler E, Brouwer A. Binding of a 3,3', 4,4'-tetra-chlorobiphenyl (CB-77) metabolite to fetal transthyretin and effects on fetal thyroid hormone levels in mice. Toxicology. 1996;106:105–114.

59. Langer P, Tajtakova M, Kocan A, Petrik J, Koska J, Ksinantova L, Radikova Z, Ukropec J, Imrich R, Huckova M, Chovancova J, Drobna B, Jursa S, Vlcek M, Bergman A, Athanasiadou M, Hovander L, Shishiba Y, Trnovec T, Sebokova E, Klimes I. Thyroid ultrasound volume, structure and function after long-term high exposure of large population to polychlorinated biphenyls, pesticides and dioxin. Chemosphere. 2007;69:118–127.

60. Schell LM, Gallo MV, Ravenscroft J, DeCaprio AP. Persistent organic pollutants and anti-thyroid peroxidase levels in Akwesasne Mohawk young adults. Environ Res. 2009;109:86–92.

61. Koopman-Esseboom C, Morse DC, Weisglas-Kuperus N, Lutkeschipholt IJ, Tuinstra LG, Brouwer A, Sauer PJ. Effects of dioxins and polychlorinated biphenyls on thyroid hormone status of pregnant women and their infants. Pediatr Res. 1994;36:468–473.

62. Zhou T, Taylor MM, DeVito MJ, Crofton KM. Developmental exposure to brominated diphenyl ethers results in thyroid hormone disruption. Toxicol Sci. 2002;66:105–116.

63. Kuriyama SN, Wanner A, Fidalgo-Neto AA, Talsness CE, Koerner W, Chahoud I. Developmental exposure to low-dose PBDE-99: tissue distribution and thyroid hormone levels. Toxicology. 2007;242:80–90.

64. Thibodeaux JR, Hanson RG, Rogers JM, Grey BE, Barbee BD, Richards JH, Butenhoff JL, Stevenson LA, Lau C. Exposure to perfluorooctane sulfonate during pregnancy in rat and mouse. I: maternal and prenatal evaluations. Toxicol Sci. 2003;74:369–781.

65. Lau C, Thibodeaux JR, Hanson RG, Rogers JM, Grey BE, Stanton ME, Butenhoff JL, Stevenson LA. Exposure to perfluorooctane sulfonate during pregnancy in rat and mouse. II: postnatal evaluation. Toxicol Sci. 2003;74:382–392.

66. Chang SC, Thibodeaux JR, Eastvold ML, Ehresman DJ, Bjork JA, Froehlich JW, Lau C, Singh RJ, Wallace KB, Butenhoff JL. Thyroid hormone status and pituitary

function in adult rats given oral doses of perfluorooctanesulfonate (PFOS) Toxicology. 2008;243:330–339.

67. O'Connor JC, Frame SR, Ladics GS. Evaluation of a 15-day screening assay using intact male rats for identifying antiandrogens. Toxicol Sci. 2002;69:92–108.

68. Howarth JA, Price SC, Dobrota M, Kentish PA, Hinton RH. Effects on male rats of di-(2-ethylhexyl) phthalate and di-n-hexylphthalate administered alone or in combination. Toxicol Lett. 2001;12:35–43.

69. Huang PC, Kuo PL, Guo YL, Liao PC, Lee CC. Associations between urinary phthalate monoesters and thyroid hormones in pregnant women. Hum Reprod. 2007;22:2715–2722.

70. Zoeller RT, Bansal R, Parris C. Bisphenol-A, an environmental contaminant that acts as a thyroid hormone receptor antagonist in vitro, increases serum thyroxine, and alters RC3/neurogranin expression in the developing rat brain. Endocrinology. 2005;146:607–612.

71. Xu X, Liu Y, Sadamatsu M, Tsutsumi S, Akaike M, Ushijima H, Kato N. Perinatal bisphenol A affects the behavior and SRC-1 expression of male pups but does not influence on the thyroid hormone receptors and its responsive gene. Neurosci Res. 2007;58:149–155.

72. Smink A, Ribas-Fito N, Garcia R, Torrent M, Mendez MA, Grimalt JO, et al. Exposure to hexachlorobenzene during pregnancy increases the risk of overweight in children aged 6 years. Acta Paediatr. 2008;97:1465–1469.

73. Bay K, Asklund C, Skakkebaek NE, Andersson AM. Testicular dysgenesis syndrome: possible role of endocrine disrupters. Best Pract Res Clin Endocrinol Metab. 2006;20:77–90.

74. Cao Y, Calafat AM, Doerge DR, Umbach DM, Bernbaum JC, Twaddle NC, Ye X, Rogan WJ. Isoflavones in urine, saliva, and blood of infants: data from a pilot study on the estrogenic activity of soy formula. J Expo Sci Environ Epidemiol. 2009;19:223–234.

75. Divi RL, Chang HC, Doerge DR. Anti-thyroid isoflavones from soybean: isolation, characterization, and mechanisms of action. Biochem Pharmacol. 1997;54:1087–1096.

PART II

AUTISM

CHAPTER 6

A RESEARCH STRATEGY TO DISCOVER THE ENVIRONMENTAL CAUSES OF AUTISM AND NEURODEVELOPMENTAL DISABILITIES

PHILIP J. LANDRIGAN, LUCA LAMBERTINI, AND LINDA S. BIRNBAUM

Autism, attention deficit/hyperactivity disorder (ADHD), mental retardation, dyslexia, and other biologically based disorders of brain development affect between 400,000 and 600,000 of the 4 million children born in the United States each year. The Centers for Disease Control and Prevention (CDC) has reported that autism spectrum disorder (ASD) now affects 1.13% (1 of 88) of American children (CDC 2012) and ADHD affects 14% (CDC 2005; Pastor and Reuben 2008). Treatment of these disorders is difficult; the disabilities they cause can last lifelong, and they are devastating to families. In addition, these disorders place enormous economic burdens on society (Trasande and Liu 2011).

Although discovery research to identify the potentially preventable causes of neuro-developmental disorders (NDDs) has increased in recent

Reproduced with permission from Environmental Health Perspectives. Landrigan PJ, Lambertini L, and Birnbaum LS. A Research Strategy to Discover the Environmental Causes of Autism and Neurodevelopmental Disabilities. Environmental Health Perspectives *120,7 (2012); doi:10.1289/ehp.1104285.*

years, more research is urgently needed. This research encompasses both genetic and environmental studies.

Genetic research has received particular investment and attention (Autism Genome Project Consortium et al. 2007; Buxbaum and Hof 2011; Fernandez et al. 2012; O'Roak et al. 2011; Sakurai et al. 2011) and has demonstrated that ASD and certain other NDDs have a strong hereditary component (Buxbaum and Hof 2011; Sakurai et al. 2011). Linkage studies have identified candidate autism susceptibility genes at multiple loci, most consistently on chromosomes 7q, 15q, and 16p (Autism Genome Project Consortium et al. 2007; Sakurai et al. 2011). Exome sequencing in sporadic cases of autism has detected new mutations (O'Roak et al. 2011), and copy number variant studies have identified several hundred copy number variants putatively linked to autism (Fernandez et al. 2012). The candidate genes most strongly implicated in NDD causation encode for proteins involved in synaptic architecture, neuro-transmitter synthesis (e.g., ©-amino-butyric acid serotonin), oxytocin receptors, and cation trafficking (Sakurai et al. 2011). No single anomaly predominates. Instead, autism appears to be a family of diseases with common pheno-types linked to a series of genetic anomalies, each of which is responsible for no more than 2–3% of cases. The total fraction of ASD attributable to genetic inheri-tance may be about 30–40%.

Exploration of the environmental causes of autism and other NDDs has been catalyzed by growing recognition of the exquisite sensitivity of the developing human brain to toxic chemicals (Grandjean and Landrigan 2006). This susceptibility is greatest during unique "windows of vulner-ability" that open only in embryonic and fetal life and have no later coun-ter-part (Miodovnik 2011). "Proof of the principle" that early exposures can cause autism comes from studies linking ASD to medications taken in the first trimester of pregnancy—thalidomide, misoprostol, and valproic acid—and to first-trimester rubella infection (Arndt et al. 2005; Daniels 2006).

This "proof-of-principle" evidence for environmental causation is sup-ported further by findings from prospective birth cohort epidemiological studies, many of them supported by the National Institute of Environmen-tal Health Sciences (NIEHS). These studies enroll women during pregnan-cy, measure prenatal exposures in real time as they occur, and then follow children longitudinally with periodic direct examinations to assess growth, development, and the presence of disease. Prospective studies are powerful engines for the discovery of etiologic associations between prenatal exposures and NDDs. They have linked autistic behaviors with prenatal exposures to the organophosphate insecticide chlorpyrifos (Eskenazi et al. 2007) and also with prenatal exposures to phthalates (Miodovnik et al. 2011). Additional prospective studies have linked loss of cognition (IQ), dyslexia, and ADHD to lead (Jusko et al. 2008), methyl-mercury (Oken et al. 2008), organophosphate insecticides (London et al. 2012), organochlorine insecticides (Eskenazi et al. 2008), polychlorinated biphenyls (Winneke 2011), arsenic (Wasserman et al. 2007), manganese (Khan et al. 2011), polycyclic aromatic hydrocarbons (Perera et al. 2009), bisphenol A (Braun et al. 2011), brominated flame retardants (Herbstman et al. 2010), and perfluorinated compounds (Stein and Savitz 2011).

Toxic chemicals likely cause injury to the developing human brain either through direct toxicity or inter-actions with the genome. An expert committee convened by the U.S. National Academy of Sciences (NAS) estimated that 3% of neuro-behavioral disorders are caused directly by toxic environ-mental exposures and that another 25% are caused by inter-actions between environmental factors, defined broadly, and inherited susceptibilities (National Research Council 2000). Epigenetic modification of gene expression by toxic chemicals that results in DNA methyla-tion, histone modification, or changes in activity levels of non-protein-coding RNA (ncRNAs) may be a mechanism of such gene–environment interaction (Grafodatskaya et al. 2010). Epigenetic "marks" have been shown to be able to influence gene expression and alter high-order DNA structure (Anway and Skinner 2006; Waterland and Jirtle 2004).

A major unanswered question is whether there are still undiscovered environ-mental causes of autism or other NDDs among the thousands of chemicals currently in wide use in the United States. In the past 50 years, > 80,000 new synthetic chemicals have been developed (Landrigan and Goldman 2011). The U.S. Environmental Protection Agency has identified 3,000 "high production volume" (HPV) chemicals that are in widest use and thus pose greatest potential for human exposure (Goldman 1998). These HPV chemicals are used today in millions of consumer products. Children and pregnant women are exposed extensively to them, and CDC surveys detect quantifiable levels of nearly 200 HPV chemicals in the bodies of virtually all Americans, including pregnant women (Woodruff et al. 2011).

The significance of early chemical exposures for children's health is not yet fully understood. A great concern is that a large number of the chemicals in widest use have not undergone even minimal assessment of potential toxicity, and only about 20% have been screened for potential toxicity during early development (Landrigan and Goldman 2011). Unless studies specifically examine developmental consequences of early exposures to untested chemicals, sub-clinical dysfunction caused by these exposures can go unrecognized for years. One example is the "silent epidemic" of childhood lead poisoning: From the 1940s to the 1980s, millions of American children were exposed to excessive levels of lead from paint and gasoline, resulting in reduced average intelligence by 2–5 IQ points (Grosse et al. 2002). The late David Rall, former director of NIEHS, once observed that "If thalidomide had caused a 10-point loss of IQ instead of birth defects of the limbs, it would likely still be on the market" (Weiss 1982).

To begin formulation of a systematic strategy for discovery of potentially preventable environmental causes of autism and other NDDs, the Mount Sinai Children's Environmental Health Center, with the support of the NIEHS and Autism Speaks, convened a workshop on "Exploring the Environmental Causes of Autism and Learning Disabilities." This workshop produced a series of papers by leading researchers, some of which are published in this issue of Environmental Health Perspectives. It also generated a list of 10 chemi-cals and mixtures widely distributed in the environment that are already suspected of causing developmental neurotoxicity:

- Lead (Jusko et al. 2008)
- Methylmercury (Oken et al. 2008)
- Polychlorinated biphenyls (Winneke 2011)
- Organophosphate pesticides (Eskenazi et al. 2007; London et al. 2012)
- Organochlorine pesticides (Eskenazi et al. 2008)
- Endocrine disruptors (Braun et al. 2011; Miodovnik et al. 2011)
- Automotive exhaust (Volk et al. 2011)
- Polycyclic aromatic hydrocarbons (Perera et al. 2009)
- Brominated flame retardants (Herbstman et al. 2010)
- Perfluorinated compounds (Stein and Savitz 2011).

This list is not exhaustive and will almost certainly expand in the years ahead as new science emerges. It is intended to focus research in environmental causation of NDDs on a short list of chemicals where concentrated study has high potential to generate actionable findings in the near future. Its ultimate purpose is to catalyze new evidence-based programs for prevention of disease in America's children.

REFERENCES

1. Anway MD, Skinner MK. Epigenetic transgenerational actions of endocrine disruptors. Endocrinology. 2006;147(6) suppl:S43–S49.
2. Arndt TL, Stodgell CJ, Rodier PM. The teratology of autism. Int J Dev Neurosci. 2005;23:189–199.
3. Autism Genome Project Consortium , Szatmari P, Paterson AD, Zwaigenbaum L, Roberts W, Brian J, et al2007. Mapping autism risk loci using genetic linkage and chromosomal rearrangements. Nat Genet 39319–328.328
4. Braun JM, Kalkbrenner AE, Calafat AM, Yolton K, Ye X, Dietrich KN, et al. Impact of early-life bisphenol A exposure on behavior and executive function in children. Pediatrics. 2011;128(5):873–882.
5. Buxbaum JD, Hof PR. The emerging neuroscience of autism spectrum disorders. Brain Res. 2011;1380:1–2.
6. CDC (Centers for Disease Control and Prevention)2005. Mental health in the United States. Prevalence of diagnosis and medication treatment for attention-deficit/hyperactivity disorder–United States, 2003. MMWR Morb Mortal Wkly Rep 54842–847.847
7. CDC (Centers for Disease Control and Prevention)2012. Prevalence of autism spectrum disorders—autism and developmental disabilities monitoring network, 14 sites, United States, 2008. MMWR Surveill Summ 6131–19.19
8. Daniels JL. Autism and the environment. Environ Health Perspect. 2006;114:A396.
9. Eskenazi B, Marks AR, Bradman A, Harley K, Barr DB, Johnson C, et al. Organophosphate pesticide exposure and neurodevelopment in young Mexican-American children. Environ Health Perspect. 2007;115:792–798.
10. Eskenazi B, Rosas LG, Marks AR, Bradman A, Harley K, Holland N, et al. Pesticide toxicity and the developing brain. Basic Clin Pharmacol Toxicol. 2008;102(2):228–236.
11. Fernandez TV, Sanders SJ, Yurkiewicz IR, Ercan-Sencicek AG, Kim YS, Fishman DO, et al. Rare copy number variants in tourette syndrome disrupt genes in histaminergic pathways and overlap with autism. Biol Psychiatry. 2012;71(5):392–402.
12. Goldman LR. Chemicals and children's environment: what we don't know about risks. Environ Health Perspect. 1998;106(suppl 3):875–880.
13. Grafodatskaya D, Chung B, Szatmari P, Weksberg R. Autism spectrum disorders and epigenetics. J Am Acad Child Adolesc Psychiatry. 2010;49(8):794–809.

14. Grandjean P, Landrigan PJ. Developmental neurotoxicity of industrial chemicals: a silent pandemic. Lancet. 2006;368(9553):2167–2178.

15. Grosse SD, Matte TD, Schwartz J, Jackson RJ. Economic gains resulting from the reduction in children's exposure to lead in the United States. Environ Health Perspect. 2002;110:563–569.

16. Herbstman JB, Sjödin A, Kurzon M, Lederman SA, Jones RS, Rauh V, et al. Prenatal exposure to PBDEs and neurodevelopment. Environ Health Perspect. 2010;118:712–719.

17. Jusko TA, Henderson CR, Jr, Lanphear BP, Cory-Slechta DA, Parsons PJ, Canfield RL. Blood lead concentrations < 10 µg/dL and child intelligence at 6 years of age. Environ Health Perspect. 2008;116:243–248.

18. Khan K, Factor-Litvak P, Wasserman GA, Liu X, Ahmed E, Parvez F, et al. Manganese exposure from drinking water and children's classroom behavior in Bangladesh. Environ Health Perspect. 2011;119:1501–1506.

19. Landrigan PJ, Goldman LR. Children's vulnerability to toxic chemicals: a challenge and opportunity to strengthen health and environmental policy. Health Aff. 2011;30(5):842–850.

20. London L, Beseler C, Bouchard MF, Bellinger DC, Colosio C, Grandjean P, et al. Neurobehavioral and neurodevelopmental effects of pesticide exposures. Neurotoxicology. 2012. http://dx.doi.org/10.1016/j.neuro.2012.01.004 [Online 17 January 2012].

21. Miodovnik A. Environmental neurotoxicants and developing brain. Mt Sinai J Med. 2011;78(1):58–77.

22. Miodovnik A, Engel SM, Zhu C, Ye X, Soorya LV, Silva MJ, et al. Endocrine disruptors and childhood social impairment. Neurotoxicology. 2011;32(2):261–267.

23. National Research Council. Washington, DC:National Academy Press: 2000. Scientific Frontiers in Developmental Toxicology and Risk Assessment.

24. Oken E, Radesky JS, Wright RO, Bellinger DC, Amarasiriwardena CJ, Kleinman KP, et al. Maternal fish intake during pregnancy, blood mercury levels, and child cognition at age 3 years in a US cohort. Am J Epidemiol. 2008;167(10):1171–1181.

25. O'Roak BJ, Deriziotis P, Lee C, Vives L, Schwartz JJ, Girirajan S, et al. Exome sequencing in sporadic autism spectrum disorders identifies severe de novo mutations. Nat Genet. 2011;43:585–589.

26. Pastor PN, Reuben CA. Diagnosed attention deficit hyperactivity disorder and learning disability: United States, 2004–2006. Vital Health Stat 10. 2008;(237):1–14.

27. Perera FP, Li Z, Whyatt R, Hoepner L, Wang S, Camann D, et al. 2009. Prenatal airborne polycyclic aromatic hydrocarbon exposure and child IQ at age 5 years. Pediatrics 1242e195–e202.e202; doi:[Online 20 July 2009]10.1542/peds.2008-3506

28. Sakurai T, Cai G, Grice DE, Buxbaum JD. In: Textbook of Autism Spectrum Disorders (Hollander E, Kolevzon A, Coyle JT. eds) Washington, DC:American Psychiatric Publishing: 2011. Genomic architecture of autism spectrum disorders. pp. 281–298.

29. Stein CR, Savitz DA. Serum perfluorinated compound concentration and attention deficit/hyperactivity disorder in children 5–18 years of age. Environ Health Perspect. 2011;119:1466–1471.

30. Trasande L, Liu Y. Reducing the staggering costs of environmental disease in children, estimated at $76.6 billion in 2008. Health Aff. 2011;30(5):863–870.

31. Volk HE, Hertz-Picciotto I, Delwiche L, Lurmann F, McConnell R. Residential proximity to freeways and autism in the CHARGE Study. Environ Health Perspect. 2011;119:873–877.

32. Wasserman GA, Liu X, Parvez F, Ahsan H, Factor-Litvak P, Kline J, et al. Water arsenic exposure and intellectual function in 6-year-old children in Araihazar, Bangladesh. Environ Health Perspect. 2007;115:285–289.

33. Waterland RA, Jirtle RL. Early nutrition, epigenetic changes at transposons and imprinted genes, and enhanced susceptibility to adult chronic diseases. Nutrition. 2004;20:63–68.

34. Weiss B. Food additives and environmental chemicals as sources of childhood behavior disorders. J Am Acad Child Psychiatry. 1982;21:144–152.

35. Winneke G. Developmental aspects of environmental neurotoxicology: lessons from lead and polychlorinated biphenyls. J Neurol Sci. 2011;308(1-2):9–15.

36. Woodruff TJ, Zota AR, Schwartz JM. Environmental chemicals in pregnant women in the United States: NHANES 2003–2004. Environ Health Perspect. 2011;119:878–885.

CHAPTER 7

A KEY ROLE FOR AN IMPAIRED DETOXIFICATION MECHANISM IN THE ETIOLOGY AND SEVERITY OF AUTISM SPECTRUM DISORDERS

ALTAF ALABDALI, LAILA AL-AYADHI, AND AFAF EL-ANSARY

7.1 INTRODUCTION

Autism is characterized by a set of repetitious behavior in combination with social, cognitive and communication deficits [1]. An emerging hypothesis states that autism may result from a combination of genetic susceptibility and exposure to environmental toxins at critical periods during brain development [2]. Neurotoxins and associated inflammation of the brain tissue are often the focus of therapies for patients with autism. However, if body detoxification is impaired, neuroinflammation will not efficiently improve unless the overall body issues are addressed. Xenobiotics are neurotoxins of external origin, such as chemicals and pollutants in the air, water, food additives and drugs, that can dramatically alter the health of the child. An efficient three-phase mechanism is involved in detoxifying these toxins [3]; however, several factors play a role in modulating

A Key Role for an Impaired Detoxification Mechanism in the Etiology and Severity of Autism Spectrum Disorders. © Alabdali A, Al-Ayadhi L, and El-Ansary A. Behavioral and Brain Functions 10,14 (2014); doi:10.1186/1744-9081-10-14. Licensed under Creative Commons Attribution 2.0 Generic License, http://creativecommons.org/licenses/by/2.0/.

this mechanism. For example, age, gender and diet are among the various biological and non-biological factors that modulate individual susceptibility. Additionally, genetic variability plays a critical role in individual susceptibility because variable detoxifier phenotypes result from mutations in the same gene. These range from individuals with regular enzyme and detoxification functions to poor metabolizers with low or no enzyme activity [4,5].

Glutathione-S-transferase (GST) functions in the detoxification of xenobiotics, drugs, toxins, and metabolites and is also involved in the regulation of mitogen-activated protein kinases, which are important during differentiation and development. Hg and Pb, however, are two well-known toxicants that have toxic effects on the body, with the brain being the most susceptible target organ. Exposure to Hg and Pb during pregnancy and early childhood can cause neurodevelopmental impairment and subclinical brain dysfunction because both heavy metals can cross the placenta and the blood–brain-barrier [6]. In the brain, these metals can affect critical developmental processes, including cell proliferation, migration, differentiation, synaptogenesis, myelination, and apoptosis [6].

It is well documented that patients with ASD have many statistically significant differences in their nutritional and metabolic status compared with those who do not have ASD. Some of these biomarkers are indicative of vitamin E insufficiency, increased oxidative stress, and poor detoxification and are associated with the severity of the disorder [7-10]. A recent study found that impaired xenobiotic detoxification is correlated with increased gut permeability (leaky gut) and neuroinflammation, two accepted pathological phenomena in ASD [3].

These findings prompted us to search for biochemical correlations related to the detoxification mechanism and neurobiological processes and the severity and social functioning of patients with ASD measured by the CARS and SRS. We selected Hg and Pb as two environmental toxicants involved in the etiology of ASD, together with GST and vitamin E as enzymatic and non-enzymatic antioxidants with high activity in terminating lipid peroxidation and environmental toxicity. We hypothesized that confirming the relationship between impaired detoxification mechanism and severity of ASD could enhance efforts at early prevention, diagnosis, and intervention and, thus, may play a role in decreasing the prevalence of autism.

7.2 MATERIAL AND METHODS

7.2.1 SUBJECTS

This cross-sectional study was conducted on 52 autistic male children who were recruited from the Autism Research and Treatment Center, Faculty of Medicine, King Saud University, Riyadh, Saudi Arabia. Of these children, 40 were nonverbal, and 12 were verbal. Their ages ranged between 3 and 12 years (mean SD $= 7.0 \pm 2.34$ years). The control group was comprised of 30 age- and sex-matched apparently healthy children with a mean age of 7.2 ± 2.14 years. The patients fulfilled the diagnostic criteria of autism described in the 4th edition of the Diagnostic and Statistical Manual of Mental Disorders. The controls were normally developing, healthy children who were unrelated to the autistic subjects and did not have any of the exclusion criteria. The control children were the healthy older siblings of healthy infants who were attending the Well Baby Clinic at King Khalid University Hospital for routine check-ups of their growth parameters. They had no clinical indications of infectious diseases or neuropsychiatric disorders. All participants had normal results for urine analysis and sedimentation rate. The local Ethical Committee of the Faculty of Medicine, King Saud University, Riyadh, Saudi Arabia, approved this study. In addition, an informed written consent of participation for this study was signed by the parents or the legal guardians of the investigated subjects, according to the Helsinki principles. The selected sample of participants was based on how convenient and readily available the group of participants was (i.e., convenience sampling). Participants were excluded from the study if they had a diagnosis of fragile X syndrome, epileptic seizures, obsessive–compulsive disorder, affective disorders, or any additional psychiatric or neurological diagnoses.

TABLE 1: Mercury (µg/L), lead (µg/dl), GST (µmol/l) and vitamin E (nmol/L) levels in the control & autistic groups

Parameters	Group	N	Mean ± S.D.	P value[a]	P value[b]
Mercury (µg/L)	Control	32	5.12 ± 0.83		
	Patients with autism	58	6.99 ± 0.94		0.001
	Autism (mild to moderate in CARS)	29	6.49 ± 0.65	0.042	0.001
	Autism (severe in CARS)	28	7.31 ± 0.49	0.001	
	Autism (mild to moderate in SRS)	22	7.02 ± 0.85	0.050	0.001
	Autism (severe in SRS)	22	7.46 ± 0.59	0.001	
Lead (µg/dl)	Control	32	4.73 ± 0.67		
	Patients with autism	58	6.79 ± 0.97		0.001
	Autism (mild to moderate in CARS)	29	6.34 ± 0.82	0.041	0.001
	Autism (severe in CARS)	28	6.80 ± 0.83		0.001
	Autism (mild to moderate in SRS)	22	6.42 ± 0.84	0.040	0.001
	Autism (severe in SRS)	22	6.95 ± 0.81		0.001
GST (µmol/min/ml)	Control	30	0.61 ± 0.17		
	Patients with autism	30	0.30 ± 0.08		0.001
	Autism (mild to moderate in CARS)	18	0.31 ± 0.07	0.043	0.001
	Autism (severe in CARS)	12	0.26 ± 0.07	0.001	
	Autism (mild to moderate in SRS)	8	0.32 ± 0.07	0.027	0.001
	Autism (severe in SRS)	18	0.25 ± 0.06	0.001	
Vitamin E (nmol/L)	Control	27	25.44 ± 2.62		
	Patients with autism	28	14.45 ± 2.28		0.001
	Autism (mild to moderate in CARS)	11	14.56 ± 1.58	0.048	0.001
	Autism (severe in CARS)	17	13.36 ± 1.47	0.001	
	Autism (mild to moderate in SRS)	11	14.85 ± 1.36	0.044	0.001
	Autism (severe in SRS)	12	13.35 ± 1.14	0.001	

[a]*P value between mild to moderate and severe in CARS and SRS.* [b]*P value between control and autistic groups.*

7.2.1.1 MEASUREMENT OF AUTISM SEVERITY SCALES (CARS AND SRS)

The Childhood Autism Rating Scale (CARS) score, which is a measurement of the severity of the disease, rates the child on a scale from one to four in each of fifteen areas (relating to people's emotional response; imitation; body use; object use; listening response; fear or nervousness; verbal communication; non-verbal communication; activity level; level and reliability of intellectual response; adaptation to change; visual response; taste, smell and touch response and general impressions). According to the scale, children who scored 30–36 had mild to moderate autism (n=23), while those with scores ranging between 37 and 60 points had severe autism (n=27) [11,12].

To calculate a score for the Social Responsiveness Scale, a questionnaire was completed in 15 to 20 minutes. A total score of 76 or higher was considered severe and strongly associated with a clinical diagnosis of autistic disorder. A score of 60–75 was interpreted as falling in the mild to moderate range of social impairment [13].

7.2.2 SAMPLE COLLECTION

After an overnight fast, 10-ml blood samples, from both groups of children, were collected in test tubes containing sodium heparin as an anticoagulant. The tubes were centrifuged at 3500 rpm for 15 minutes at room temperature. Plasma and red blood cells were separated and stored at - 80°C until required for analysis.

7.2.3 BIOCHEMICAL ANALYSIS

Plasma is a complex bodily fluid containing proteins, peptides, lipids and metabolites and can reflect physiological activity and pathology in various body organs, including the CNS. In humans, approximately 500 ml of CSF is absorbed into the blood daily, making blood a suitable source of biomarkers of neurodegenerative or neurodevelopmental diseases [14]. All biochemical assays were performed in duplicate and blinded to the clinical status of the participants.

7.2.3.1 MEASUREMENT OF MERCURY

The concentration of inorganic mercury (Hg) in red blood cells was determined by the method described by Magos [15] using a flameless atomic-absorption method. The red blood cells were diluted with saline to 20 ml, followed by the addition of 1 ml of a 1% cysteine solution, 10 ml of 8 M H_2SO_4 and 1 ml of $SnCl_2$ (100 mg/ml). The sample was subjected to immediate aeration at a constant rate of 2.5 l/min through the reaction vessel, and 20 ml of a 45% NaOH was added. The $SnCl_2$ reagent was used to release all of the inorganic mercury from the samples. Aeration was discontinued after the recorder pen had settled back to within a few chart divisions (2 or 3) of its original baseline, which was approximately 1 to 1.5 min, depending on the actual aeration rate. The concentration of mercury was measured using a flameless atomic-absorption method, and the concentration was calculated using a standard calibration curve prepared using a standard Hg concentration.

7.2.3.2 MEASUREMENT OF PB

Lead levels were measured in red blood cells using adaptations of the methods described by Miller et al. [16] and Parsons and Slavin [17]. Briefly, RBCs (0.1 ml) were resuspended and digested in 3.9 ml of 0.5 N nitric acid. Lead quantification was based on the measurement of light absorbed at 283.3 nm by the ground-state atoms of Pb from a hollow cathode lamp (HCl) source.

7.2.3.3 DETERMINATION OF GLUTATHIONE-S-TRANSFERASE ACTIVITY (GST)

GST activity was assessed in the plasma using an assay kit (Biovision, USA). The kit is based on a GST-catalyzed reaction between GSH and the GST substrate, CDNB (1-chloro-2, 4-dinitrobenzene). The GST-catalyzed formation of GS-DNB produces a dinitrophenyl thioether, which can be detected by a spectrophotometer at 340 nm. GST activity was expressed as μmole/min/ml plasma.

7.2.3.4 VITAMIN E ASSAY (α -TOCOPHEROL)

Plasma vitamin E was assessed using high pressure liquid chromatography (HPLC) as described by Driskell et al. [18]. The separation via HPLC follows an isocratic method at 30°C using a "reversed phase" column; one run lasts 15 minutes. The detection was performed with a UV detector at 290 nm. The quantification was performed with the delivered standard solution; the concentration was calculated via the integration of the peak areas in the internal standard calibration mode.

7.2.4 STATISTICAL ANALYSIS

The Statistical Package for the Social Sciences (SPSS) computer program was used. The results were expressed as the mean±SD, and all statistical comparisons were made by means of independent t-tests, with $P \leq 0.05$ considered as significant. ROC analysis was performed. Areas under the curve and cut off values were selected by the program. The degree of specificity and sensitivity were calculated. Moreover, the predictiveness diagrams of the four measured parameters were drawn using a Biostat 16 computer program in which the x axis represents percentile rank of the biomarker, the y axis represents the probability of identifying the disease and the horizontal line is the prevalence of the disease. Enter and stepwise multiple regression analyses were performed using CARS and SRS as two dependent variables and Hg, Pb, GST and vitamin E as independent variables.

TABLE 2: ROC-curve of mercury (µg/L), lead (µg/dl), GST (µmol/l) and vitamin E (nmol/L) levels in the autistic groups

Parameters		Autistic patients	CARS		SRS	
			Mild to moderate	Severe	Mild to moderate	Severe
Mercury	Area under the curve	0.926	0.961	1.000	0.935	0.997
	Best cutoff value	6.018	6.018	6.316	6.105	6.346
	Sensitivity %	84.5%	93.1%	100.0%	86.4%	95.5%
	Specificity %	93.8%	93.8%	100.0%	96.9%	100.0%
Lead	Area under the curve	0.953	0.917	0.980	0.923	0.980
	Best cutoff value	5.586	5.590	6.132	6.132	6.321
	Sensitivity %	89.7%	79.3%	89.3%	72.7%	86.4%
	Specificity %	87.5%	87.5%	96.9%	96.9%	100.0%
GST	Area under the curve	0.980	0.974	1.000	0.983	1.000
	Best cutoff value	0.443	0.443	0.320	0.443	0.320
	Sensitivity %	100.0%	100.0%	100.0%	100.0%	100.0%
	Specificity %	93.3%	93.3%	100.0%	93.3%	100.0%
Vitamin E	Area under the curve	0.999	1.000	1.000	1.000	1.000
	Best cutoff value	19.254	18.718	18.089	18.718	17.953
	Sensitivity %	96.4%	100.0%	100.0%	100.0%	100.0%
	Specificity %	100.0%	100.0%	100.0%	100.0%	100.0%

7.3 RESULTS

Table 1 and Figure 1 present the mean±SD of Hg, Pb and plasma GST and vitamin E levels in RBCs of the control, severe autistic and mild-moderate autistic patients with different CARS and SRS scores. Mercury and Pb were significantly elevated in the autistic patients compared with the controls, with increases of 36.58% and 43.34%, respectively. GST and vitamin E levels decreased by 50.71% and 43.18% percent, respectively (Figure 2).

Table 2 and Figure 3 show the ROC analysis of the four measured parameters. The area under the curve (AUC), specificity and sensitivity are illustrated. Figure 4 shows the predictiveness curves of the four measured parameters exhibiting high and low risk in relation to the prevalence of autism in Saudi Arabia. Table 3 shows positive and negative correlations between the four measured parameters in this study. The results showed that while Pb and Hg were positively correlated with each other, both metals were negatively correlated with GST and vitamin E as enzymatic and non-enzymatic detoxifiers.

TABLE 2: ROC-curve of mercury (μg/L), lead (μg/dl), GST (μmol/l) and vitamin E (nmol/L) levels in the autistic groups

Parameters	R (Person correlation)	Sig.	
GST~Mercury	-0.613	0.001**	N[b]
GST~Lead	-0.588	0.001**	N[b]
GST~Vitamin E	0.696	0.001**	P[a]
Mercury~Lead	0.761	0.001**	P[a]
Mercury~Vitamin E	-0.710	0.001**	N[b]
Lead~Vitamin E	-0.715	0.001**	N[b]

[a]*Positive correlation.* [b]*Negative correlation.* **Correlation is significant at the 0.01 level (2-tailed).*

TABLE 3: Statistically significant Pearson's correlation between the four measured parameters

Parameters	R (Person correlation)	Sig.	
GST~Mercury	-0.613	0.001**	N[b]
GST~Lead	-0.588	0.001**	N[b]
GST~Vitamin E	0.696	0.001**	P[a]
Mercury~Lead	0.761	0.001**	P[a]
Mercury~Vitamin E	-0.710	0.001**	N[b]
Lead~Vitamin E	-0.715	0.001**	N[b]

[a]*Positive correlation.* [b]*Negative correlation.* **Correlation is significant at the 0.01 level (2-tailed).*

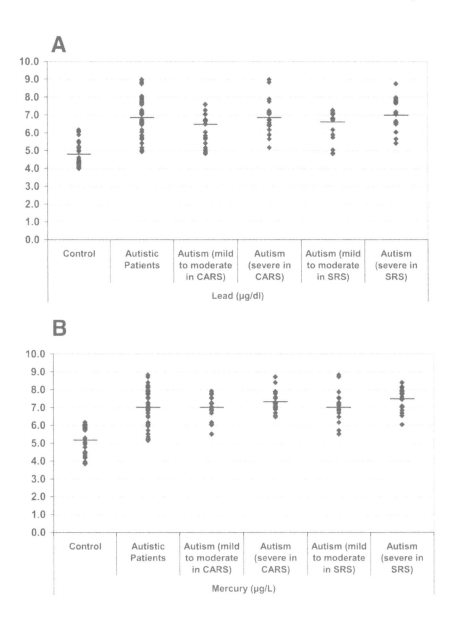

FIGURE 1: Mean levels of A) mercury (µg/L), B) lead (µg/L), C) GST (µmol/min/ml) and D) vitamin E (nmol/L) of the autistic groups compared with age- and sex-matched controls. The mean value for each group is designated by a line.

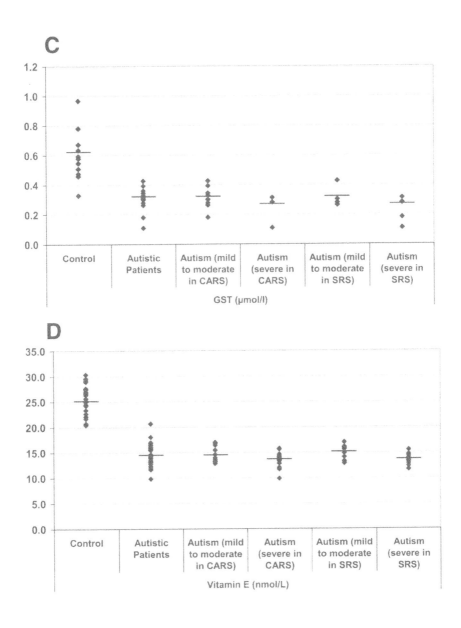

FIGURE 1: *Cont.*

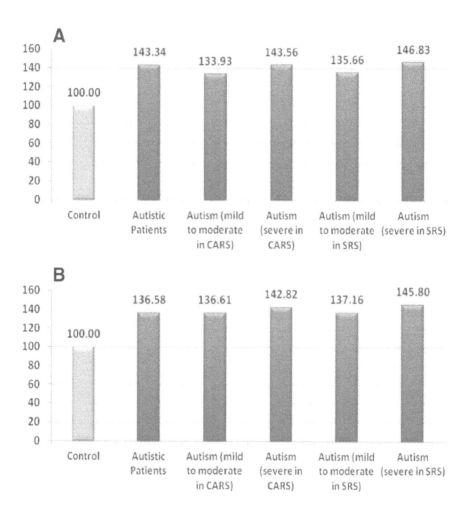

FIGURE 2: Percentage change of A) mercury, B) lead, C) GST and D) vitamin E in the autistic group relative to the control group, which is represented as 100%.

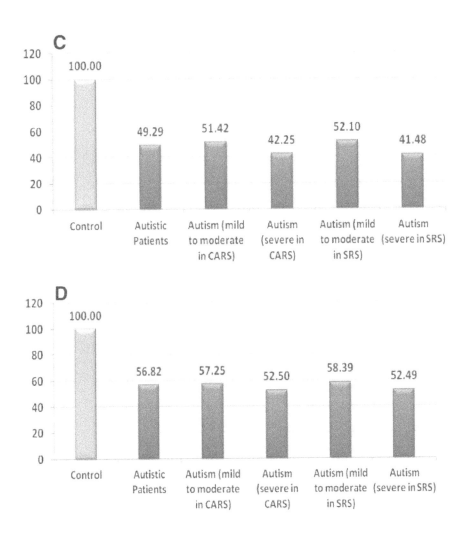

FIGURE 2: *Cont.*

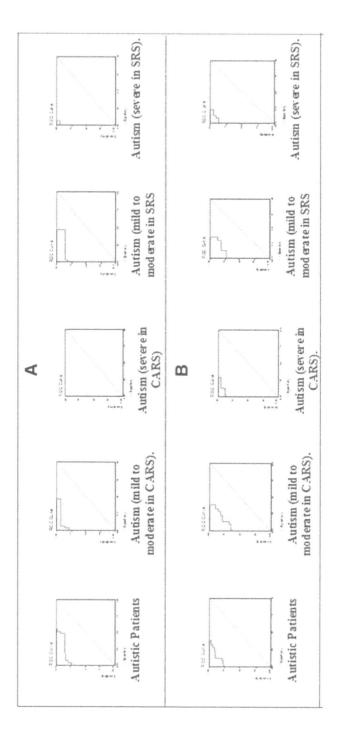

FIGURE 3: ROC-curves for A) mercury, B) lead, C) GST and D) vitamin E in the autistic groups.

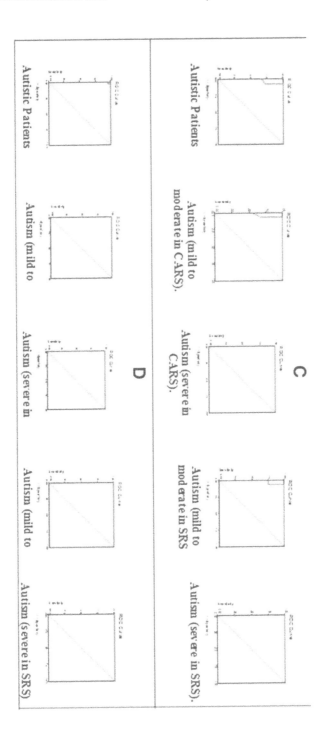

FIGURE 3: *Cont.*

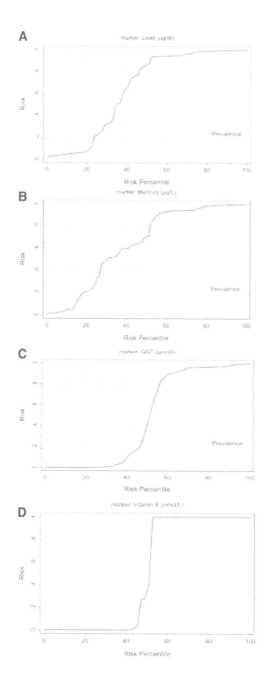

FIGURE 4: Predictiveness curve for A) mercury, B) lead, C) GST and D) vitamin E in the autistic patients.

Tables 4, 5, 6 and 7 show multiple regression analysis results using the Enter method (Tables 4 & 6) and Stepwise method (Tables 5 & 7) for the CARS and SRS scores as two dependent variables, respectively. The value of R^2 shows that 0.56 or 56% of the variance of the CARS scores and almost 40% of the variance of the SRS scores were explained by the regression of the four measured parameters, with GST and vitamin E being more predictive (stepwise regression as presented in Tables 5 & 7).

TABLE 4: Multiple regression using the enter method for CARS as a dependent variable

Model	Beta	P value	Adjusted R^2	Model	
				F value	P value
(Constant)	3.038	0.005	0.564	25.907	0.001
Mercury (µg/L)	0.161	0.139			
Lead (µg/dl)	0.004	0.971			
GST (µmol/l)	-1.159	0.081			
Vitamin E (nmol/L)	-0.082	0.002			

TABLE 5: Multiple regression using the stepwise method for CARS as a dependent variable

Model	Beta	P value	Adjusted R^2	Model	
				F value	P value
(Constant)	4.517	0.001	0.560	49.909	0.001
Vitamin E (nmol/L)	-0.103	0.001			
GST (µmol/l)	-1.383	0.035			

TABLE 6: Multiple regression using the enter method for SRS as a dependent variable

Model	Beta	P value	Adjusted R^2	Model	
				F value	P value
(Constant)	4.844	0.028	0.391	12.867	0.001
Mercury (µg/L)	0.261	0.248			
Lead (µg/dl)	0.117	0.575			
GST (µmol/l)	-1.890	0.185			
Vitamin E (nmol/L)	-0.134	0.012			

Table 7. Multiple regression using the stepwise method for SRS as a dependent variable

Model	Beta	P value	Adjusted R²	Model	
				F value	P value
(Constant)	6.298	0.001	0.384	47.167	0.001
Vitamin E (nmol/L)	-0.202	0.001			

7.4 DISCUSSION

Exposure to even low levels of lead (Pb) early in life has adverse effects on a variety of cognitive and behavioral functions and neurochemical systems, resulting in deficits in learning, memory and attention that may persist into adulthood [19-22]. Persistent effects of Pb exposure early in life can produce changes that arise from physiological re-programming [23]. In this study, there was a significant increase in Pb levels in patients with ASD compared with the control group, coupled with a correlation between Pb concentration and the severity of SRS and CARS scores. These observations support a recent study on patients with ASD by Schneider et al. (2013) [24], who suggested potential epigenetic effects of developmental Pb exposure on DNA methylation. These effects were mediated at least partially through the dysregulation of methyltransferases as multiple forms of proteins, at least some of which are potentially involved in cognition [25], and the resulting abnormalities were recorded in patients with ASD [26].

The reported elevation of Hg and Pb in the RBCs of patients with ASD compared with the control subjects (Table 1 and Figure 1A&B) can be related to and support a previous study by Al-Yafee et al. [27] in which Saudi patients with ASD were described as poor detoxifiers with a lower GSH/GSSG ratio and remarkably less active GST and thioredoxin reductase as markers of the detoxification mechanism. It is well known that GSH and GST are both critical for the detoxification of mercury [28]. While GSH carries Hg through biliary transport for excretion, Hg^{2+} rapidly oxidizes glutathione [28]. This observation is correlated with the previous work of

Al-Gadani et al. [8] who reported lower GSH in the plasma of Saudi patients with ASD. Additionally, the increase of Hg and Pb recorded in this study is consistent with previous studies. For example, Blaurock-Busch et al. [29] found a significant increase of both toxicants in the hair of autistic children compared with non-autistic children. This observation may indicate an impaired detoxification mechanism as a risk factor that significantly contributes to the etiology of autism. The exposure of patients with ASD in early childhood to mercury vapor, methylmercury and ethylmercury may occur through dental amalgams, fish intake and vaccinations [30-32].

Furthermore, in this study, remarkably higher levels of Hg and Pb were recorded in patients with severe social and cognition impairment (SRS & CARS) compared with those with mild-moderate abnormalities. This observation suggests that heavy metal toxicity is closely related to the pathophysiology of autism. This outcome does not concur with a study by Elsheshtawy et al. in which Hg, but not Pb, was found in the hair of autistic patients as a biochemical correlate to disease severity (CARS) [33]. However, our results are consistent with the recent work of Adams et al. [34] who reported that children with autism have higher average levels of several toxic metals, among which Hg and Pb are strongly associated with variations in the severity of the disorder. However, in their study, Adams et al. found a non-significant difference of Hg in children with autism vs. neurotypical children. This could be attributed to differences in geographic exposure to mercury (Saudi Arabia vs. Arizona). Patients with autism are poor detoxifiers (i.e., unable to detoxify mercury when it reaches a certain level) [27]. Therefore, this could indicate a higher rate of exposure to Hg in the Saudi population compared with the population in Arizona.

Face recognition is a core deficit of social impairment in autism. A number of studies indicate that norepinephrine (NE) and dopamine (DA) modulate and reduce behavioral responses to changes in the social environment [35,36]. In addition, serotonin (5HT) transporter binding appears to be reduced in certain brain regions known to play an important role in social cognition and behavior [37], and 5HT binding potential is negatively correlated with social impairment. Therefore, recording Pb as a correlate to severity of SRS and CARS scores in the present study is consistent with the recent findings of El-Ansary et al. [38] in which a positive association was observed between chronic Pb toxicity and lower levels of neurotransmitters as markers of neurologic injury in autistic brains in a Saudi population. Alternately, the biochemical correlation between Pb and the severity of autism is in agreement with other studies. Szkup-Jabłońska et al. [39] and Blaurock-Busch et al. [40] reported a significant correlation between Pb and fear, nervousness, verbal and nonverbal communication, social activity level, and consistency of intellectual response. Moreover, the positive correlation between elevated Pb toxicity and both autistic scales could be supported by the fact that Pb exposure affects multiple health outcomes and physiological systems [41]. These include behavioral/cognitive/IQ effects, nerve conductive effects, hearing loss, reproduction and development effects and death from encephalopathy. Long-term trends in population exposure to Pb (indexed through use of leaded petrol and paint) were remarkably consistent with the link between IQ and social behavior [42].

The significant reduction in plasma GST in Saudi patients with autism compared with controls is documented in this study (Table 1 and Figure 1C&D). This could be related to the significant depletion of GSH as a substrate of GST in the plasma of patients with ASD compared with control subjects [8,43,44]. The reduction in this essential detoxifying enzyme can explain the poor detoxification in patients with ASD, leading to the Hg and Pb toxicity discussed above.

In our study, there was an inverse relationship between decreased levels of plasma GST and the severity of autism, as measured by the SRS and CARS. Severely autistic cases had a remarkably lower GST activity compared to mild-moderate cases of autism. These outcomes concur with Geier et al. [45], who also found a significant inverse relationship between blood GSH levels and autism severity measured with the CARS. Mercury aggravates impaired glutathione synthesis by depleting glutathione in lymphocytes and monocytes, leading to an increased risk of immuno and cytotoxic effects.

Although, the roles and importance of various forms of vitamin E are still unclear [46], it has been suggested that the most important function of α-tocopherol is as a signaling molecule playing an important role in protecting neurons from damage [47]. As an antioxidant, vitamin E may prevent or reduce the propagation of free radicals, which are associated with physical decline, in the human body. This may help reduce muscle or DNA damage and prevent the development of pathological conditions, such as autism [48]. Table 1 and Figure 1D demonstrate the significantly reduced levels of vitamin E in the plasma of patients with ASD compared with the control group. Herndon et al. [49] also found decreased vitamin E levels in autistic patients. The brain contains high levels of oxidizable lipids that must be protected by antioxidants; hence, the supplementation of ASD patients with vitamin E as a major lipophilic antioxidant could be helpful [7,50]. The highly significant correlation between vitamin E depletion and severity of autism, as measured by the SRS and CARS, supports its critical role in protecting against the toxic effects of Pb and Hg. This is consistent with a previous report by Adams et al. [7] that showed a significant association between vitamin E insufficiency and the severity of the Autism Scale (SAS).

ROC analyses of Pb, Hg, GST and vitamin E are presented in Table 2 and Figure 3(A-D). All measured parameters demonstrated almost 100% sensitivity and very high specificity, which also confirmed the hypothesis that autistic patients are poor detoxifiers, unable to readily excrete toxic substances (e.g., Hg and Pb), and suggests that reduced GST activity and depleted vitamin E are two critical factors related to poor detoxification.

Lead, Hg, GST and vitamin E show perfect predictiveness curves (Figure 4A-D). Excellent predictiveness curves for the four parameters reflect the possibility of using any of these parameters to follow up an antioxidant-related treatment strategy. A successful treatment could be followed through a remarkable elevation of plasma vitamin E, the activation of GST or both in autistic patients. Alternately, efficacious treatment could occur through a reduction in Pb and Hg levels. In addition, the relationship between vitamin E deficiency and the etiology of autism could be ascertained by the high specificity, sensitivity and AUC, as shown with the ROC analysis (Table 2).

The negative correlations between Hg & Pb and vitamin E & GST (Table 3) suggest the use of vitamin E as a non-enzymatic antioxidant in treating patients with autism. This suggestion is supported by the multiple regression analysis results (Tables 4, 5, 6 and 7), confirming that higher levels of Hg and Pb, together with lower levels of GST and vitamin E, can be used to predict cognitive and social impairment with the regression of both antioxidant parameters, which is more related to abnormalities of both.

7.5 CONCLUSION

The high values of both sensitivity and specificity recorded for Pb, Hg, GST and vitamin E, together with the good predictiveness curves; suggest that these can be used as biomarkers for measuring the severity of SRS and CARS scores in a Saudi population. This study confirmed the impaired antioxidant and detoxification mechanisms in Saudi autistic patients. Hence, early intervention through the supplementation of good quality and safe antioxidants, including vitamin E, carnosine and selenium, can be helpful in decreasing the burden of heavy metal toxicity. Vitamin E exists in eight different forms: four tocopherols and four tocotrienols. The measured form of vitamin E, α –tocopherol, is one of the forms that regulate signal transduction pathways by mechanisms that are independent of its antioxidant properties, and its use as a supplement can be effective in reducing the toxicity burden in these patients. Autistic children who undergo intensive intervention have better social interaction than children who do not.

REFERENCES

1. American Psychiatric Association: Diagnostic and Statistical Manual of Mental Disorders (fourth, text revision ed.). Washington, DC: American Psychiatric Association; 2000.
2. Garrecht M, Austin DW: The plausibility of a role for mercury in the etiology of autism: a cellular perspective. Toxicol Environ Chem 2011, 93(5-6):1251-1273.
3. El-Ansary A: Detoxification mechanisms in autism spectrum disorders. OA Autism 2013, 1(2):19.
4. Koch L: Cancer: polymorphisms in detoxification genes increase in HMTC and match tumor phenotype. Nat Rev Endocrinol 2013, 9:128.
5. McFadden SA: Phenotypic variation in xenobiotic metabolism and adverse environmental response: focus on sulfur-dependent detoxification pathways. Toxicology 1996, 111(1–3):43-65.
6. Grandjean P, Landrigan P: Developmental neurotoxicity of industrial chemicals. Lancet 2006, 368:2167-2178.

7. Adams JB, Audhya T, McDonough-Means S, Rubin RA, Quig D, Geis E, Gehn E, Loresto M, Mitchell J, Atwood S, Barnhouse S, Lee W: Nutritional and metabolic status of children with autism vs. neurotypical children, and the association with autism severity. Nutr Metab 2011, 8:34.

8. Al-Gadani Y, El-Ansary A, Attas O, Al-Ayadhi L: Metabolic biomarkers related to oxidative stress and antioxidant status in Saudi autistic children. Clin Biochem 2009, 42:1032-1040.

9. Krajkovicova-Kudlackova M, Valachovicova C, Mislanova Z, Hudecova Sudstrova M, Ostatnikova D: Plasma concentration of selected anti-oxidants in autistic children and adolescents. Bratisl Lek Listy 2009, 110:247-250.

10. Al-Gadani Y, Al-Ansary A, Al-Attas O, Al-Ayadhi L: Oxidative stress andantioxidant status in Saudi autistic children. Clin Biochem 2009, 24:1032-1040.

11. Schopler E, Reichler RJ, Rochen Renner B: The childhood autism rating scale. Los Angeles: Western Psychology Services; 2007.

12. Castelloe P, Dawson G: Sub classification of children with autism and pervasive developmental disorder: A questionnaire based on Wing's subgrouping scheme. J Autism Dev Disord 1993, 23:229-241.

13. Constantino JN, Gruber CP: Social Responsiveness Scale. Los Angeles: Western Psychological Services; 2005.

14. Hye A, Lynham S, Thambisetty M, Causevic M, Campbell J, Byers HL, Hooper C, Rijsdijk F, Tabrizi SJ, Banner S, Shaw CE, Foy C, Poppe M, Archer N, Hamilton G, Powell J, Brown RG, Sham P, Ward M, Lovestone S: Proteome-based plasma biomarkers for Alzheimer's disease. Brain 2006, 129:3042-3050.

15. Magos L: Selective atomic-absorption determination of inorganic mercury and methylmercury in undigested biological samples. Analyst 1971, 96:847-853.

16. Miller DT, Paschal DC, Gunter EW, Stroud PE, D'Angelo J: Determination of blood lead with electrothermal atomic absorption using a L'vov platform and matrix modifier. Analyst 1987, 112:1701-1704.

17. Parsons PJ, Slavin W: A rapid Zeeman graphite furnace atomic absorption spectrometric method for the determination of lead in blood. Spectrochim Acta 1993, 48B(6/7):925-939.

18. Driskell WJ, Neese WJ, Bryant CC, Bashor MM: Measurement of vitamin A and vitamin E in human serum by high performance liquid chromatography. J Chromatogr 1982, 231:439-444.

19. Nigg JT, Nikolas M, Mark Knottnerus G, Cavanagh K, Friderici K: Confirmation and extension of association of blood lead with attentiondeficit/ hyperactivity disorder (ADHD) and ADHD symptom domains at population-typical exposure levels. J Child Psychol Psychiatry 2010, 51:58-65.

20. Surkan PJ, Zhang A, Trachtenberg F, Daniel DB, McKinlay S, Bellinger DC: Neuropsychological function in children with blood lead levels <10 microg/dL. Neurotoxicology 2007, 28:1170-1177.

21. Mazumdar M, Bellinger DC, Gregas M, Abanilla K, Bacic J, Needleman HL: Low-level environmental lead exposure in childhood and adult intellectual function: a follow-up study. Environ Health 2011, 10:24.

22. Cecil KM, Brubaker CJ, Adler CM, Dietrich KN, Altaye M, Egelhoff JC, Wessel S, Elangovan I, Hornung R, Jarvis K, Lanphear BP: Decreased brain volume in adults with childhood lead exposure. PLoS Med 2008, 5:e112.

23. Cottrell EC, Seckl JR: Prenatal stress, glucocorticoids and the programming of adult disease. Front Behav Neurosci 2009, 3:19.

24. Schneider JS, Kidd SK, Anderson DW: Influence of developmental lead exposure on expression of DNA methyltransferases and methyl cytosine-binding proteins in hippocampus. Toxicol Lett 2013, 217(1):75-81.

25. Rudenko A, Tsai LH: Epigenetic regulation in memory and cognitive disorders. Neuroscience 2013.

26. Depienne C, Moreno-De-Luca D, Heron D, Bouteiller D, Gennetier A, Delorme R, Chaste P, Siffroi JP, Chantot-Bastaraud S, Benyahia B, Rouillard TO, Nygren G, Kopp S, Johansson M, Rastam M, Burglen L, Leguern E, Verloes A, Leboyer M, Brice A, Gillberg C, Betancur C: Screening for genomic rearrangements and methylation abnormalities of the 15q11-q13 region in autism spectrum disorders. Biol Psychiatry 2009, 66(4):349-359.

27. Al-Yafee YA, Al-Ayadhi LY, Haq SH, El-Ansary AK: Novel metabolic biomarkers related to sulfur-dependent detoxification pathways in autistic patients of Saudi Arabia. BMC Neurol 2011, 11:139.

28. Hyman MH: The impact of mercury on human health and the environment. Altern Ther Health Med 2004, 10(6):70-75.

29. Blaurock-Busch E, Amin OR, Dessoki HH, Rabah T: Toxic metals and essential elements in hair and severity of symptoms among children with Autism. Maedica (Buchar) 2012, 7(1):38-48.

30. Takahashi Y, Tsuruta S, Honda A, Fujiwara Y, Satoh M, Yasutake A: Effect of dental amalgam on gene expression profiles in rat cerebrum, cerebellum, liver and kidney. J Toxicol Sci 2012, 37(3):663-666.

31. Mania M, Wojciechowska-Mazurek M, Starska K, Rebeniak M, Postupolski J: Fish and seafood as a source of human exposure to methylmercury. Rocz Panstw Zakl Hig 2012, 63(3):257-264.

32. Aschner M, Ceccatelli S: Are neuropathological conditions relevant to ethyl mercury exposure? Neurotox Res 2010, 18(1):59-68.

33. Elsheshtawy E, Tobar S, Sherra K, Atallah S, Elkasaby R: Study of some biomarkers in hair of children with autism. Middle East Curr Psychiatry 2011, 18:6-10.

34. Adams JB, Audhya T, McDonough-Means S, Rubin RA, Quig D, Geis E, Gehn E, Loresto M, Mitchell J, Atwood S, Barnhouse S, Lee W: Toxicological status of children with autism vs. neurotypical children and the association with autism severity. Biol Trace Elem Res 2013, 151(2):171-180.

35. Marino MD, Bourdelat-Parks BN, Liles LC, Weinshenker D: Genetic reduction of noradrenergic function alters social memory and reduces aggression in mice. Behav Brain Res 2005, 161:197-203.

36. Stone JM, Morrison PD, Pilowsky LS: Glutamate and dopamine dysregulation in schizophrenia-a synthesis and selective review. J Psychopharmacol 2007, 21:440-452.

37. Makkonen I, Riikonen R, Kokki H, Airaksinen MM, Kuikka JT: Serotonin and do-pamine transporter binding in children with autism determined by SPECT. Dev Med Child Neurol 2008, 50:593-597.

38. El-Ansary AK, Bacha AB, Ayahdi LY: Relationship between chronic lead toxicity and plasma neurotransmitters in autistic patients from Saudi Arabia. Clin Biochem 2011, 44:1116-1120.

39. Szkup-Jabłońska M, Karakiewicz B, Grochans E, Jurczak A, Zaremba-Pechmann L, Rotter I, Nowak-Starz G, Samochowiec J: The effects of lead level in the blood on social functioning in children with developmental disabilities. Psychiatr Pol 2011, 45(5):713-722.

40. Blaurock-Busch E, Amin OR, Rabah T: Heavy metals and trace elements in hair and urine of a sample of arab children with autistic spectrum disorder. Maedica 2011, 6:247-257.

41. ATSDR: Toxicological Profile for Lead (update). (Agency for Toxic Substances and Disease Registry). Atlanta, GA: U.S. Department of Health and Human Services; 1999.

42. Nevin R: How lead exposure relates to temporal changes in IQ, violent crime, and unwed pregnancy. Environ Res 2000, 83:1-22.

43. Geier DA, King PG, Sykes LK, Geier MR: A comprehensive review of mercury provoked autism. Indian J Med Res 2008, 128:383-411.

44. Vojdani A, Mumper E, Granpeesheh D, Mielke L, Traver D, Bock K, Hirani K, Neu-brander J, Woeller KN, O'Hara N, Usman A, Schneider C, Hebroni F, Berookhim J, McCandless J: Low natural killer cell cytotoxic activity in autism: the role of gluta-thione, IL-2 and IL-15. J Neuroimmunol 2008, 205(1–2):148-154.

45. Geier DA, Kern J, Geier MA: A prospective study of oxidative stress biomarkers in autistic disorders. Electron J Appl Psychol Innov Autism 2009, 5:2-10.

46. Atkinson A, Epand RF, Epand RM: Tocopherols and tocotrienols in membranes: a critical review. Free Radic Biol Med 2007, 44:739-764.

47. Zingg JM, Azzi A: Non-antioxidant activities of vitamin E. Curr Chem Med 2004, 11:1113-1133.

48. Azzi A: Molecular mechanism of alpha-tocopherol action. Free Radic Biol Med 2007, 43(1):16-21.

49. Herndon AC, Diguiseppi C, Johndon SL: Dose nutritional intake differs between children with autism spectrum disorder and children with typical development? Au-tism Dev Disord 2008, 6:341-349.

50. Kontush KO, Schekatolina A: Vitamin E in neurodegenerative disorder: Alzheimers disease. Ann N Y Acad Sci 2004, 1031:249-262.

CHAPTER 8

ASSESSMENT OF INFANTILE MINERAL IMBALANCES IN AUTISM SPECTRUM DISORDERS (ASDs)

HIROSHI YASUDA AND TOYOHARU TSUTSUI

8.1 INTRODUCTION

ASDs are a group of neural development disorders characterized by impairments in social interaction and communication, and by the presence of restricted and repetitive behaviours [1,2]. Clarification of the pathogenesis and effective treatment of autism spectrum disorders (ASDs) is one of the challenges today. ASDs continue to increase in prevalence up to 1 in 88 children [1,2,3] and are known to be highly heritable (~90%), and some related genes have been reported [4,5,6,7,8]. However, the underlying genetic determinants are still not clarified [1,9], and the interaction of heritable factors with uncertified lifestyle and environmental factors seem play a significant role in the pathogenesis. For example, organic mercury had been claimed one of environmental candidates causing autistic disorders [10,11,12], but its relationship remains to be established.

Assessment of Infantile Mineral Imbalances in Autism Spectrum Disorders (ASDs). © Yasuda H and Tsutsui T. International Journal of Environmental Research and Public Health *10,11 (2013); doi:10.3390/ijerph10116027. Licensed under a Creative Commons Attribution 3.0 Unported License, http://creativecommons.org/licenses/by/3.0/.*

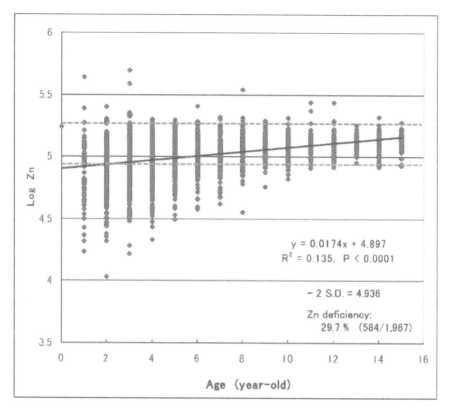

FIGURE 1: Relation of logarithmic zinc concentration with age in autistic children [33].

Recently, epigenetic alteration of gene expression by environmental factors is considered one of key events in the pathogenesis of genetic diseases [13,14], and some toxic elements such as cadmium and arsenic have been reported to be candidate factors that induce epigenetic alterations [15,16,17,18,19] and neurodevelopmental disorders [20].

Recent great advances in high-sensitive and reliable trace element analysis method using inductively coupled plasma mass spectrometry (ICP-MS) have enabled it to be applied for forensic medical research and estimating chronic toxic metal burden and mineral deficiency in the human body [21,22]. Thus, the clinical application of reliable hair mineral analysis methods based on ICP-MS has been tried to investigate the association of some diseases/symptoms with trace bio-element kinetics including toxic metals and essential minerals [23,24,25,26,27,28].

For the last seven years, we have examined the association of toxic metal burdens with autistic disorders, and reported that some of the autistic children have suffered from high accumulation of toxic metals such as cadmium, lead or aluminium [29,30,31], and recently demonstrating the association with infantile zinc deficiency [32,33].

In this overview article in which human scalp hair concentrations of 26 trace elements have been examined for 1,967 children with autistic disorders aged 0–15 years, we demonstrate that many of the patients, especially in the infants aged 0–3 years-old, are suffering from marginal to severe zinc- and magnesium-deficiency and/or high burdens of several toxic metals such as aluminium, cadmium and lead, indicating the presence of a critical term "infantile window" in neurodevelopment and probably for therapy.

8.2 MINERAL DISORDERS IN AUTISM

8.2.1 INFANTILE ZINC DEFICIENCY

The histogram of hair logarithmic zinc concentrations for 1,967 autistic children diagnosed by their physicians was non-symmetric with tailing in lower range, and 584 in 1,967 subjects (29.7%) were found to have a lower zinc concentration than—2 S.D. (standard deviation) level of the reference range (86.3–193 ppm; geometric mean = 129 ppm), estimated as zinc deficiency. The incidence rates of zinc deficiency in the age groups of 0–3, 4–9 and 10–15 years-old were estimated 43.5%, 28.1% and 3.3% in male and 52.5%, 28.7% and 3.5% in female, and a significant correlation of zinc concentration with age ($r = 0.367$, $p < 0.0001$) was observed (Figure 1), suggesting that infants are more liable to zinc deficiency than elder children. The minimum zinc concentration of 10.7 ppm was detected in a 2-year-old boy, corresponding to about 1/12 of the mean reference level. The zinc concentration of only one 0-year-old case (11 months-old) was 173 ppm in the normal range and seem to be a suspected case, because she was suffered from high burdens of aluminium (52.5 ppm), lead (9.1 ppm), iron (12.8 ppm) and copper (134 ppm). There was little marked gender difference in hair zinc concentration and incidence rate of zinc deficiency.

8.2.2 INFANTILE MAGNESIUM/CALCIUM DEFICIENCY

Following to zinc deficiency, magnesium and calcium deficiency was observed in 347 (17.6%) and 114 (5.8%) individuals in the autistic children, and for the other essential metals such as iron, chromium, manganese, copper and cobalt, their incidence rates of deficiency were 2.0% or less (Table 1). The incidence rates of magnesium deficiency in the age groups of 0–3, 4–9 and 10–15 years-old were 27.0%, 17.1% and 4.2% in male and 22.9%, 12.7% and 4.3% in female subjects, and a significant correlation of magnesium concentration with age ($r = 0.362$, $p < 0.0001$) was observed, suggesting that infants are also liable to magnesium deficiency than elder children. The minimal magnesium concentration of 3.88 ppm was detected in a 2-year-old girl, corresponding to almost 1/10 of the mean reference level (39.5 ppm). Considerable calcium deficiency rate was observed only in lower age groups less than 10 years-old.

TABLE 1: Prevalence of mineral deficiency in autistic children [33].

Mineral	Number of Cases with Deficiency	Rate (%) of Deficiency
Zn	584	29.7
Mg	347	17.6
Ca	114	5.8
Co	40	2.0
Fe	17	0.9
Cr	12	0.6
Mn	4	0.2
Cu	4	0.2

The number and incidence rate of individuals with mineral deficiency (lower than −2 S.D.) in 1,967 autistic children (1,553 males and 414 females) are shown in the table [33].

8.2.3 TOXIC METAL BURDENS

In contrast to essential metals, high body burdens of some toxic metals such as aluminium, cadmium and lead of over their +2 S.D. levels were observed in 339 (17.2%), 168 (8.5%) and 94 (4.8%) individuals, respectively, and their incidence rates of high burden were higher than that of mercury and arsenic (2.8% and 2.6%) (Table 2).

TABLE 2: Prevalence of high toxic metal burden and the maximum level in autistic children [33].

Toxic Metal	Number of Cases with High Burden	Rate (%) of High Burden	Maximum (ppm)	Ratio to Reference
Al	339	17.2	79.4	21.1
Cd	168	8.5	5.5	782.0
Pb	94	4.8	24.9	57.4
Hg	56	2.8	36.3	9.3
As	52	2.6	1.7	33.5

The number and incidence rate of individuals with high toxic metal burden (higher than +2 S.D.) in 1,967 autistic children (1,553 males and 414 females) and the maximum concentration are tabled [33].

High toxic metal burdens were more frequently observed in the infants aged 0–3 years-old: that is, the incidence rate was 20.6%, 12.1%, 7.5%, 3.2% and 2.3% for aluminium, cadmium, lead, arsenic and mercury. The detected maximal concentration of aluminium, cadmium, lead, mercury and arsenic was 79.4 ppm, 5.47 ppm, 24.9 ppm, 36.3 ppm and 1.7 ppm, respectively, corresponding to 21-, 782-, 57-, 9- and 33-fold of each mean reference level.

A high significant inverse relationship between zinc and lead concentrations ($r = -0.339$, $p < 0.0001$; Figure 2), and also aluminium ($r = -0.247$) and cadmium ($r = -0.198$) concentrations, was observed, suggesting that these toxic metal burdens associate with infantile zinc deficiency.

8.2.4 METALLOMICS PROFILES IN AUTISTIC INFANTS

There are some sub-types observed in the metallomics profiles character-istic in autistic children. Figure 3 shows a representative autistic profile in a 1-year-old boy suffering from severe zinc- and magnesium-deficiency and simultaneous high burdens of cadmium and lead. The other autistic metallomics profiles with high burdens of aluminium, mercury or arsenic are shown in Figure 4, Figure 5 and Figure 6. Figure 7 shows a unique profile with high sodium and potassium concentrations, a characteristic profile detectable in hair specimens. It remains to be clarified which type of metallomcs profiles corresponds to which type of autism spectrum dis-orders.

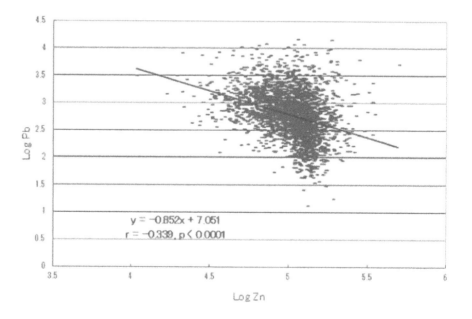

FIGURE 2: Inverse relation of zinc and lead concentration in autistic children.

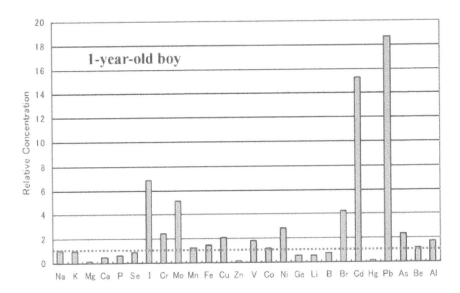

FIGURE 3: Metallomics profile of an autistic child with high cadmium and lead burdens [33].

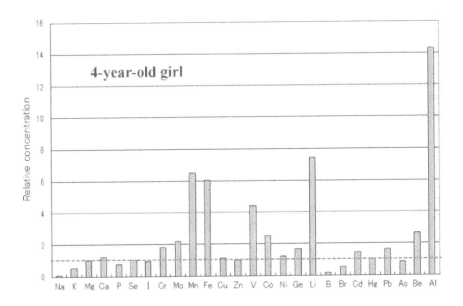

FIGURE 4: Metallomics profile of an autistic child with high aluminium burden.

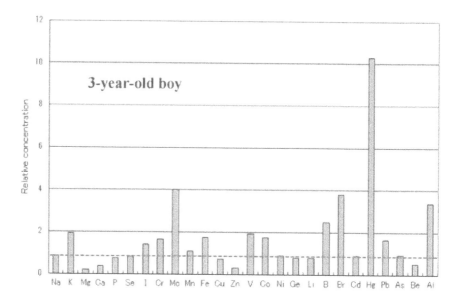

FIGURE 5: Metallomics profile of an autistic child with high mercury burden.

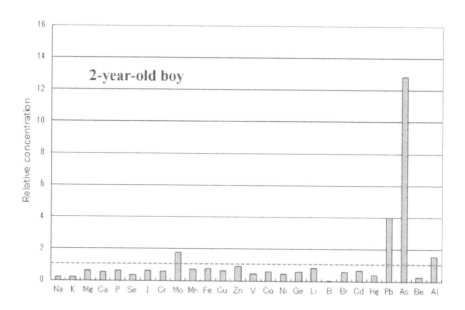

FIGURE 6: Metallomics profile of an autistic child with high arsenic burden.

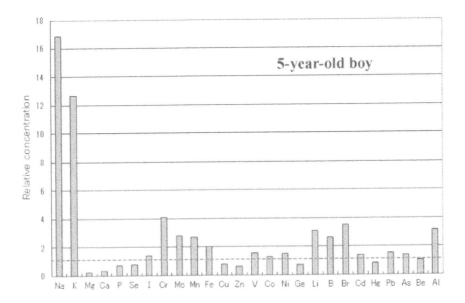

FIGURE 7: Metallome profile of an autistic child with high sodium and potassium levels

8.2.5 INFANTILE TIME WINDOW IN NEURODEVELOPMENT AND FOR THERAPY

The age at final diagnosis of autism spectrum disorders ranges from 3 to 6 years, although most cases of autism are diagnosed by the age of three and as early as 14 months [34]. In facts, zinc deficiency was detected in many of the infantile patients in the first 3 years of life (Figure 1), and high toxic metal burdens were also detected in the autistic subjects, especially in the younger children (Table 2). Thus, for treatment/prevention of autism spectrum disorders, its early screening and estimation is necessary and it is desirable to early check any metabolic and/or mineral disorders for the infants and children with autistic symptoms, though there are serious limitations of diagnosis of the younger children. It should be considered that the pathogenesis of neurodevelopment disorders might start in prenatal phase and be progressive within the time window for diagnosis.

8.2.6 AUTISM-RELATED GENES AND EPIGENETIC ALTERATION BY MINERAL DISORDERS

Zinc is a structural component of zinc-finger proteins and a transcriptional regulator, and influences some candidate genes reported to be associated with the development of autism, such as MTF1 (metal-responsive transcription factor 1), metallothionein, ZnT5 (zinc transporter 5), COMMD1 (COMM domain-containing protein 1), ERK1 (extracellular signal-regulated kinase 1), TrkB (tyrosine-related kinase B), and ProSAP/Shank (proline-rich synapse-associated protein/SH and multiple ankyrin repeat domains) that themselves are involved in zinc signalling and homeostasis [35,36,37,38,39,40]. Thus, zinc deficiency observed in the autistic subjects (Figure 1) might induce critical epigenetic alterations to provide a central mechanism of gene/environment interaction to interfere with neuronal maturation during early development [32,38,39].

In addition, high toxic metal burdens detected in the autistic patients (Table 2) might contribute to the mechanism of gene/environment interaction, because cadmium and arsenic have been reported to be candidate factors that induce epigenetic alterations [15,16,17,18,19] and neurodevelopmental disorders [20].

8.3 DISCUSSION

In this metallomics study of human scalp hair concentrations of 26 trace elements for 1,967 children with autistic disorders aged 0–15 years, we demonstrate that many of the patients, especially in the infants aged 0–3 year-old, are suffering from marginal to severe zinc- and magnesium-deficiency and/or high burdens of several toxic metals such as aluminium, cadmium and lead.

Zinc is well-accepted as essential trace element that plays important roles in nucleic acid/protein synthesis, cell replication, tissue growth and repair, especially in pregnant women and infants. In fact, zinc ions function as the active centers in more than 300 kinds of enzymes, and about 10% in the total gene-coded proteins have been known to have zinc-finger sequences [38,39,40,41,42], emphasizing the physiological importance of this trace element. In brain, especially in the hippocampus, zinc is co-stored with glutamate in pre-synaptic vesicles in the excitatory neuron terminal, is released from them and controls the activity of excitatory glutamate receptors on the post-synaptic excitable membrane [43,44]. Thus, zinc deficiency is known associated with not only various pathological conditions, including dysgeusia, delayed wound healing, impaired immunity and retarded growth, but also neurodegenerative diseases and neuro-development disorders [45,46,47,48,49].

Recently we reported that many infants with autistic disorders are suffering from marginal to severe zinc deficiency, suggesting considerable relationship of infantile zinc deficiency with autism [32]. Furthermore, we have determined scalp hair concentrations of 26 trace elements for 1,967 subjects with autism spectrum disorders and demonstrated that infantile autistic children are liable to deficiency in magnesium and calcium next to zinc, but not in the other essential metals (Table 1) [33]. These findings suggest that autistic infants and probably infants generally have a characteristic liability to zinc- and magnesium-deficiency, because larger amounts of the essential metals (per kg body weight) are needed for the development and growth.

There are numerous studies with the same theme reporting nutritional status and mineral deficiencies in autistic children [50,51,52,53,54]. However, the conclusions of their studies, in which the restricted age (over 4-years-old) of children and number of minerals were examined, were not consistent, and the critical environmental factors remained to be established. In our metallomics analysis study for the 1,967 autistic children aged 0–15 years-old, we were able to demonstrate not only the critical and environmental epigenetic factor (zinc- and magnesium-deficiency and high burdens of aluminium, cadmium, lead and so on) but also the presence of another critical factor, "infantile window" in neurodevelopment and probably for therapy [32,33].

Recently, Gebremedhin et al. [55] reported that compared to pregnant women aged 15–24 years, those aged 25–34 and 35–49 years had 1.57 (95% CL: 1.04–2.34) and 2.18 (95% CL: 1.25–3.63) times higher risk of zinc deficiency, respectively. Their study may demonstrate that old age pregnancy is negatively associated to zinc status, maybe suggesting that one of the origins of the high incidence rate of infantile zinc deficiency may be higher age pregnancy of their mothers. Recently, Kurita et al. [56] reported that zinc deficiency in utero induces foetal epigenetic alterations of histone modifications in metallothionein 2 promoter region having metal responsive elements in 1-day-old and 5-week-old mice, of which pregnant mother were fed low zinc diet from gestation day 8 until delivery.

Arnold et al. [57] reported that mean serum zinc level in children was significantly lower in attention-deficit/hyperactivity disorder (ADHD) group, and that serum zinc level correlated inversely with parent- and teacher-rated inattention in ADHD children. Furthermore, zinc treatment was reported significantly superior to placebo in reducing symptoms of hyperactivity, impulsivity and impaired socialization in ADHD patients [58,59]. Another preliminary human study showed that many children with ADHD have lower zinc concentration in comparison to healthy children and zinc supplement as an adjunct to methylphenidate has favourable effects in the treatment of ADHD children, pointing to the possible association of zinc deficiency and ADHD pathophysiology [60].

Kozielec et al. [61] have reported that in 116 hyperactive children with ADHD, magnesium deficiency was found in 95% of the subjects, most frequently in hair (77.6%), next in red-blood cells (58.6%) and in blood serum (33.6%). Furthermore, they reported that in the group of ADHD children given 6 months of magnesium supplementation, a significant decrease of hyperactivity and increase in hair magnesium contents has been achieved [62]. Mousain-Bosc et al. [63] also reported that 52 hyper-excitable children have low intra-erythrocyte magnesium levels with normal serum magnesium values, and that magnesium/vitamin B6 supplementation can restore the erythrocyte magnesium levels to normal and improve their abnormal behaviours. They also reported that thirty-three children with clinical symptoms of pervasive developmental disorder or autism (PDD) exhibit significantly lower red blood cell magnesium values, and that the combination therapy with magnesium/vitamin B6 for 6 months improved significantly PDD symptoms in 23/33 children ($p < 0.0001$) with concomitant increases in intra-erythrocyte magnesium values [64].

Recently, Ochi et al. [65] found that hair magnesium concentration, but not its serum level, was significantly ($p < 0.01$) inversely-associated with left ventricular hypertrophy in hemodialysis patients, suggesting that hair magnesium concentration is a useful intracellular biomarker independent of its serum level. In a preliminary metallomics study for healthy volunteers, we have observed a high significant correlation between whole blood levels and scalp hair levels of trace elements, but little relation between their serum levels and whole blood levels (unpublished observation). These findings suggest that as biomarker specimen representing mineral dynamics in human body, whole blood/erythrocyte and hair samples are superior to extra-cellular fluids such as serum or plasma for metallomics analysis, although it is necessary to consider that there is a problem of contamination of some trace-elements due to artificial hair treatment such as permanent and colouring.

Recently, dietary restriction-induced zinc deficiency has been reported to up-regulate intestinal zinc-importer (ZIP4) and induce the increase in ZIP4 protein located to the plasma membrane of enterocytes [66,67]. This adoptive response to zinc deficiency is known to lead to increasing in the risk of high-uptake of toxic metals such as cadmium and lead [68]. Thus, infants with zinc deficiency are liable to increased risk of absorbing high amount of toxic metals and retaining them in their bodies, as shown in Figure 4, which demonstrates a high significant inverse relationship between zinc and lead level. These findings suggest that the increased toxic metal burdens concomitant with zinc deficiency may also epigenetically contribute to the pathogenesis of this disorder.

Deficiency in magnesium/calcium seems further enhance the toxic effects of lead (Pb) on cognitive and behavioural development in children [69]. A significant inverse relationship between dietary calcium intake and blood lead concentrations was found in 3,000 American children examined as part of NHANES II [69]. Elevated blood lead levels are found in some children diagnosed with autism and are associated with the development of ADHD [70,71].

About 250,000 children in the U.S.A. were reported to have high blood lead (Pb) levels over the current Level of Concern of 10 µg/dL [72], despite significant progresses over the past half century in reducing child lead poisoning rates [73]. Therefore, the U.S. Centers for Disease Control and Prevention (CDC) has lowered the Level of Concern from 10 µg/dL to 5 µg/dL [74]. This major change in national policy is based on a large and growing body of evidence showing that even single-digit blood Pb levels have significant impacts on Intelligence Quotients, risk for Attention Deficit Hyperactivity Disorder (ADHD), cardiovascular disease, and kidney function [75,76,77,78,79].

The most common lead exposure pathway for children are ingestion or inhalation of lead-bearing road dusts, whether in the household or outdoor environment [80,81,82], and its most common sources are fossil fuels, asphalt and paints (lead chromate or lead carbonate) [82,83,84]. In addition, maternal cigarette smoking has been reported to be associated with lower zinc and higher cadmium and lead concentrations in their neonates [85,86]. These toxic metals accumulated in the maternal bone tissues are co-transferred with calcium to foetal and new-born bodies through activated bone-resorption during pregnancy and lactation [85,86,87,88]. In fact, a recent birth cohort study for new-borns in Nepal shows that the motor cluster score was inversely associated with the cord blood levels of lead and arsenic, suggesting that high exposures to Pb and As during the prenatal period may induce retardation during in-utero neurodevelopment [89].

For mercury and arsenic, the maximum burden levels of 9.3- and 33.5-fold of the reference level (Table 2) may also epigenetically play a pathogenic role in the respective autistic individuals, even though their incidence rates were 2.8% or less. It remains to be established that these mineral disorders induce the epigenetic deficits in autism-related candidate genes. In near future, we hope it will be clarified what type of metallomics profiles is associated with what disorder in various behaviour/neurological deficits in autism spectrum disorders.

It is demonstrated that many autistic infants are suffering from marginal to severe zinc- and magnesium-deficiency and/or high toxic metal burdens of aluminium, cadmium, lead and so on. These findings suggest that infantile autistic patients with mineral disorders may respond to a novel evidence-based nutritional approach which supplements deficient nutrients and detoxifies accumulated toxic metals. This evidence-based nutritional approach may yield a new vista into early screening/assessment and treatment/prevention of infantile patients with autism spectrum disorders including the suspects. Well-controlled intervention studies for this novel nutritional therapy are desired to establish the epigenetic roles of infantile mineral imbalances in the pathogenesis of neurodevelopment disorders and to develop an early screening and therapy of neurodevelopment disorders such as autism spectrum disorders, ADHD and learning disorder.

8.4 CONCLUSIONS

This overview demonstrates that many of infantile patients with autism spectrum disorders suffer from marginal to severe zinc- and magnesium-deficiency and/or high toxic metal burdens, and that these mineral disorders (mineral imbalances) in bodies may play principal, epigenetic roles as environment factors in the pathogenesis of the neurodevelopment disorders. In addition, it is suggested that there is a critical time window "infantile window" in neurodevelopment and probably for treatment and prevention of these disorders. In near future, an introduction of innovative clinical tests such as metabolomics and metallomics analysis is desired for early estimation and treatment of neurodevelopment disorders.

REFERENCES

1. Weintraub, K. Autism counts. Nature 2011, 479, 22–24.
2. Pinto, D.; Pagnamenta, A.T.; Klei, L.; Anney, R.; Merico, D.; Regan, R.; Conroy, J.; Magalhaes, T.R.; Correia, C.; Abrahams, B.S.; et al. Functional impact of global rare copy number variation in autism spectrum disorders. Nature 2010, 466, 368–372.
3. Chakrabarti, S.; Fombonne, E. Pervasive developmental disorders in preschool children: Confirmation of high prevalence. Amer. J. Psychiat. 2005, 162, 1133–1141, doi:10.1176/appi.ajp.162.6.1133.
4. Bailey, A.; le Couteur, A.; Gottesman, I.; Bolton, P.; Simonoff, E.; Yuzda, E.; Rutter, M. Autism as a strongly genetic disorder: Evidence from a British twin study. Psychol. Med. 1995, 25, 63–77, doi:10.1017/S0033291700028099.
5. Marshall, C.R.; Noor, A.; Vincent, J.B.; Lionel, A.C.; Feuk, L.; Skaug, J.; Shago, M.; Moessner, R.; Pinto, D.; Ren, Y.; et al. Structural variation of chromosomes in autism spectrum disorder. Amer. J. Hum. Genet. 2008, 82, 477–488, doi:10.1016/j.ajhg.2007.12.009.
6. Kim, S.J.; Silva, R.M.; Flores, C.G.; Jacob, S.; Guter, S.; Valcante, G.; Zaytoun, A.M.; Cook, E.H.; Badner, J.A. A quantitative association study of SLC25A12 and restricted repetitive behavior traits in autism spectrum disorders. Mol. Autism 2011, 2, doi:10.1186/2040-2392-2-8.
7. Murdoch, J.D.; State, M.W. Recent developments in the genetics of autism spectrum disorders. Curr. Opin. Genet. Dev. 2013, 23, 310–315, doi:10.1016/j.gde.2013.02.003.
8. Huguet, G.; Ey, E.; Bourgeron, T. The genetic landscapes of autism spectrum disorders. Ann. Rev. Genomics Hum. Genet. 2013, 14, 191–213, doi:10.1146/annurev-genom-091212-153431.
9. Hughes, V. Autism: Complex disorder. Nature 2012, 491, S2–S3, doi:10.1038/491S2a.

10. Dufault, R.; Schnoll, R.; Lukiw, W.J.; Leblanc, B.; Cornett, C.; Patrick, L.; Wallinga, D.; Gilbert, S.G.; Crider, R. Mercury exposure, nutritional deficiencies and metabolic disruption may affect learning in children. Behav. Brain Funct. 2009, 5, 44–58, doi:10.1186/1744-9081-5-44.

11. Palmer, R.F.; Blanchard, S.; Wood, R. Proximity to point sources of environmental mercury release as a predictor of autism prevalence. Health Place 2009, 15, 18–24, doi:10.1016/j.healthplace.2008.02.001.

12. Majewska, M.D.; Urbanowicz, E.; Rok-Bujko, P.; Namyslowska, I.; Mierzejewsky, P. Age-dependent lower or higher levels of hair mercury in autistic children than in healthy controls. Acta Neurobiol. Exp. 2010, 70, 196–208.

13. O'Rahilly, S. Human genetics illuminates the paths to metabolic disease. Nature 2009, 462, 307–314, doi:10.1038/nature08532.

14. James, S.J.; Shpyleva, S.; Melnyk, S.; Pavliv, O.; Pogribny, I.P. Complex epigenetic regulation of engrailed-2 (EN-2) homeobox gene in the autism cerebellum. Transl. Psychiat. 2013, 3, e232, doi:10.1038/tp.2013.8.

15. Jin, Y.H.; Clark, A.B.; Slebos, R.J.; Al-Refai, H.; Taylor, J.A.; Kunkel, T.A.; Resnick, M.A.; Gordenin, D.A. Cadmium is a mutagen that acts by inhibiting mismatch repair. Nat. Genet. 2003, 34, 239–241, doi:10.1038/ng0703-239.

16. Takiguchi, M.; Achanzar, W.E.; Qu, W.; Li, G.; Waalkes, M.P. Effects of cadmium on DNA-(cytosine-5) methyltransferase activity and DNA methylation status during cadmium-induced cellular transformation. Exp. Cell Res. 2003, 286, 355–365, doi:10.1016/S0014-4827(03)00062-4.

17. Arita, A.; Costa, M. Epigenetics in metal carcinogenesis: Nickel, arsenic, chromium and cadmium. Metallomics 2009, 1, 222–228, doi:10.1039/b903049b.

18. Perera, F.; Herbstman, J. Prenatal environmental exposure, epigenetics, and disease. Reprod. Toxicol. 2011, 31, 363–373, doi:10.1016/j.reprotox.2010.12.055.

19. Jakovcevski, M.; Akbarian, S. Epigenetic mechanisms in neurological disease. Nat. Med. 2012, 18, 1194–1204, doi:10.1038/nm.2828.

20. Ciesielski, T.; Weuve, J.; Bellinger, D.C.; Schwartz, J.; Lanphear, B.; Wright, R.O. Cadmium exposure and neurodevelopmental outcomes in U.S. children. Environ. Health Perspect. 2012, 120, 758–763, doi:10.1289/ehp.1104152.

21. Rodushkin, I.; Axelsson, M.D. Application of double focusing sector field ICP-MS for multi elemental characterization of human hair and nails. Part I. Analytical methodology. Sci. Total Environ. 2000, 250, 83–100, doi:10.1016/S0048-9697(00)00369-7.

22. Goulle, J.P.; Mahieu, L.; Castermant, J.; Neveu, N.; Bonneau, L.; Lainé, G.; Bouige, D.; Lacroix, C. Metal and metalloid multi-elementary ICP-MS validation in whole blood, plasma, urine and hair: Reference values. Forensic Sci. Int. 2005, 153, 39–44, doi:10.1016/j.forsciint.2005.04.020.

23. Wang, C.T.; Chang, W.T.; Zeng, W.F.; Lin, C.H. Concentrations of calcium, copper, iron, magnesium, potassium, sodium and zinc in adult female hair with different body mass indexes in Taiwan. Clin. Chem. Lab. Med. 2005, 43, 389–393.

24. Munakata, M.; Onuma, A.; Kobayashi, Y.; Haginoya, K.; Yokoyama, H.; Fujiwara, I.; Yasuda, H.; Tsutsui, T.; Iinuma, K. A preliminary analysis of trace elements in the scalp hair of patients with severe motor disabilities receiving enteral nutrition. Brain Dev. 2006, 28, 521–525, doi:10.1016/j.braindev.2006.02.004.

25. Yasuda, H.; Yonashiro, T.; Yoshida, K.; Ishii, T.; Tsutsui, T. Mineral imbalance in children with autistic disorders. Biomed. Res. Trace Elem. 2005, 16, 285–291.

26. Yasuda, H.; Yonashiro, T.; Yoshida, K.; Ishii, T.; Tsutsui, T. Relationship between body mass index and minerals in male Japanese adults. Biomed. Res. Trace Elem. 2006, 17, 316–321.

27. Yasuda, H.; Yoshida, K.; Segawa, M.; Tokuda, R.; Tsutsui, T.; Yasuda, Y.; Magara, S. Metallomics study using hair mineral analysis and multiple logistic regression analysis: Relationship between cancer and minerals. Environ. Health Prev. Med. 2009, 14, 261–266, doi:10.1007/s12199-009-0092-y.

28. Ochi, A.; Ishimura, E.; Tsujimoto, Y.; Kakiya, R.; Tabata, T.; Mori, K.; Tahara, H.; Shoji, T.; Yasuda, H.; Nishizawa, Y.; et al. Elemental concentrations in scalp hair, nutritional status and health-related quality of life in haemodialysis patients. Ther. Apher. Dial. 2012, 16, 127–133, doi:10.1111/j.1744-9987.2011.01043.x.

29. Yasuda, H.; Yonashiro, T.; Yoshida, K.; Ishii, T.; Tsutsui, T. High toxic metal levels in scalp hair of infants and children. Biomed. Res. Trace Elem. 2005, 16, 39–45.

30. Yasuda, H.; Yoshida, K.; Segawa, M.; Tokuda, R.; Yasuda, Y.; Tsutsui, T. High accumulation of aluminium in hairs of infants and children. Biomed. Res. Trace Elem. 2008, 19, 57–62.

31. Yasuda, H.; Yoshida, K.; Yasuda, Y.; Tsutsui, T. Two age-related accumulation profiles of toxic metals. Curr. Aging Sci. 2012, 5, 105–111, doi:10.2174/18746098112 05020105.

32. Yasuda, H.; Yoshida, K.; Yasuda, Y.; Tsutsui, T. Infantile zinc deficiency: Association with autism spectrum disorders. Sci. Rep. 2011, 1, doi:10.1038/srep00129.

33. Yasuda, H.; Yasuda, Y.; Tsutsui, T. Estimation of autistic children by metallomics analysis. Sci. Rep. 2013, 3, ep01199, doi:10.1038/srep01199.

34. Landa, R.J. Diagnosis of autism spectrum disorders in the first 3 years of life. Nat. Clin. Pract. Neurol. 2008, 4, 138–147, doi:10.1038/ncpneuro0731.

35. Huang, Y.Z.; Pan, E.; Xiong, Z.Q.; McNamara, J.O. Zinc-mediated transactivation of TrkB potentiates the hippocampal mossy fiber-CA3 pyramidal synapse. Neuron 2008, 57, 546–558, doi:10.1016/j.neuron.2007.11.026.

36. O'Roak, B.J.; Deriziotis, P.; Lee, C.; Vives, L.; Schwartz, J.J.; Girirajan, S.; Karakoc, E.; Mackenzie, A.P.; Ng, S.B.; Baker, C.; et al. Exome sequencing in sporadic autism spectrum disorders identifies severe de novo mutations. Nat. Genet. 2011, 43, 585–589, doi:10.1038/ng.835.

37. Sanders, S.J.; Murtha, M.T.; Gupta, A.R.; Murdoch, J.D.; Raubeson, M.J.; Willsey, A.J.; Ercan-Sencicek, A.G.; DiLullo, N.M.; Parikshak, N.N.; Stein, J.L.; et al. De novo mutations revealed by whole exome sequencing are strongly associated with autism. Nature 2012, 485, 237–241, doi:10.1038/nature10945.

38. Grabrucker, A.M. Environmental factors in autism. Front. Psychist. 2013, 3, 1–13.

39. Dufault, R.; Lukiw, W.J.; Crider, R.; Schnoll, R.; Wallinga, D.; Deth, R. A macroepigenetic approach to identify factors responsible for the autism epidemic in the United States. Clin. Epigenetics 2012, 4, 6, doi:10.1186/1868-7083-4-6.

40. Grabrucker, A.M. A role for synaptic zinc in ProSAP/Shank PSD scaffold malformation in autism spectrum disorders. Dev. Neurobiol. 2013, doi:10.1002/dneu.22089.

41. Fukada, T.; Yamasaki, S.; Nishida, K.; Murakami, M.; Hirano, T. Zinc homeostasis and signalling in health and diseases: Zinc signalling. J. Biol. Inorg. Chem. 2011, 16, 1123–1134, doi:10.1007/s00775-011-0797-4.

42. Andreini, C.; Banci, L.; Bertini, I.; Rosato, A. Counting the zinc-proteins encoded in the human genome. J. Proteome Res. 2006, 5, 196–201, doi:10.1021/pr050361j.

43. Takeda, A. Movement of zinc and its functional significance in the brain. Brain Res. Rev. 2000, 34, 137–148, doi:10.1016/S0165-0173(00)00044-8.

44. Takeda, A.; Nakamura, M.; Fujii, H.; Tamano, H. Synaptic Zn(2+) homeostasis and its significance. Metallomics 2013, 5, 417–423, doi:10.1039/c3mt20269k.

45. Prasad, A.S. Impact of the discovery of human zinc deficiency on health. J. Am. Coll. Nutr. 2009, 28, 257–265, doi:10.1080/07315724.2009.10719780.

46. Arnold, L.E.; di Silvestro, R.A. Zinc in attention-deficit/hyperactivity disorder. J. Child Adolesc. Psychopharmacol. 2005, 15, 619–627, doi:10.1089/cap.2005.15.619.

47. di Girolamo, A.M.; Raminez-Zea, M. Role of zinc in maternal and child mental health. Amer. J. Clin. Nutr. 2009, 89, S940–S945, doi:10.3945/ajcn.2008.26692C.

48. Scheplyagina, L.A. Impact of the mother's zinc deficiency on the woman's and new-borns health status. J. Trace Elem. Med. Biol. 2005, 19, 29–35, doi:10.1016/j.jtemb.2005.07.008.

49. Plum, L.M.; Rink, L.; Haase, H. The essential toxin: Impact of zinc on human health. Int. J. Environ. Res. Public Health 2010, 7, 1342–1365, doi:10.3390/ijerph7041342.

50. Yorbik, O.; Akay, C.; Sayal, A.; Cansever, A.; Sohmen, T.; Cavdar, A.O. Zinc status in autistic children. J. Trace Elem. Exp. Med. 2004, 17, 101–107, doi:10.1002/jtra.20002.

51. Fido, A.; Al-Saad, S. Toxic trace elements in the hair of children with autism. Autism 2005, 9, 290–298, doi:10.1177/1362361305053255.

52. Adams, J.B.; Holloway, C.E.; George, F.; Quig, D. Analyses of toxic metals and essential minerals in the hair of Arizona children with autism and associated conditions, and their mothers. Biol. Trace Elem. Res. 2006, 110, 193–209, doi:10.1385/BTER:110:3:193.

53. Faber, S.; Zinn, G.M.; Kern, J.C.; Kingston, H.M. The plasma zinc/serum copper ratio as a biomarker in children with autism spectrum disorders. Biomarkers 2009, 14, 171–180, doi:10.1080/13547500902783747.

54. Priya, M.D.L.; Geetha, A. Level of trace elements (copper, zinc, magnesium and selenium) and toxic elements (lead and mercury) in the hair and nail of children with autism. Biol. Trace Elem. Res. 2011, 142, 148–158, doi:10.1007/s12011-010-8766-2.

55. Gebremedhin, S.; Enquselassie, F.; Umeta, M. Prevalence of prenatal zinc deficiency and its association with socio-demographic, dietary and health care related factors in Rural Sidama, Southern Ethiopia: A cross-sectional study. BMC Public Health 2011, 11, 898–907, doi:10.1186/1471-2458-11-898.

56. Kurita, H.; Ohsako, S.; Hashimoto, S.; Yoshinaga, J.; Tohyama, C. Prenatal zinc deficiency-dependent epigenetic alterations of mouse metallothionein-2 gene. J. Nutr. Biochem. 2013, 24, 256–266, doi:10.1016/j.jnutbio.2012.05.013.

57. Arnold, L.E.; Bozzolo, H.; Hollway, J.; Cook, A.; di Silvestro, R.A.; Bozzolo, D.R.; Crowl, L.; Ramadan, Y.; Williams, C. Serum zinc correlates with parent- and teach-

er- rated inattention in children with attention-deficit/hyperactivity disorder. J. Child Adoles. Psychopharmacol. 2005, 15, 628–636, doi:10.1089/cap.2005.15.628.

58. Yorbik, O.; Ozdag, M.F.; Olgun, A.; Senol, M.G.; Bek, S.; Akman, S. Potential effects of zinc on information processing in boys with attention deficit hyper-activity disorder. Prog. Neuropsychopharmacol. Biol. Psychiatry 2008, 32, 662–667, doi:10.1016/j.pnpbp.2007.11.009.

59. di Girolamo, A.M.; Ramirez-Zea, M.; Wang, M.; Flores-Ayala, R.; Martorell, R.; Neufeld, L.M.; Ramakrishnan, U.; Sellen, D.; Black, M.M.; Stein, A.D. Randomized trial of the effect of zinc supplementation on the mental health of school-age children in Guatemala. Am. J. Clin. Nutr. 2010, 92, 1241–1250, doi:10.3945/ajcn.2010.29686.

60. Akhondzadeh, S.; Mohammadi, M.R.; Khademi, M. Zinc sulfate as an adjunct to methylphenidate for the treatment of attention deficit hyperactivity disorder in children: A double blind and randomised trial [ISRCTN64132371]. BMC Psychiatry 2004, 4, 9–14, doi:10.1186/1471-244X-4-9.

61. Kozielec, T.; Starobrat-Hermelin, B. Assessment of magnesium levels in children with attention deficit hyperactivity disorder (ADHD). Magnes. Res. 1997, 10, 143–148.

62. Starobrat-Hermelin, B.; Kozielec, T. The effects of magnesium physiological supplementation on hyperactivity in children with attention deficit hyperactivity disorder (ADHD). Positive response to magnesium oral loading test. Magnes. Res. 1997, 10, 149–156.

63. Mousain-Bose, M.; Roche, M.; Rapin, J.; Bali, J.P. Magnesium VitB6 intake reduces central nervous system hyperexcitability in children. J. Amer. Coll. Nutr. 2004, 23, S545–S548, doi:10.1080/07315724.2004.10719400.

64. Mousain-Bose, M.; Roche, M.; Polge, A.; Pradal-Prat, D.; Rapin, J.; Bali, J.P. Improvement of neurobehavioral disorders in children supplemented with magnesium-vitanin B6 II. Pervasive developmental disorder-autism. Magnes. Res. 2006, 19, 53–62.

65. Ochi, A.; Ishimura, E.; Tsujimoto, Y.; Kakiya, R.; Tabata, T.; Mori, K.; Fukumoto, S.; Tahara, H.; Shoji, T.; Yasuda, H.; et al. Hair magnesium, but not serum magnesium, is associated with left ventricular wall thickness in hemodialysis patients. Circ. J. 2013, doi:10.1253/circj.CJ-13-0347.

66. Dufner-Beattie, J.; Kuo, Y.M.; Gitschier, J.; Andrews, G.K. The adaptive response to dietary zinc in mice involves the differential cellular localization and zinc regulation of the zinc transporters ZIP4 and ZIP5. J. Biol. Chem. 2004, 279, 49082–49090, doi:10.1074/jbc.M409962200.

67. Lichten, L.A.; Cousins, R.J. Mammalian zinc transporters: Nutritional and physiologic regulation. Ann. Rev. Nutr. 2009, 29, 153–176, doi:10.1146/annurev-nutr-033009-083312.

68. Goyer, R.A. Toxic and essential metal interactions. Ann. Rev. Nutr. 1997, 17, 37–50, doi:10.1146/annurev.nutr.17.1.37.

69. Mahaffey, K.R.; Gartside, P.S.; Glueck, C.J. Blood lead levels and dietary calcium intake in 1 to 11 year-old children: The second national health and nutrition examination survey, 1976 to 1980. Pediatrics 1986, 78, 257–262.

70. Shannon, M.; Graef, J.W. Lead intoxication in children with pervasive developmental disorders. J. Toxicol. Clin. Toxicol. 1996, 34, 177–181, doi:10.3109/15563659609013767.

71. Eubig, P.A.; Agular, A.; Schantz, S.L. Lead and PCBs as risk factors for attention deficit/hyperactivity disorder. Environ. Health Perspect. 2010, 118, 1654–1667, doi:10.1289/ehp.0901852.

72. Centers for Disease Control and Prevention (CDC). CDC National Surveillance Data (1997–2009), National Centers for Environmental Health 2012. Available online: http://www.cdc.gov/nceh/lead/data/national.htm. (accessed on 6 November 2013).

73. Jones, R.L.; Homa, D.M.; Meyer, P.A.; Brody, D.J.; Caldwell, K.L.; Pirkle, J.L.; Brown, M.J. Trends in blood lead levels and blood testing among US children aged 1 to 5 years, 1988–2004. Pediatrics 2009, 123, 376–385, doi:10.1542/peds.2007-3608.

74. Advisory Committee on Childhood Lead Poisoning Prevention, of the Centers for Disease Control and Prevention. Low Level Lead Exposure Harms Children: A Renewed Call for Primary Prevention: Report to the CDCP; ACCLPP: Atlanta, GA, USA, 2012; pp. 1–54.

75. Needleman, H.L.; Schell, A.; Bellinger, D.; Leviton, A.; Allred, E.N. The long-term effects of exposure to low doses of lead in childhood. An 11-year follow up report. N. Engl. J. Med. 1990, 322, 83–88, doi:10.1056/NEJM199001113220203.

76. Binns, H.J.; Campbell, C.; Brown, M.J. Interpreting and managing blood lead levels of less than 10 micro g/dL in children and reducing childhood exposure to lead: Recommendations of the centers for disease control and prevention advisory committee on childhood lead poisoning prevention. Pediatrics 2007, 120, e1285–e1298, doi:10.1542/peds.2005-1770.

77. Bellinger, D.C. Lead neurotoxicity and socioeconomic status: Conceptual and analytical issues. Neurotoxicology 2008, 29, 828–832, doi:10.1016/j.neuro.2008.04.005.

78. Gump, B.B.; Stewart, P.; Reihman, J.; Lonky, E.; Darvill, T.; Parsons, P.J.; Granger, D.A. Low-level prenatal and postnatal blood lead (Pb) exposure and adrenocortical responses to acute stress in children. Environ. Health Perspect. 2008, 116, 249–255.

79. Nigg, J.T.; Knottnerus, G.M.; Martel, M.M.; Nikoas, M.; Cavanagh, V.; Karmaus, W.; Rappley, M.D. Low blood lead levels associated with clinically diagnosed attention-deficit/hyperactivity disorder and mediated by weak cognitive control. Biol. Psychiatry 2008, 63, 325–331, doi:10.1016/j.biopsych.2007.07.013.

80. Dixon, S.L.; Gaitens, J.M.; Jacobs, D.E.; Strauss, W.; Nagaraja, L.; Pivetz, T.; Wilson, J.W.; Ashley, P.J. Exposure of U.S. children to residential dust lead, 1999–2004: II. The contribution of lead-contaminated dust to children's blood lead levels. Environ. Health Perspect. 2009, 117, 468–474.

81. American Academy of Pediatrics. Lead exposure in children: Prevention, detection, and management: Statement of policy reaffirmation. Psychiatry 2009, 123, 1421–1422.

82. Deocampo, D.M.; Reed, P.J.; Kalenuik, A.P. Road dust lead (Pb) in two neighbourhoods of urban Atlanta, (GA, USA). Int. J. Environ. Res. Public Health 2012, 9, 2020–2030, doi:10.3390/ijerph9062020.

83. Hall, G.; Tinklenberg, J. Determination of Ti, Zn, and Pb in lead-based house paints by EDXRF. J. Anal. At. Spectrom. 2003, 18, 775–778, doi:10.1039/b300597f.

84. Lewis, P.A. Inorganic Colored Pigments. In Paint and Coating Testing Manual, 14th ed.; Koleske, J.V., Ed.; ASTM: West Conshohocken, PA, USA, 1995; pp. 1–950.

85. Symanski, E.; Hertz-Picciotto, I. Blood lead levels in relation to menopause, smoking, and pregnancy history. Amer. J. Epidemiol. 1995, 141, 1047–1058.

86. Razagui, I.B.; Ghribi, I. Maternal and neonatal scalp hair concentrations of zinc, cadmium, and lead: Relationship to some lifestyle factors. Biol. Trace Elem. Res. 2005, 106, 1–28, doi:10.1385/BTER:106:1:001.

87. Gulson, B.L.; Jameson, C.W.; Mahaffey, K.R.; Mizon, K.J.; Korsch, M.J.; Vimpani, G. Pregnancy increases mobilization of lead from maternal skeleton. J. Lab. Clin. Med. 1997, 130, 51–62, doi:10.1016/S0022-2143(97)90058-5.

88. Sanders, A.P.; Flood, K.; Chiang, S.; Herring, A.H.; Wolf, L.; Fry, R.C. Towards prenatal biomonitoring in North Carolina: Assessing arsenic, cadmium, mercury and lead levels in pregnant women. PLoS One 2012, 7, e31354, doi:10.1371/journal.pone.0031354.

89. Parajuli, R.P.; Fujiwara, T.; Umezaki, M.; Watanabe, C. Association of cord blood levels of lead, arsenic, and zinc with neurodevelopmental indicators in newborns: A birth cohort study in Chitwan Valley, Nepal. Environ. Res. 2012, 10, 509–519.

CHAPTER 9

URINARY PORPHYRIN EXCRETION IN NEUROTYPICAL AND AUTISTIC CHILDREN

JAMES S. WOODS, SARAH E. ARMEL, DENISE I. FULTON, JASON ALLEN, KRISTINE WESSELS, P. LYNNE SIMMONDS, DOREEN GRANPEESHEH, ELIZABETH MUMPER5, J. JEFFREY BRADSTREET, DIANA ECHEVERRIA, NICHOLAS J. HEYER, AND JAMES P. K. ROONEY

Porphyrins are formed as intermediates in the biosynthesis of heme, a process that proceeds in essentially all eukaryotic tissues. In humans and other mammals, porphyrins with 8,7,6,5, and 4 carboxyl groups are commonly formed in excess of that required for heme biosynthesis and are excreted in the urine in a well-established pattern (Bowers et al. 1992; Woods et al. 1993). In previous studies we described specific changes in the urinary porphyrin excretion pattern (porphyrin profile) associated with prolonged exposure to mercury (Hg) in either organic or elemental forms (Pingree et al. 2001a; Woods et al. 1991, 1993). These changes are characterized by dose- and time-related increases in urinary concentrations of

Reproduced with permission from Environmental Health Perspectives. Woods JS, Armel SE, Fulton DI, Allen J, Wessels K, Simmonds PL, Granpeesheh D, Mumper E, Bradstreet JJ, Echeverria D, Heyer NJ, Rooney JPK. Microbial Diversity of Vermicompost Bacteria that Exhibit Useful Agricultural Traits and Waste Management Potential. Environmental Health Perspectives **118** (2010); http://dx.doi.org/10.1289/ehp.0901713

pentacarboxyl (5-carboxyl) and copro- (4-carboxyl) porphyrins and also by the appearance of precoproporphyrin, an atypical porphyrin [molecular weight (mw) = 668] that elutes on high-performance liquid chromatography (HPLC) prior to coproporphyrin (mw = 655) (Woods et al. 1991). The potential utility of these porphyrin changes as a biomarker of Hg exposure and body burden in adults with occupational exposure to elemental mercury (Hg^0) has been described (Bowers et al. 1992; Gonzalez-Ramirez et al. 1995; Woods 1995; Woods et al. 1993)

Autism (AU), or autistic spectrum disorder (ASD), represents a serious neurodevelopmental disorder that afflicts as many as 1 in 110 children in the United States (Rice 2009). Although genetic factors likely play a principal role in the etiology of autism, a number of studies suggest that environmental exposures, occurring especially at critical periods of neurological development, may trigger events etiologic in AU/ASD among some children. In this respect, several reports (Kern et al. 2007; Mutter et al. 2005; Windham et al. 2006) have implicated prenatal and/or postnatal Hg exposure as associated with autism, in terms of frequency of exposure as well as total body burden. Notably, important mechanistic and toxicokinetic distinctions between different forms of Hg (Burbacher et al. 2005) or in child-specific factors (Faustman et al. 2000) that might affect susceptibility to Hg in autism remain to be fully considered in studies of this association. Nonetheless, some of the neuropsychiatric disturbances associated particularly with Hg^0 exposure, such as cognition and communication deficits, sensory dysfunction, and impaired motor coordination, are notably similar to those observed in autism and ASD (Echeverria et al. 1998; Kolevzon et al. 2007).

In this context, Nataf et al. (2006) reported that a majority of > 100 French children with clinically confirmed autism displayed a urinary porphyrin excretion pattern comparable with that which we have observed in adult subjects with occupational Hg^0 exposure and, moreover, that elevated porphyrin levels in these autistic children declined after chelation treatment, also comparable with that seen in occupationally exposed adults (Gonzalez-Ramirez et al. 1995; Woods et al. 1993). Similar findings have been reported among autistic children in the United States (Geier and Geier 2007) and Australia (Austin and Shandley 2008). Although Hg levels or exposure histories of the children involved in those studies were not reported, the precise change in the porphyrin excretion pattern that we observed in association with occupational Hg^0 exposure in adult subjects implies that exposure to Hg may underlie this response among at least a subset children with autism. A principal concern with respect to these findings, however, is that urinary porphyrin levels in autistic children were commonly evaluated in relation to porphyrin concentrations for older control children or adults, which potentially could be misleading in light of finding that urinary porphyrin concentrations vary substantially with age among children and adolescents (Woods et al. 2009b). Moreover, no reference ranges for all typically excreted porphyrins for children < 8 years of age are currently available. Of additional concern is the common attribution in those studies of elevated porphyrins levels observed among autistic children to increased metal body burden when, in fact, direct measures of metal exposure were not reported.

We undertook the present exploratory study to address several issues associated with the use of urinary porphyrin changes as a diagnostic biomarker of Hg exposure among children and, in particular, those with autism. As the first objective, we measured urinary porphyrin concentrations for neurotypical (NT) children between 2 and 12 years of age against which porphyrin levels in same-age autistic children could be compared. Additionally, we sought to determine if differences in urinary porphyrin levels existed between NT and autistic children of the same age and, if so, if they were consistent with recent Hg exposure as assessed by urinary Hg levels and/or past Hg exposure determined from information acquired online at the time of registration.

9.1 MATERIALS AND METHODS

The study population. The principal source of subjects for this study was approximately 600 families with autistic children who subscribe to the informational services of the Autism Research Institute (ARI), Lacey, Washington (USA). We recruited a convenience sample of subjects [NT, AU, and pervasive developmental disorder-not otherwise specified (PDD-NOS) children, ages 2–12 years] into the study via a flyer and sent instructions by the study coordinator at the ARI to all subscribing ARI families, informing them about the study and inviting them to participate. The flyer directed interested parents/caregivers to respond by e-mail or telephone regarding their interest in participating. The study coordinator then contacted interested parents to describe the study and obtain consent. Consenting participants were asked to complete an online enrollment form and to provide a urine sample from the child/children in their families. The estimated participation rate for the ARI was 37%.

The online enrollment form contained detailed questions pertaining to the child's diagnosis, including diagnostic criteria, diagnosing facility, name of diagnosing clinician, month/year of diagnosis, and diagnostic procedure(s) used. Additional questions were asked regarding dietary practices, drug exposures including chelation history, dental amalgam history, and child's inoculation history. The number of vaccinations was collected as a potential source of Hg exposure; a distinction was made between total vaccinations and vaccinations prior to the year 2002 when thimerosal, a preservative containing an organomercurial moiety, was eliminated from many vaccines. In addition, to estimate maternal exposures to Hg during the 9 months of the index pregnancy, a count of dental amalgam tooth fillings (a potential source of Hg0 exposure) and an estimate of fish meals per week (a potential source of methylmercury exposure) for the mother were obtained for this time period.

Urine samples were collected in the home, transferred to the ARI by hand, and assigned a coded identification (ID) number by the ARI. They were then sent to the University of Washington for analysis, identified only by ID number, age, sex, and diagnosis. Data derived from these studies were evaluated in relation to the diagnostic information provided online to establish mean porphyrin levels for NT children and to determine the association of urinary porphyrin concentrations with autism or related neurobehavioral disorders.

To augment the number of subjects for whom porphyrin comparisons could be made, we analyzed porphyrin concentrations in urine samples acquired from an additional 41 subjects recruited through the Center for Autism and Related Disorders (CARD) in Tarzana, California, and 24 subjects, also through the CARD, from the Rimland Center for Integrative Medicine in Lynchburg, Virginia. CARD subjects were restricted to 2- to 12-year-old NT or AU males who had never undergone chelation treatment and were without amalgam dental fillings. CARD subjects were recruited prior to the initiation of the ARI study and hence did not complete the online enrollment questionnaire used by ARI participants. The estimated participation rate for the CARD was 31%.

TABLE 1: Distributions for all subjects.

Total Subjects	NT (n = 117)	AU (n = 100)	PDD (n = 27)	Other (n = 34)	Total (n = 278)
Males	61 (52)	93 (93)	22 (81)	25 (74)	201 (72)
Females	56 (48)	7 (7)	5 (19)	8 (24)	77 (28)
Chelated	3 (3)	36 (36)	8 (30)	8 (24)	55 (20)
Age (years)	6.67 ± 2.96	6.33 ± 2.36	6.88 ± 3.07	7.78 ± 2.60	6.70 ± 2.75

Values are n (%) or mean ± SD

Methods of subject recruitment as well as timing and manner of urine collection and processing were comparable between the CARD and ARI cohorts, and preliminary analyses of mean urinary porphyrin and Hg levels by subject source indicated no significant differences within age groupings. Therefore, data from both sources were pooled for porphyrin and Hg analyses. Overall, we enrolled 278 children in the study. After 55 children who had been previously chelated were excluded, 197 children were eligible for analysis. Final statistical models were performed using males only and included 59 NT, 59 AU, and 15 PDD-NOS subjects.

Human subjects considerations. The study protocol was approved by the institutional review boards at the University of Washington and the CARD. Human subjects approval of the ARI was conferred via an individual investigator agreement between the study coordinator at the ARI and the University of Washington. All parents/caretakers gave written consent for themselves and their children prior to enrollment in the study.

Diagnostic procedures. For children enrolled through the ARI, diagnosis of autism or other neurodevelopmental disorder was performed by established autism diagnostic and treatment centers that included the University of Washington Autism Center, the Seattle Children's Autism Center [formerly the Autism Spectrum Treatment and Research Center

(ASTAR)], and other pediatric neurology clinics throughout the Pacific Northwest. The diagnosis of AU, PDD-NOS, or other disorder at these centers was made using a multidisciplinary approach that combines a clinical evaluation using the Diagnostic and Statistical Manual of Mental Disorders, 4th Edition, Text Revision (DSM-IV-TR) (American Psychiatric Association 2000) criteria, along with a psychological evaluation using the Autism Diagnostic Observation Schedule (ADOS) (Lord et al. 2000), and other established diagnostic procedures such as the Autism Diagnostic Interview-Revised (Lord et al. 1994) or the Childhood Autism Rating Scale (Schopler et al. 1993). Verification of AU status by further psychological testing of children enrolled through the ARI was not feasible in this study. However, comparison of dates of AU diagnosis revealed that > 90% of subjects had been diagnosed since 2003, that is, within the immediate 5-year period since inception of this study, supporting continuity in the methods and procedures used and, therefore, homogeneity in the AU diagnosis. These observations further serve to verify the distinction between diagnoses of AU and other neurodevelopmental disorders, particularly PDD-NOS, as the same testing procedures and treatment centers were employed to diagnose PDD-NOS, most also occurring since 2003. No subjects were diagnosed before 2001.

For subjects enrolled through the CARD, all diagnosed children were fully evaluated by a trained psychologist and met the International Classification of Diseases, 9th Revision (World Health Organization 1975) and DSM-IV-TR (American Psychiatric Association 2000) criteria for autism. All diagnoses were verified by obtaining copies of the diagnoses and subsequently validated by additional evaluations at the CARD using the ADOS and other diagnostic procedures cited above.

Participants recruited through the ARI were invited to enroll children with a previous diagnosis of autism or other neurodevelopmental disorder as well as their typically developing siblings. Children whose parents responded "No" to the question "Is this child diagnosed with any neurodevelopmental disorder?" were designated NT. However, verification of NT status through further psychological testing of children enrolled through this process was not conducted. NT subjects enrolled through the CARD were children of CARD employees, all of whom were trained observers and aware of their children's development. In this respect, all children designated as NT met all developmental milestones, had no symptoms of ASD, ADHD (attention deficit hyperactivity disorder), or (other) learning disabilities, and were seen to be performing successfully in school or preschool with normal peer play. Opportunities for misclassification, therefore, were minimal. The possibility exists that siblings may differ from unrelated controls from the same source population in their genetic contribution to specific inherited disorders such as those affecting porphyrin metabolism. We note in this regard that genetic variation in porphyrin metabolism, particularly that affecting urinary porphyrin excretion, is exceedingly rare especially within the U.S. population, affecting, in the case of the most prevalent form, < 1 in 100,000 individuals (0.001%) (Health Grades, Inc. 2010). Although the absence of differences in genetic variance in related and unrelated NT subjects in this study was not verified, it is unlikely that siblings and unrelated controls differed significantly in this respect.

Procedures for urine collection and measurement of urinary porphyrins, Hg, and creatinine concentrations. Urine samples (~ 50 mL, first or second morning voids when possible) were collected by parents/caregivers in clean glass containers and then transferred to Nalgene Nunc 60-mL, wide-mouth polyethylene bottles with screw-on lids (Item 2106–0002; Fisher Scientific, Seattle, WA). Samples were delivered frozen to the ARI, where they were logged, assigned an ID number, and shipped in batch in frozen ice packs by overnight express service to the University of Washington. A comparable protocol was followed by the CARD. For analyses, a 10-mL aliquot was removed and acidified with 1 N HCl for Hg analysis by continuous-flow, cold-vapor spectrofluorometry (Pingree et al. 2001b). Porphyrins were quantified in the remaining unacidified portion of the urine sample by HPLC-spectrofluorometric analysis, as previously described (Bowers et al. 1992; Woods et al. 1991). Urinary creatinine concentrations were also measured in unacidified urine using a standard colorimetric procedure (Sigma, St. Louis, MO, USA). Urinary porphyrin concentrations were first creatinine adjusted (nanomoles per gram) and then transformed using the natural logarithm because of the wide variation and skewed distribution. Hg values below the detection limit (LOD) (0.02 μg/L) were assigned $LOD/\sqrt{-2}$.

TABLE 2: Demographic and potential risk factors among nonchelated subjects in study.

Nonchelated subjects	Sex	NT (n = 114)	AU (n = 64)	PDD (n = 19)	Total (n = 197)
No.	M	59 (52)	59 (92)	15 (79)	133 (67)
	F	55 (48)	5 (8)	4 (21)	64 (33)
Age (years)	M	6.39 ± 3.06	6.01 ± 2.14	6.16 ± 3.03	6.19 ± 2.67
	F	6.93 ± 2.85	4.60 ± 1.82	8.73 ± 4.98	6.86 ± 3.00
Urinary Hg (µg/L)	M	0.29 ± 0.53	0.36 ± 0.62	0.27 ± 0.26	0.32 ± 0.55
	F	0.21 ± 0.45	0.09 ± 0.10	0.30 ± 0.48	0.21 ± 0.43
Urinary Hg (µg/g creatinine)	M	0.28 ± 0.43	0.40 ± 0.66	0.32 ± 0.33	0.34 ± 0.53
	F	0.21 ± 0.48	0.12 ± 0.14	0.29 ± 0.51	0.21 ± 0.46
Creatinine (g/Lr)	M	1.01 ± 0.48	0.95 ± 0.38	0.96 ± 0.41	0.98 ± 0.43
	F	1.03 ± 0.40	0.86 ± 0.30	1.51 ± 0.75	1.04 ± 0.43
Amalgams in child	M	0.18 ± 0.6	0.20 ± 1.1	0.53 ± 1.3	0.25 ± 0.9
	F	0.23 ± 1.2	0.0 ± 0.0	0.0 ± 0.0	0.19 ± 1.1
Amalgams in mother when pregnant	M	2.9 ± 4.2	4.3 ± 5.3	4.0 ± 4.4	3.6 ± 4.6
	F	4.1 ± 4.6	4.6 ± 2.7	3.7 ± 0.6	4.2 ± 4.3
Total vaccines	M	6.5 ± 6.9	10.1 ± 7.8	6.5 ± 6.9	7.9 ± 7.4
	F	8.9 ± 7.1	12.2 ± 3.3	5.8 ± 8.0	8.9 ± 6.9
Vaccines before 2002	M	3.5 ± 5.2	1.8 ± 3.9	1.5 ± 4.1	2.5 ± 4.6
	F	4.1 ± 5.5	2.0 ± 3.5	0.0 ± 0.0	3.6 ± 5.2
Restricted diet (%)	M	24	48	60	41
	F	25	80	100	36
Eat fish (%)	M	59	40	25	55
	F	70	58	53	62

Values are n(%), mean ± SD, or %

Statistical procedures. Statistical analyses were conducted using PASW Statistics 17.0 (formerly SPSS) (Chicago, IL). Descriptive assessments first eliminated statistical outliers (values ≥ 3 SD in both directions) and then used cross-tabulations and one-way analysis of variance (ANOVA) procedures to compare nonchelated children from the three confirmed diagnostic groups [AU (n = 64), PDD-NOS (n = 19), and NT (n = 114)] with regard to sex, age, potential sources of Hg exposure, and mean (± SD) urinary Hg and porphyrin levels. The small number of five females in the AU group precluded subsequent statistical analyses for each sex. Thus, we examined potential determinants of diagnostic status among only the 133 male children (59 AU, 15 PDD-NOS, and 59 NT).

In males, logistic regression models that controlled for age initially tested potential associations between diagnosis and sources of exposure to Hg from the number of dental amalgam tooth fillings in the child and the mother, the number of vaccines that the child was reported to have received, the number of fish meals per month, and urinary Hg concentrations. The mean (± SD) of each porphyrin was also stratified by diagnosis, age, and sex, where an ANOVA F-test was applied separately for each sex to identify statistically significant differences between diagnostic groups.

Logistic regression analyses were also used to evaluate potential associations among males between porphyrins and the risk of having a diagnosis of AU or PDD-NOS, using NT as controls. Statistical measures included regression coefficients, their SDs, and estimates of the strength of association expressed as odds ratios (ORs) and 95% confidence intervals (CIs) for each porphyrin model. A statistically significant association was accepted if $p < 0.05$. Apart from the expected effect of age and age-squared, which were retained in final models, the only covariate that approached statistical significance was a restricted diet ($p < 0.065$). This variable was more reasonably attributed to response to diagnosis rather than to etiology or causal association and therefore was not retained in the analyses. The analyses also evaluated the combination of the three lesser carboxyl porphyrins (hexa-, penta-, and copro-) for potential association with AU or PDD-NOS. Urinary porphyrin concentrations corrected for creatinine (nanomoles per gram), along with the natural logs of these values, were tested in the analyses.

9.2 RESULTS

The study population. Table 1 describes the demographic distributions for the study population by diagnosis category. Among all children enrolled, 278 had urinary measures of porphyrins and Hg. Among these subjects,

117 were determined to have NT development, 100 met the criteria for AU, and 27 were determined to have PDD-NOS. An additional 34 had other neurodevelopmental diagnoses that included Rett syndrome (n = 1), Asperger's syndrome (n = 4), attention deficit hypersensitivity disorder (ADD/ADHD) (n = 12), sensory integration disorder (n = 5), and language and speech delay (n = 3). Fifty-five subjects had undergone chelation therapy, including 3 NT, 36 AU, 8 PDD-NOS, and 8 other. Only the 197 children who had not been chelated and who had diagnoses of NT, AU, or PDD-NOS were included in further analyses, depicted in Table 2. Only five AU and four PDD-NOS cases were girls, consistent with the much lower frequency of autism and related disorders among females. Therefore, although female subjects are included in descriptive analyses of porphyrin levels (Table 3), they were not included in the logistic regression analyses. Thus, logistic regression analyses (Table 4) were conducted among the group of 133 male children that included 59 AU, 15 PDD-NOS, and 59 NT.

As noted in Table 2, age distributions by diagnosis were similar among male subjects. In addition, most covariates were not statistically different between diagnostic groups. In particular, mean urinary past Hg levels, whether unadjusted (micrograms per liter) or adjusted for creatinine (micrograms per gram), were not significantly different between groups. This was also true for the potential sources of Hg exposure, including the mean number of amalgam fillings (both currently in the child or in the mother over the course of pregnancy) and the mean sum of vaccines administered to the child in total, or before 2002.

Urinary porphyrin concentrations in children. The distribution of six urinary porphyrins is presented in Table 3 and Figures 1 and 2. Table 3 presents the mean (± SD) creatinine-adjusted porphyrin concentrations by sex for all nonchelated NT and AU subjects. Values were stratified by 2-year age groups between 2 and 12 years of age. Figures 1 and 2 show the variation in these porphyrin levels by age for males only.

Average concentrations of most porphyrins were elevated in two NT male subjects < 2 years of age compared with older NT males (Table 3). No AU children < 2 years of age were included in the study. Among males in the 2- to 12-year age groups, the mean concentrations of hexacarboxyl- ($p < 0.01$), pentacarboxyl- ($p < 0.001$), and copro- ($p < 0.009$) porphyrins

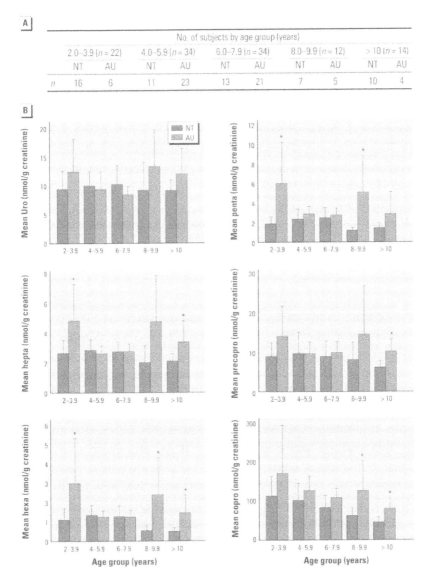

FIGURE 1: Distributions of urinary porphyrins by age (mean and 95% CI). (A) Table describes number of subjects by age group. (B) Bar graphs represent mean and 95% CIs of individual creatinine-adjusted urinary porphyrins (nmol/g) by age group for nonchelated NT (n = 57) and AU (n = 59) boys, age 2–12 years. Graphs depict substantial excess and variable excretion of most porphyrins among AU compared with NT. Porphyrins were evaluated as described under "Materials and Methods." *NT significantly (p ≤ 0.05) different from same-age AU.

were significantly higher among AU compared with NT groups based on ANOVA F-test values, whereas the heptacarboxyl porphyrin was more of borderline significance ($p < 0.06$). Uro- and precoproporphyrins did not differ significantly between AU and NT groups.

We observed substantial variation in creatinine-adjusted urinary porphyrin levels among AU males as well as decreasing concentrations of heptacarboxyl-, hexacarboxyl-, pentacarboxyl-, and coproporphyrins with increasing age among NT males (Figure 1). Scatterplots with simple linear regression fit lines show inverse associations between age and porphyrins among NT males, while also demonstrating that this pattern is disrupted among those with AU (Figure 2).

Urinary porphyrins and risk of autism. Logistic regression models of age-adjusted associations between porphyrin levels and AU, AU plus PDD-NOS, and PDD-NOS alone (all vs. NT) in males indicated significant associations of hexacarboxyl-, pentacarboxyl-, and coproporphyrins with AU (Table 4). A one-unit increase in the natural log of the creatinine-adjusted value for coproporphyrin is associated with a 2-fold risk for AU (OR = 2.03; 95% CI, 1.15–3.57). Similar associations were observed with pentacarboxyl porphyrin (OR = 2.36; 95% CI, 1.3–4.07) and with hexacarboxyl-, pentacarboxyl-, and coproporphyrins combined (OR = 2.38; 95% CI, 1.42–3.97). In contrast, porphyrin levels did not differ between PDD-NOS and NT males in this study; consequently, combining PDD-NOS and AU subjects weakened associations. Thus, this analysis seems to indicate that AU is a distinct entity from PDD-NOS in terms of being associated with altered porphyrin excretion. Alternatively, too few PDD-NOS subjects were available to this exploratory study to demonstrate an association with PDD-NOS as a less markedly affected portion of the autistic spectrum. Further studies involving greater numbers of subjects with PDD-NOS as well as other recognized disorders of the autistic spectrum are required to determine the extent to which the strength of the association varies with the degree of ASD. Urinary Hg and other Hg-related measures were not significantly associated with AU based on logistic models with and without adjustment for porphyrins (data not shown).

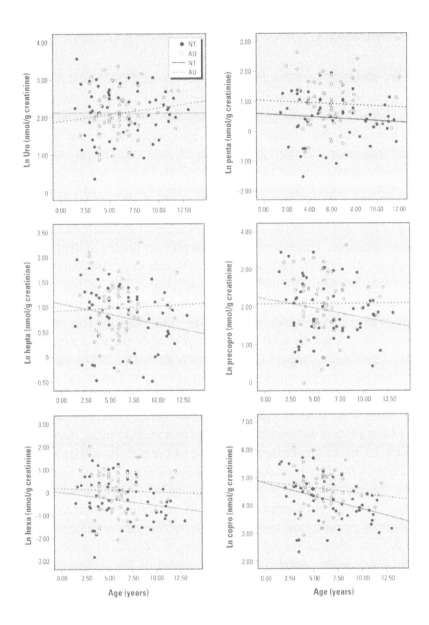

FIGURE 2: Association between urinary porphyrins and age. Scatterplots and simple linear regression fit lines of natural logs of individual creatinine-adjusted urinary porphyrins by age group for nonchelated NT (n = 57) and AU (n = 59) boys, age 2–12 years. Graphs clearly depict decreasing porphyrin concentrations with age among NT and disruption of that effect among AU.

9.3 DISCUSSION

Urinary porphyrins are naturally elevated in young children. We describe here mean urinary porphyrin concentrations for children in the age range of 2–12 years who participated in the present study. Of particular note is the observation that younger children have inherently higher porphyrin concentrations, particularly of uro-, hepta-, and coproporphyrins, which decline by as much as 2.5 times over the 2- to 12-year age range. Also of interest is the finding that precoproporphyrin, an atypical porphyrin previously identified only in adult humans and animals with prolonged exposure to Hg or Hg compounds, is present in substantial concentrations in urine of younger children. This is a novel and unexpected finding in light of previous observations from studies in animals (Woods et al. 1991) showing that precoproporphyrin is formed as a consequence of Hg inhibition of uroporphyrinogen decarboxylase in the kidney during prolonged exposure, producing excess pentacarboxylporphyrinogen, which then competes with coproporphyrinogen as a substrate for coproporphyrinogen oxidase as the basis of precoproporphyrin formation (Woods et al. 2005). The etiology of this atypical porphyrin in the urine of young children in the presumed absence of prolonged Hg exposure as observed here remains unknown. One possible explanation may be the consequence of accelerated hepatic heme biosynthesis that occurs during the period of perinatal development (Woods 1976). In this respect, formation of precoproporphyrin would be consistent with the observation that the specific activity of hepatic uroporphyrinogen decarboxylase in perinatal rat liver greatly exceeds that of the adult (Woods and Kardish 1983), likely generating comparably greater amounts of pentacarboxylporphyrinogen to compete with coproporphyrinogen as a substrate for coproporphyrinogen oxidase, as proposed in the etiology of precoproporphyrin in the presence of Hg exposure in adults (Woods et al. 2005). Further research is required to confirm this prospect.

   Comparison of urinary porphyrins in NT and AU children. Our findings suggest that mean concentrations of uro- and precoproporphyrins are comparable between NT and AU children of the same age ranges. In contrast, the concentrations of all remaining porphyrins, particularly hexacarboxyl-, pentacarboxyl-, and coproporphyrins, were significantly higher in AU children than NT children, especially in older age groups. Several possibilities might account for these differences. Of initial concern, Hg exposure appears unlikely to play a role in this effect, because no significant differences were observed between NT and AU subjects for indices of past exposure to Hg from dental or medical sources, as reported by parents/ caregivers. Additionally, urinary Hg concentrations, measures of recent Hg exposure, were very low among all subjects in this study (Table 2), and no significant differences between diagnostic groups were observed. As noted recently (Woods et al. 2009a), incipient although statistically nonsignificant changes in urinary porphyrin concentrations were seen among children with urinary Hg concentrations derived from prolonged dental amalgam Hg exposure on the order of 3.2 µg/g creatinine. This is nearly 10 times the mean urinary Hg concentration observed among children in this study. Similar findings describing very low blood Hg levels and insignificant differences between NT and AU children have recently been reported (Hertz-Picciotto et al. 2010). These observations do not preclude a possible role of Hg exposure from sources not measured or validated in the present study, especially during the perinatal period, in the etiology of autism or related neurodevelopmental disorders in some children, particularly in relation to genetic variation that may predispose to increased risk of the neurotoxic effects of Hg as Hg0 as reported in adults (Echeverria et al. 2005, 2006, 2010; Heyer et al. 2009). Our findings indicate instead that porphyrin metabolism, particularly in preadolescent children, may be too disordered or differently regulated to permit detection of the Hg-mediated changes in urinary porphyrin excretion apparent in adult subjects. Further studies using a substantially larger population, such as the National Children's Study now in progress (National Children's Study 2010), are required to resolve this question.

Another factor that may account for the differences in urinary porphyrin levels between AU and NT children is mitochondrial dysfunction, a disorder commonly associated with autism (Correia et al. 2006; Oliveira et al. 2005; Pons et al. 2004). Of particular interest in this respect is the prospect of deficient mitochondrial porphyrin uptake mediated by the recently identified mammalian mitochondrial porphyrin transporter Abcb6 (Krishnamurthy et al. 2006). Abcb6, one of several identified ATP-binding cassette transporters, is located in the outer mitochondrial membrane and has a particularly high affinity for coproporphyrinogen III. Defects in Abcb6 gene expression or in Abcb6 activity could predispose to impaired mitochondrial porphyrin uptake, leading to cellular accumulation and aberrant porphyrin metabolism and excretion. Similarly, defects in the mitochondrial transmembrane domain that mediates the binding of porphyrins with the Abcb6 transporter could restrict normal porphyrin metabolism, contributing to the disordered porphyrin excretion observed (Krishnamurthy et al. 2006, 2007). Although the association of Abcb6 with autism has yet to be investigated, numerous validated missense mutations of the Abcb6 gene have been reported (National Center for Biotechnology Information 2010).

Finally, although genetic susceptibility studies were not included as part of the present investigation, previous studies identified a polymorphism in the gene encoding corproporphyrinogen oxidase (CPOX, EC 1.3.3.3) (Li and Woods 2009; Woods et al. 2005) that may predispose to impaired heme biosynthesis and subsequent heme-dependent neurological functions (Chernova et al. 2006; Echeverria et al. 2006). Genotyping studies of 100 DNA samples from autistic children acquired through the University of Washington Autism Center revealed more than double the expected frequency of the homozygous variant of this polymorphism (CPOX4) (rs1131857). An intriguing notion rests on the possibility that mitochondrial respiratory chain disorder associated with CPOX4, which itself is linked to the mitochondrial inner membrane (Grandchamp et al. 1978), could account for exaggerated porphyrin excretion as observed here among at least a subgroup of those with autism. Future studies involving a larger cohort of subjects are required to confirm these findings and to define the genetic and/or metabolic factors associated with altered porphyrin excretion in autism.

Strengths and limitations. A principal limitation of this exploratory study is the relatively small population of NT and AU subjects among whom we sought to define and differentiate excretion levels of metabolites (urinary porphyrins) that can exhibit substantial intraindividual (e.g., diurnal) and interindividual variability, especially in children. Despite this shortcoming, the findings demonstrate significant differences both with age among NT and between NT and AU of the same age, suggesting disordered porphyrin excretion as a metabolic characteristic among at least some AU subjects. Although these findings must be confirmed through larger studies, these preliminary observations provide a context for better understanding and interpreting altered porphyrin excretion among children with AU/ASD.

An additional limitation is potential misclassification of case (AU) or control (NT) status for subjects enrolled through the ARI. We view the possibility of AU misclassification as unlikely, however, because of the multidisciplinary evaluation protocol employed by the neurodevelopmental diagnostic and treatment centers from which subjects were recruited. We note also likely continuity in the diagnostic procedures employed for most subjects enrolled in the study, supporting homogeneity in the AU, PDD-NOS, and NT diagnoses. Nonetheless, our inability to confirm each diagnosis by outside review of subjects' records is a potential limitation of the present exploratory investigation. Future studies in which subjects are identified through established registries such as the Autism Treatment Network (2010) or that developed by the CHARGE study (Hertz-Picciotto et al. 2006) will minimize prospects of this concern.

Although we made direct measurements of urinary Hg levels as indices of recent Hg exposure, there was the potential for measurement error based on participants' recall of past Hg exposures from dietary, medical, and dental sources, which could not be fully validated in this study. Such exposures may be of concern in relation to perinatal events that can be accurately assessed only in the context of a prospective study design. Moreover, potential exposures to Hg from other environmental or occupational sources were not assessed and therefore could not be controlled in the present analysis. Thus, although we found few significant differences between AU and NT in reported measures of past Hg exposure, the possibility of exposure misclassification remains a limitation of this study.

Principal strengths of this study were the availability of urine samples for porphyrin and Hg analyses from all study participants and our established capabilities for accurately measuring and interpreting these constituents in the context of this study. Notably, the urinary porphyrin levels reported herein among NT children ≥ 8 years of age are comparable with normative values recently described for children and adolescents of the same ages who were participants in a large clinical trial (Woods et al. 2009b), supporting the generalizability of these findings. The urinary Hg levels measured in this study were also comparable with those reported for a nationally representative sample of children 6–11 years of age acquired as part of the 2003–2004 U.S. National Health and Nutrition Examination Survey [geometric mean = 0.245; 95% CI, 0.213–0.304) (Centers for Disease Control and Prevention 2007)]. Finally, despite the small number of cases, the results were consistent across age groups with significant differences in porphyrin levels between the diagnostic groups, suggesting that further consideration of this observation may be warranted.

9.4 CONCLUSIONS

Mean urinary porphyrin concentrations are inherently high in young children compared with those in adults and decline by as much as 2.5 times between ages 2 and 12 years. Coproporphyrin and heptacarboxyl-, hexacarboxyl-, and pentacarboxylporphyrins were generally elevated among autistic children compared with NT children of the same age. Elevated porphyrin levels among AU children were not associated with measures of past or current Hg exposure, and a porphyrin pattern consistent with that seen in adults with prolonged Hg exposure was not apparent. These findings suggest that disordered porphyrin metabolism may be a salient characteristic of autism and encourage further investigation of genetic, metabolic, and/or environmental factors that may explain this association.

REFERENCES

1. American Psychiatric Association 2000. Diagnostic and Statistical Manual of Mental Disorders. 4th ed. Text Revision. Washington, DC:American Psychiatric Press.
2. Austin DW, Shandley K. 2008. An investigation of porphyrinuria in Australian children with autism. J Toxicol Environ Health 71:1349–1351.
3. Autism Treatment Network 2010. Homepage. Available: http://www.autismspeaks.org/science/programs/atn/index.php#ATN [accessed 22 June 2010]
4. Bowers MA, Aicher LD, Davis HA, Woods JS. 1992. Quantitative determination of porphyrins in rat and human urine and evaluation of urinary porphyrin profiles during mercury and lead exposures. J Lab Clin Med 120:272–281.
5. Burbacher TM, Shen DD, Liberato N, Grant KS, Cernichiari E, Clarkson T. 2005. Comparison of blood and brain mercury levels in infant monkeys exposed to meth-

ylmercury or vaccines containing thimerosal. Environ Health Perspect 113:1015–1021.

6. Centers for Disease Control and Prevention 2007. National Health and Nutrition Examination Survey. Available: http://www.cdc.gov/nchs/nhanes.htm [accessed 21 June 2010]

7. Chernova T, Nicotera P, Smith AG. 2006. Heme deficiency is associated with senescence and causes suppression of N-methyl-D-aspartate receptor subunits expression in primary cortical neurons. Mol Pharmacol 69:697–705.

8. Correia C, Coutinho AM, Diogo L, Grazina M, Marques C, Miguel T, et al. 2006. Brief report: high frequency of biochemical markers for mitochondrial dysfunction in autism: no association with the mitochondrial aspartate/glutamate carrier SLC25A12 gene. J Autism Dev Disord 36:1137–1140.

9. Echeverria D, Aposhian HV, Woods JS, Heyer NJ, Aposhian MM, Bittner AC, et al. 1998. Neurobehavioral effects from exposure to dental amalgam Hg0: new distinctions between recent exposure and Hg body burden. FASEB J 12:971–980.

10. Echeverria D, Woods JS, Heyer NJ, Martin MD, Rholman D, Farin FM, et al. 2010. The association between serotonin transporter gene promoter polymorphism (5-HT-TLPR) and elemental mercury exposure on mood and behavior in humans. J Toxicol Environ Health 73:552–569.

11. Echeverria D, Woods JS, Heyer NJ, Rholman D, Farin FM, Bittner AC Jr, et al. 2005. Chronic low-level mercury exposure, BDNF polymorphism, and associations with memory, attention and motor function. Neurotoxicol Teratol 27:781–796.

12. Echeverria D, Woods JS, Heyer NJ, Rholman D, Farin FM, Li T, et al. 2006. The association between a genetic polymorphism of coproporphyrinogen oxidase, dental mercury exposure, and neurobehavioral response in humans. Neurotoxicol Teratol 28:39–48.

13. Faustman EM, Silbernagel SM, Fenske RA, Burbacher TM, Ponce RA. 2000. Mechanisms underlying children's susceptibility to environmental toxicants. Environ Health Perspect 108: suppl 113–21.

14. Geier DA, Geier MR. 2007. A prospective study of mercury toxicity biomarkers in autistic spectrum disorders. J Toxicol Environ Health 70:1723–1730.

15. Gonzalez-Ramirez D, Maiorino RM, Zuniga-Charles M, Xu ZF, Hurlbut KM, Junco-Munoz P, et al. 1995. Dimaval challenge test for mercury in humans. II. Urinary mercury and porphyrin levels and neurobehavioral testing of dental workers in Monterrey, Mexico. J Pharmacol Exp Ther 272:264–274.

16. Grandchamp B, Phung N, Nordmann Y.. 1978. The mitochondrial localization of coproporphyrinogen III oxidase. Biochem J 176:97–102.

17. Health Grades, Inc 2010. WrongDiagnosis.com. Prevalence and incidence of Porphyria cutanea tarda, familial type. Available: http://www.wrongdiagnosis.com/p/porphyria_cutanea_tarda_familial_type/prevalence.htm [accessed 21 June 2010]

18. Hertz-Picciotto I, Croen LA, Hansen R, Jones CR, van de Water J, Pessah IN. 2006. The CHARGE study: an epidemiologic investigation of genetic and environmental factors contributing to autism. Environ Health Perspect 114:1119–1125.

19. Hertz-Picciotto I, Green PG, Delwiche L, Hansen R, Walker C, Pessah IN. 2010. Blood mercury concentration in CHARGE Study children with and without autism. Environ Health Perspect 118:161–166.

20. Heyer NJ, Echeverria D, Martin MD, Farin FM, Woods JS. 2009. Catechol-O-methyltransferase (COMT) Val158Met functional polymorphism, dental mercury exposure, and self-reported symptoms and mood. J Toxicol Environ Health 72:599–609.

21. Kern JK, Grannemann BD, Trivedi MH, Adams JB. 2007. Sulfhydryl-reactive metals in autism. J Toxicol Environ Health 70:715–721.

22. Kolevzon A, Gross R, Reichenberg A.. 2007. Prenatal and perinatal risk factors for autism. A review and integration of findings. Arch Pediatr Adolesc Med 161:326–333.

23. Krishnamurthy P, Du G, Fukuda Y, Sun D, Sampath J, Mercer KE, et al. 2006. Identification of a mammalian mitochondrial porphyrin transporter. Nature 443:586–589.

24. Krishnamurthy P, Xie T, Schuetz JD. 2007. The role of transporters in cellular heme and porphyrin homeostasis. Pharmacol Ther 114:345–358.

25. Li T, Woods JS. 2009. Cloning, expression, and biochemical properties of CPOX4, a genetic variant of coproporphyrinogen oxidase that affects susceptibility to mercury toxicity in humans. Toxicol Sci 109:228–236.

26. Lord C, Risi S, Lambrecht L, Cook EH Jr, Leventhal BL, DiLavore PC, et al. 2000. The autism diagnostic observation schedule-generic: a standard measure of social and communication deficits associated with the spectrum of autism. J Autism Dev Disord 30:205–223.

27. Lord C, Rutter M, Le Couteur A.. 1994. Autism Diagnostic Interview-Revised: a revised version of a diagnostic interview for caregivers of individuals with possible pervasive developmental disorders. J Autism Dev Disord 24:659–685.

28. Mutter J, Naumann J, Schneider R, Walach H, Haley B.. 2005. Mercury and autism: accelerating evidence? Neuro Endocrinol Lett 26:439–446.

29. Nataf R, Skorupka C, Amet L, Lam A, Sorubgbett A, Lathe R.. 2006. Porphyrinuria in childhood autistic disorder: implications for environmental toxicity. Toxicol Appl Pharmacol 214:99–108.

30. National Center for Biotechnology Information 2010. SNP linked to Gene ABCB6(geneID:10058) Via Contig Annotation. Available: http://www.ncbi.nlm.nih.gov/projects/SNP/snp_ref.cgi?chooseRs=all&go=Go&locusId=10058 [accessed 21 June 2010]

31. National Children's Study 2010. Homepage. Available: http://www.nationalchildrensstudy.gov/Pages/default.aspx [accessed 21 June 2010]

32. Oliveira G, Diogo L, Grazina M, Garcia P, Ataide A, Marques C, et al. 2005. Mitochondrial dysfunction in autism spectrum disorders: a population-based study. Dev Med Child Neurol 47:185–189.

33. Pingree SD, Simmonds PL, Rummel KT, Woods JS. 2001.. Quantitative evaluation of urinary porphyrins as a measure of kidney mercury content and mercury body burden during prolonged methylmercury exposure in rats. Toxicol Sci 61:234–240.

34. Pingree SD, Simmonds PL, Woods JS. 2001.. Effects of 2,3-dimercapto-1-propane-sulfonic acid (DMPS) on tissue and urine mercury levels following prolonged methylmercury exposure in rats. Toxicol Sci 61:224–233.

35. Pons R, Antoni AL, Checcarelli N, Vila MR, Engelstaf K, Sue CM, et al. 2004. Mitochondrial DNA abnormalities and autistic spectrum disorders. J Pediatr 144:81–85.

36. Rice C.. 2009. Prevalence of autistic spectrum disorders–autism and developmental disabilities monitoring network, United States, 2006. MMWR Morb Mortal Wkly Rep 58(SS10):1–20.
37. Windham GC, Zhang L, Gunier R, Croen LA, Grether JK. 2006. Autism spectrum disorders in relation to distribution of hazardous air pollutants in the San Francisco Bay Area. Environ Health Perspect 114:1438–1444.
38. Woods JS. 1976. Developmental aspects of hepatic heme biosynthetic capability and hematotoxicity. Biochem Pharmacol 25:2147–2152.
39. Woods JS. 1995. Porphyrin metabolism as indicator of metal exposure and toxicity. In: Handbook of Experimental Pharmacology: Toxicology of Metals-Biochemical Aspects (Goyer RA, Cherian MG, eds). Vol 115. Berlin:Springer-Verlag. pp. 19–52.
40. Woods JS, Bowers MA, Davis HA. 1991. Urinary porphyrin profiles as biomarkers of trace metal exposure and toxicity: studies on urinary porphyrin excretion patterns in rats during prolonged exposure to methyl mercury. Toxicol Appl Pharmacol 110:464–476.
41. Woods JS, Echeverria D, Heyer NJ, Simmonds PL, Wilkerson J, Farin FM. 2005. The association between genetic polymorphisms of coproporphyrinogen oxidase and an atypical porphyrinogenic response to mercury exposure in humans. Toxicol Appl Pharmacol 206:113–120.
42. Woods JS, Kardish RM. 1983. Developmental aspects of hepatic heme biosynthetic capability and hematotoxicity. II. Studies on uroporphyrinogen decarboxylase. Biochem Pharmacol 32:73–78.
43. Woods JS, Martin MD, Leroux BG, DeRouen TA, Bernardo MF, Luis HS, et al. 2009. . Urinary porphyrin excretion in children with mercury amalgam treatment: findings from the Casa Pia Children's Dental Amalgam Trial. J Toxicol Environ Health 72:891–896.
44. Woods JS, Martin MD, Leroux BG, DeRouen TA, Bernardo MF, Luis HS, et al. 2009. . Urinary porphyrin excretion in normal children and adolescents. Clin Chim Acta 405:104–109.
45. Woods JS, Martin MD, Naleway CA, Echeverria D. 1993. Urinary porphyrin profiles as a biomarker of mercury exposure: studies on dentists with occupational exposure to mercury vapor. J Toxicol Environ Health 40:235–246.
46. World Health Organization 1975. International Classification of Diseases. 9th Revision. Geneva:World Health Organization.

There are two tables that are not available in this version of the article. To view them, please use the citation on the first page of this chapter.

CHAPTER 10

B-LYMPHOCYTES FROM A POPULATION OF CHILDREN WITH AUTISM SPECTRUM DISORDER AND THEIR UNAFFECTED SIBLINGS EXHIBIT HYPERSENSITIVITY TO THIMEROSAL

MARTYN A. SHARPE, TAYLOR L. GIST, AND DAVID S. BASKIN

10.1 INTRODUCTION

Autism spectrum disorder (ASD) is a complex developmental disorder characterized by abnormalities of verbal and nonverbal communication, stereotyped restricted interests, repetitive behavioral patterns, and impairment of socialization. ASD now affects 1 in 88 children in the USA [1, 2]. In Great Britain, the costs of supporting children with ASD amount to be £2.7 bil/yr, while for adults these costs amount to £25 bil/year [3]. Recent studies have estimated that the lifetime cost to care for an individual with an ASD is $3.2 mil [4]. In the USA individuals with ASD have medical expenditures 4.1–6.2x greater than those without ASD, with median ex-

B-Lymphocytes from a Population of Children with Autism Spectrum Disorder and Their Unaffected Siblings Exhibit Hypersensitivity to Thimerosal. © Sharpe MA, Gist TL, and Baskin DS. Journal of Toxicology **2013** (2013); http://dx.doi.org/10.1155/2013/801517. Licensed under Creative Commons Attribution 3.0 Unported License, http://creativecommons.org/licenses/by/3.0/.

penditures being almost 9 times greater [5, 6]. ASD is usually diagnosed before 4 years of age and has a 5 : 1 male to female gender bias. Although it is believed that multiple interacting genetic and environmental factors influence individual vulnerability to ASD, none have been reproducibly identified in more than a fraction of cases. In addition to complex gene-environment interactions, the heterogeneous presentation of behavioral symptoms within the spectrum of autistic disorders suggests a variable and multifactorial pathogenesis.

Mercury. Mercury is a ubiquitous environmental contaminant, that is, transformed into the volatile neurotoxins methylmercury and ethylmercury. In the United States, more than 8500 water bodies in 45 states and territories are listed as impaired for Hg in water, sediments, and/or fish tissue, including many sites lacking a point source of Hg pollution [7]. In addition to the environmental inorganic/organic mercury assaults many children have been exposed to ethylmercury in the form of thimerosal (called thiomersal in the UK, marketed as Merthiolate in the USA) has been used as a preservative agent for vaccines and toxoids [8]. The relationship between thimerosal and ASD has become a very debated topic over the last decade and some researchers have suspected a causal link [9–12]. Large-scale epidemiological surveys have disputed a causal link between ASD and thimerosal exposure [8, 13–16]. The concentration of mercury in the blood of infants and children receiving vaccines with thimerosal has been reported to be very low and without any effects [11]. Therefore, thimerosal is still recommended as a cheap and stable vaccine preservative in some countries.

Mitochondria. Evidence that an underlying mitochondrial encephalopathy is associated with ASD has been produced by a number of studies [17–20], although the connection is not universally accepted [21, 22]. A disturbed bioenergetic metabolism underlying autism has been suggested by the detection of high lactate levels in many ASD patients, indicating a mitochondrial oxidative phosphorylation dysfunction in these children. Reduced levels of respiratory mitochondrial enzymes, ultrastructural mitochondrial abnormalities, and a broad range of mitochondrial DNA mutations suggest a linkage between autism and mitochondrial disorders [2]. In addition, markers indicative of elevated steady state levels of oxidative stress are found in the body fluids of ASD individuals and in vitro cell studies [23–27]. Recent media attention has been focused on the case of Hannah Poling, a young girl with mitochondrial encephalopathy and autistic features, whose parents won compensation under the United States National Vaccine Injury Compensation Program [28]. It is clearly important to know if a subpopulation of children were/are hypersensitive to the toxic effects of mercury and its compounds.

Cell Growth or Cell Death? ASD is a disease associated with a neurological deficit that may be caused by neurodegeneration during development or by a lack of cell growth during brain development, either in utero or post-utero [1]. While some studies have suggested that the brains of children with autism are oversized [29], many have demonstrated diminished populations of cells such as the Purkinje cells in the cerebellum [30], defects in white matter [31], and functional connectivity [32]. A large number of stressors have been implicated as causative agents in ASD, but only two, valproate and thalidomide, have been definitely shown to cause ASD in both humans and in animal models of ASD. What is so interesting about these two very different compounds is that valproate [33, 34] and thalidomide [35–37] both inhibit mammalian cell proliferation. We designed our growth study to identify if there was a differential effect of thimerosal on B-cell growth, drawn from the families with an affected child, compared with the general population.

10.2 MATERIALS AND METHODS

B-cells from ASD individuals, their unaffected fraternal twins, and their unaffected nontwin siblings were obtained from the Autism Genetic Resource Exchange collection (AGRE; Los Angeles, CA, USA). Unaffected sex and age matched external controls were obtained from the Coriell collection (Coriell Cell Repository, Camden, NJ, USA). This design was chosen to allow comparison of the familial ASD genotype with external controls and to also allow comparison between same and different in utero environments on the development of ASD. Many potential environmental triggers of ASD have been examined in a toxicological setting. We have elected to monitor cell growth as our metric so we could identify if ethyl-mercury, in the form of thimerosal, significantly inhibited cell growth in cells drawn from ASD familial genotypes with respect to non-ASD controls.

Cells were grown in 96-well plates where 84 wells were inoculated with 270 μL of 100,000 cells/mL in the presence of 0, 25, 50, 100, 250, 500, and 1000 nM thimerosal. 10 μL of thimerosal was added to each well as an ethanolic solution, some 60 minutes prior to inoculation, and the ethanol was allowed to evaporate. We use one series of 12 wells as internal controls for the assays and these were filled with 270 μL of growth medium. On each plate we grew three ASD, twin, sibling, and Coriell controls at each of the thimerosal concentration. On day 0, 7 plates were inoculated and 6 were placed in an incubator. Each day a plate was removed from the incubator and underwent the following analysis.

LDH Assay. 2 × 30 μL of cell suspension was assayed for the levels of lactate dehydrogenase activity in the absence and presence of detergent [38–40]. The final assay mixture was comprised of 110 mM lactate, 3.35 mM NAD+, 350 μM resazurin and 2.2 units/mL of diaphorase in 3 mM Tris/30 mM HEPES/10 mM NaCl buffer (pH 7.4), and 0.45% Triton X-100 for total LDH. The resorufin formed was measured over the course of 15 minutes in a plate reader using 530/25 nm ex and 590/35 nm em. The rate of resorufin formation is proportional to the level of LDH. Total cellular LDH was recorded in the presence of detergent, whereas dead/dying cells were recorded in the absence of detergent. The relationship between cell numbers and LDH levels is calculated by measuring LDH and comparing this to the number of cells counted in a cell counter.

XTT Assay. 1 × 40 μL of cell suspension was withdrawn to be assayed for mitochondrial function/number using the XTT (2,3-Bis(2-methoxy-4-nitro-5-sulfophenyl)-2H-tetrazolium-5-carboxanilide) assay method [41–43]. This assay consists of adding cell suspension to 40 μL of XTT (1 mg/mL) diluted in media and the XTT is then converted to formazan by the mitochondrial reductase in metabolically intact cells. After 30 minutes of incubation, 40 μL of stop solution (40% SDS in 1 : 1 water : ethanol) was added and the formazan product was measured at 570 minus 650 nm. The signal was quantified using authentic XTT formazan.

ROS Basal/Antioxidant Levels. 4 mL of cell suspension was grown for 5 days in 5 mL wells and then washed in 2xPBS. They were assayed for protein and then resuspended on PBS/15 mM glucose and plated into wells at 30 μL of 0.5 mg/mL. Cells from 96-well plates were washed once in PBS and were diluted to ≈500,000 cells per mL. 2 × 30 μL of cell suspension was assayed for the ability to oxidize 2',7'-dichlorofluorescein diacetate (DCFH-DA). 30 μL of cell suspension was added to 60 μL of 120 uM DCFH-DA in PDB/15 mM glucose, in the presence and absence of 900 μM hydrogen peroxide. The kinetics of dichlorofluorescein generation is monitored at 428/20 nm ex and 528/20 nm em, for 2 hours and for 15 minutes, respectively. The signal is quantified using authentic dichlorofluorescein.

Lactate. 50 μL samples of cell media were acidified using TCA to a final concentration of 400 mM in order to precipitate protein, the plates were then centrifuged, and 40 μL samples were removed and neutralized with 400 mM NaOH. 50 μL aliquots were then removed and added to 50 μL of LDH assay mixture containing 3.1 mM NAD+, 130 uM hydrazine sulphate, and LDH 20.8 U/mL, in PBS. The formation of NADH was monitored at 340–380 nm over 40 minutes.

10.3 RESULTS

10.3.1 REPRESENTATIVE GROWTH CURVES AND THE CALCULATION OF LDH-G50 AND XTT-G50

Figure 1 shows a typical dataset from one family, Family B. Figure 1(a) shows % LDH levels for the ASD, Twin, Sib, and control cells with respect to thimerosal concentration. The arrows indicate the LDH-G50 values, ASD = 314 nM (Black), Twin = 648 nM (Red), Sib = 373 nM (Blue), and Cont = 1000 nM (Green); the same color scheme for each cell line is used throughout this paper. In Figure 1(b), the XTT-G_{50} values obtained using the mitochondrial XTT assay are shown. At <250 nM thimerosal one observes an increase in the levels of XTT reduction compared with the untreated cells. This upregulation is a feature of low thimerosal treatment and is present in >70% of the cells examined. It is also obvious from Figure 1(b) that the calculation of the XTT-G_{50} is problematic when it is >1000 nM, and estimates of XTT-G50 >1000 nM obtained from semilog plots have to be treated with caution. Figure 1(c) shows the percentage of cellular LDH, that is, accessible to lactate (i.e., percentage of dead and dying cells). While the death rate correlates well with both of the G_{50}s, at neither G_{50} concentration is there an equal number of dead and living cells. Thus, thimerosal is inhibiting cell proliferation as well as causing cell death. The LD_{50} for thimerosal in the ASD cells is 680 nM, more than twice the LDH-G_{50} value of 314 nM and a third larger than the XTT-G_{50}. This means that concentrations of thimerosal that do not induce significant cell death can profoundly affect cell proliferation. The cells shown in Figure 1 have a background death rate between 7 and 10%. Increasing this rate to 20% leads to a growth reduction of 60% of the control in the ASD cells, 45% of control in the Twin cells, 25% of control in the Sib cells, and, by projection, to 30% of control in the Coriell control cells. Finally, in Figure 1(d) we show the relationship between cell numbers and XTT reduction rate in the four cells types as a function of thimerosal concentration. These plots exhibit "hockey stick" slopes, where low thimerosal appears to cause the B-cells to restrict their proliferation and use their resources to upregulate their mitochondrial numbers. After this reallocation of resources in response to low levels of thimerosal, there is a steady fall in the cell population which tracks mitochondria function as the concentration of thimerosal is increased.

10.3.2 THE DISTRIBUTION OF THIMEROSAL SENSITIVITY IN THE FOUR CELL TYPES

In Figure 2 the LDH-G_{50}s obtained for all 44 cell lines are shown. It is also apparent that there are two populations of cells: those hypersensitive to thimerosal, like the ASD and Sib shown in Figure 1, and a more robust hyposensitive population, like the Twin and Cont of Figure 1. The population distribution of the LDH-G_{50}, that is, generated by varying thimerosal concentrations is shown in Figure 2, measured on Day 5 postinoculation. In Figure 2(a) we have ranked the color-coded cells in terms of sensitivity to thimerosal and have highlighted four family groups: A, B, C, and D. Underlined letters denote cell lines believed to have a heightened sensitivity to thimerosal. Figure 2(b) shows the distribution of the four cells types within the four quartiles of ranked distribution. It is quite evident

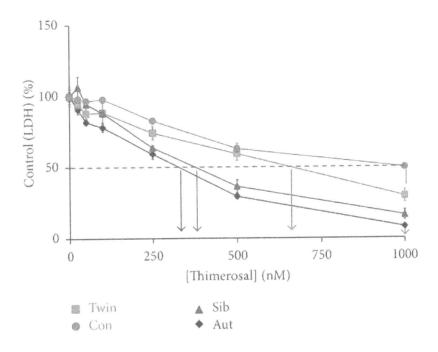

FIGURE 1: This figure shows the typical responses of a family of cells to thimerosal, measured on day 5 postinoculation. ASD = diamonds, Twin = squares, Sibling = triangles, Control = circles. (a) The percent control LDH values are plotted against increasing thimerosal concentrations for the 4 cell types. Arrows indicate LDH-G50 values with ASD = 314 nM, Twin = 648 nM, Sib = 373 nM, and Cont = 1000 nM. (b) The percent control XTT values are plotted against increasing thimerosal concentrations. XTT-G50 values are obtained using the mitochondrial XTT assay. (c) The percentage of cellular LDH that is accessible to lactate (i.e., percentage of dead and dying cells) is plotted against thimerosal. (d) Cell number and XTT reduction rates as a function of increasing thimerosal concentrations are shown. The plots obtained are "hockey stick" in shape.

that ASD cells are very much overrepresented on the left hand side of the ranked plot and controls on the right hand side. Also evident from the distribution of the controls for family groups A to D is the possibility of a systemic error to the distribution, indicating that low G50s in cells from the hypersensitive ASD families have low scoring external controls. Such an error could be caused, for instance, by differences in different batches of growth media which predispose cells to thimerosal sensitivity or, hypothetically, a difference in the amount of thimerosal added to each growth well. To test for a systematic error, the difference data was plotted (e.g., ASD A-Cont A, Twin A-Cont A) and tested to see if there was a difference in the three populations with respect to the control. Figure 2(c) shows the average and standard deviation of the difference between the appropriate age/sex matched control and each of the ASD familial LDH-G50. The positive values indicate that cells from the affected families are more sensitive to thimerosal than the external controls. The P values indicate that the whole ASD and Twin populations are significantly different from the controls.

The Statistics of the LDH-G_{50} Distribution. The Coriell control cells for the other 7 families (i.e., families E–K, those families not having autistic B-cell LDH-G_{50}s less than 2 standard deviations below the mean) have a mean LDH-G_{50} of 1026 nM, with a SD of 295 nM, and the 21 hyposensitive cell lines (ASD, Twin, and Sib) of families E to K have a mean G_{50} of 985 nM, with a SD of 259 nM. In contrast, the 12 cell lines (ASD, Twin, and Sib) of families A to D have a statistically different mean LDH-G_{50} of 452 nM and a SD of 167 nM. The distribution of cells is best split into two types (hyper- and hyposensitive) with four ASD individuals (Families A to D), two twins (Families A and D), and two siblings (B and D) being hypersensitive to thimerosal, with all the other cells being the same as the control population (see Figure 2 in Supplementary Material available online at http://dx.doi.org/10.1155/2013/801517 for plotted data). One-tailed t-tests to determine if these individuals belong to a more sensitive population, with respect to the Coriell controls, give P values of 0.0003, 0.003, and 0.007 for ASD, Twin, and Sib, respectively.

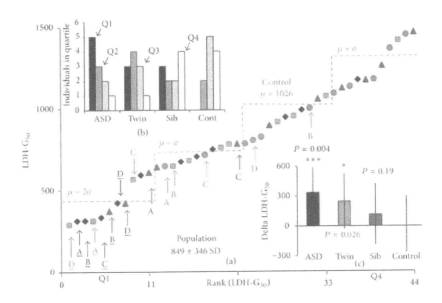

FIGURE 2: (a) shows the thimerosal concentration that induced a 50% growth inhibition at day 5, measured by the LDH method (LDH-G50). In (a) the color-coded cells are ranked in terms of sensitivity to thimerosal. Four family groups are shown whose autistic B-cell LDH-G50's fall greater than 2 standard deviations below the mean: A, B, C, and D. Underlined letters denote those cells believed to have a heightened sensitivity to thimerosal (i.e., those falling outside two standard deviations of the control population). The distribution of the control population is indicated by the green lines showing mean + SD, mean, mean – SD, and mean − 2SD. Distribution of Cells Types. In the upper insert, (b) we show the distribution of the four cells types: ASD, unaffected Twin, unaffected Sibling, and external age/sex matched control, in the four quartiles of the ranked distribution. It is noteworthy that the ASD derived cells are more clustered in the left hand side of the distribution and the external controls are distributed to the right hand side. Test for Systemic Errors. In the second insert, (c) we show that there is no systemic correlation between low LDH-G50's in cells drawn from families from an ASD background and their respective controls. The graph in (c) shows the average and standard deviation of the difference between the appropriate age/sex matched control and each of the ASD familial LDH-G50. The positive values indicate that cells from the affected families are more sensitive than the external controls. The P values indicate the results from a one-tailed t-test, n = 11, with, (*) indicating <0.05, and (***) indicating <0.005.

What Is n? The population was further tested for the degree of bimodalism and for the size of the sensitive population, n, in two ways. Firstly, a pseudo-Jackknife statistical procedure was performed whereby the means and standard deviations of the ranked data were calculated for increasing sizes of hypersensitive population n; that is, for a hypersensitive population of n =8, the hyposensitive population is 36. The two standard deviations/means were then plotted against the size of the hypersensitive population (Figure 3(a)). This treatment of the data gives a visual demonstration of the methodology of Holzmann-Vollmer Test for bimodality [44]. In Figure 3(a) it is apparent that as the size of the hypersensitive population is increased its σ/μ ratio rises and the σ/μ ratio of the hyposensitive population falls. In the (hyposensitive) Coriell controls the σ/μ ratio is 0.29 and that value is reached for the hyposensitive population when n = 8. At n = 10, the two σ/μ ratios are equal, indicating that at this point the two hypo/hypersensitive populations have the same Gaussian distribution, and the only difference in the populations is the means.

In the insert of Figure 3(a) the same σ/μ ratio data is shown, but in this case the two ratios are plotted against each other. It is evident that $8 \leq n \leq 10$ as this is the inflection point of the plot.

It is clear from the two plots shown in Figure 3(a) that there are two populations of cells with differing thimerosal sensitivity.

We also attempted to define n using simulation. We fitted the LDH-G_{50} curve presented in Figure 2 with two normal distributions where the two σ/μ ratios were allowed to vary between 0.1 and 0.6. We found that by simulation, the best fit occurred when n =9, Figure 3(b). When n was increased >9 the σ/μ ratio of the hypersensitive population became unreasonably large, and at n < 9 the σ/μ ratio of the hypersensitive population became unreasonably small.

If n =9, then the LDH-G_{50} of the hypersensitive population is 372 nM and has a standard deviation of 87 nM and the hyposensitive population has a mean of 972 nM and a standard deviation of 272 nM. Given the size of the two populations, 9 and 35, and the two distributions we expect that in the first quartile of the ranked data there would be all 9 hypersensitive cell lines and 2 hyposensitive cell lines.

The Statistics of the XTT-G_{50} Distribution. A similar effect of thimerosal on the ability of cellular mitochondrial complexes to reduce XTT was

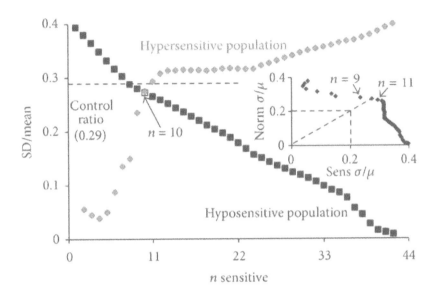

FIGURE 3: This figure shows two methods to estimate the size of the thimerosal sensitive population, by using a pseudo-Jackknife statistical procedure (a) and by simulation (b). In (a) the ranked data set shown in Figure 2 was treated as a bimodal population. We calculate the mean and standard deviation where the size of the hypersensitive population, n, was increased from 0 to 44 and the bulk population fell from 44 to 0. The ratios of the two SDs divided by their means were plotted against n. The dashed line is the ratio of the SD/mean of the control population. The insert shows the line-shape generated when the two ratios are plotted against each other. This pseudo-Jackknifing procedure indicates that the size of the hypersensitive population is at least 8 and could be as high as 11. The ranked data were also fitted by simulation to two populations with means of ≈380 and ≈100 nM, respectively. The simulations indicated that the two populations had the same population distribution when n was 9, (b).

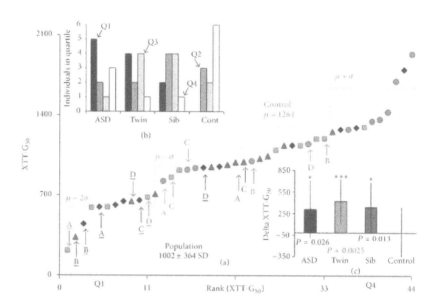

FIGURE 4: This figure shows the concentration of thimerosal which induced a 50% inhibition of growth at day 5, measured by the XTT method (XTT-G$_{50}$). In (a) we have ranked the color-coded cells in terms of sensitivity to thimerosal and have highlighted four family groups: A, B, C, and D. Underlined letters denote cell lines we believe have a heightened sensitivity to thimerosal. The distribution of the control population is indicated by the green line that indicated mean + SD, mean, mean – SD, and mean – 2SD. Distribution of Cells Types. In the upper insert, (b) we show the distribution of the four cells types, ASD, unaffected Twin, unaffected Sibling, and external age/sex matched control, in the four quartiles of the ranked distribution. There is less clustering of the ASD derived cells, but as with the LDH assay, the external controls are distributed to the right hand side of the rankings. Test for Systemic Errors. In the second insert, (c) we show that there is no systemic correlation between low XTT-G$_{50}$'s in cells drawn from families from an ASD background and their respective controls. The plot in (c) shows the average and standard deviation of the difference between the appropriate age/sex matched control and each of the ASD familial XTT-G$_{50}$. The positive values indicate that cells from the affected families are more sensitive than the external controls. The P values indicate the results from a one-tailed t-test, n = 11, with (*) indicating <0.05 and (***) indicating <0.005.

also found. In Figure 4, the XTT-G_{50} obtained for all 44 cell lines is shown with $8 \leq n \leq 10$ cell lines again shown to be hypersensitive to thimerosal. The population distribution of the XTT-G_{50}, measured on day 5 postinoculation is shown in Figure 4(a) and again the different cell types are color-coded. Figure 4(b) shows the distribution of the four cell types within the four quartiles of the ranked distribution. ASD cells are again very much over-represented on the left hand side of the plot and controls on the right hand side. Figure 4(c) shows the average and standard deviation of the difference between the appropriate age/sex matched control and each of the ASD familial XTT-G_{50}. The positive values indicate that cells from the affected families are more sensitive to thimerosal than the external controls. The P values indicate that all three types of cell lines from the ASD families are significantly more sensitive to thimerosal than are the controls drawn from the general population.

Are Mitochondria the Target in the Hypersensitive Population? It is quite clear from Figures 1, 3, and 4 that the ability of cells to be able to reduce XTT is linked to their growth. This can be more easily seen in Figure 4 Supplementary Material where the ranked ratio of LDH-G_{50}/XTT-G_{50} is shown. The cells identified as hypersensitive to thimerosal have a much greater LDH-G_{50}/XTT-G_{50} than the controls and also to other cells drawn from ASD families. There is no difference in the distributions of the n = 11 ASD, Twin, and Sibs, when compared to controls. However, if the 8 ASD, Twin, and Sibs we have previously identified as being hypersensitive to thimerosal are compared to the remaining 36 cells, we find that they are statistically significant with a P value of 0.024 in a t-test. However, the ability of mitochondria to reduce XTT does not directly track either LDH-G_{50} or cell death. We appear to see an upregulation of mitochondrial activity at low thimerosal levels and then a decline in the ability to reduce XTT at higher thimerosal levels.

In Figure 5, data that shows mitochondria are the primary target of thimerosal in the hypersensitive populations is presented. Figure 5(a) shows the rate of XTT reduction per million cells versus the % cell growth for increasing thimerosal concentrations. These data are of Family B and are part of the same data set presented in Figure 1. What is evident is that there is an initial upregulation of mitochondria, followed by a collapse in both cells and mitochondria, in the sensitive cells. The cells can also generate ATP by glycolysis, producing lactate. Figure 5(b) shows how the levels of lactate per cell are increased in the hypersensitive cells, in response to increasing levels of thimerosal. Moreover, it is evident that the ASD cells have a higher proportion of their energy generation from glycolysis than the other cells. This is best seen by examining the ratio of XTT reduction divided by lactate generation versus cell growth, Figure 5(c). A low XTT/lactate ratio is indicative of a high rate of glycolysis and a low rate of oxidative phosphorylation. Both hypersensitive cells (ASD and Sib) have a crash in their XTT/lactate ratios that correlates with the onset of falling growth, the increase in cell death (Figure 1(c)), and the manifestation of markers of oxidative stress. Figure 5(d) shows the levels of protein carbonyls, measured using the dinitrophenyl hydrazine method, with respect to thimerosal concentration. Again, both of the hypersensitive cells show an increase in oxidized protein levels, with the ASD cells being severely damaged at LDH-G50 levels. What is also very interesting is that the background levels of the two hypersensitive cells were higher than the two hyposensitive cells. The Coriell controls and Twin reported background levels of 48.37 ± 1.2 and 48.1 ± 1.43 nM/mg protein, respectively, whereas the Sib and ASD reported 54.05 ± 5.9 and 62.34 ± 12.39 nM/mg protein, respectively ($n = 6$). This is consistent with either an increase in the rate of reactive oxygen species production, as was reported in ASD cells drawn from AGRE versus controls from Coriell by James et al. [27], or a decrease in the rate of ROS detoxification, as measured by the DCFH-DA method.

Similar measurements were performed in two families, Family B and Family H. The latter family of cells was picked as they were the most representative of the Coriell control population with a LDH-G$_{50}$ of and a XTT-G$_{50}$ of 1102 ± 340, giving SD/mean ratios of 0.34 and 0.31. Table 1 shows the rate of DCFH oxidation for cells drawn from Families B and H. Twelve independent measurements were taken for each family and averaged to yield the means (μ) and standard deviations (σ) shown. A statistically significant difference in the steady state oxidant levels is seen only in the ASD cells drawn from Family B, $P = 0.000121$. There is also a rise in the background of the (hypersensitive) Sib, but it is not statistically significant. This is rather similar to, but less than, the increase in the oxidant levels observed in the two cell types by James et al. [27].

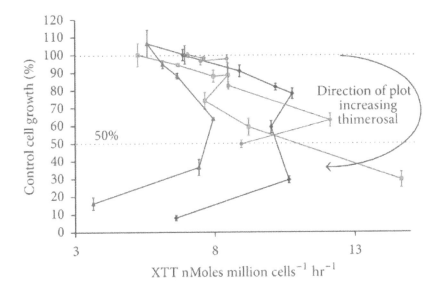

FIGURE 5: This figure shows data from Family B only, part of the same data set presented in Figure 1. (a) shows the rate of XTT reduction per million cells versus the % control cell growth for increasing thimerosal concentrations. (b) shows the rate of lactate production per million cells versus the % control cell growth for increasing thimerosal concentrations. (c) shows the XTT/lactate ratio versus % control cell growth for increasing thimerosal concentrations. (d) shows the amount of nMoles of carbonyl per mg of protein produced versus the % control cell growth for increasing thimerosal concentrations.

TABLE 1: The rate of DCFH oxidation for cells drawn from Families B and H. Twelve independent measurements were taken for each family and averaged to yield the means (μ) and standard deviations (σ) shown. The ASD cell type was the only cell type that differed significantly between the two families ($P = 0.000121$).

Cell Type	DCFH Oxidation nMole mg^{-1}hr^{-1}					
	Fam B	Fam H	Fam B	Fam H	% Coriell B	% Coriell H
ASD	3.56 ***	2.52	0.237	0.121	148	87
Twin	2.44	2.14	0.170	0.076	101	74
Sib	2.65	2.52	0.088	0.093	110	87
Cont	2.42	2.90	0.107	0.080	100	100

That the basal level of oxidant levels in these ASD cells is 50% higher than in the controls does not inform as to whether the cells are generating more oxidants, if they have worse antioxidant defenses, or if they have a combination of both. To dissect out the intrinsic difference in the rate at which oxidants are generated by a particular cell type and the state of their antioxidant defenses due to thimerosal, the rate of DCFH oxidation in the presence of a hydrogen peroxide load was measured. Cells were grown in either the absence or presence of 250 nM thimerosal, washed, and then loaded with DCFH and presented with an oxidative insult in the form of a 100 µM H_2O_2 addition (see Table 2). In this experiment, the level of DCFH generation is independent of the low levels of oxidants generated by the cells and is only dependent on the activity of the various antioxidant defenses. A cell with robust antioxidants will generate less fluorescent oxidized DCFH than will cells with an antioxidant defect. Family H, which appears hyposensitive to thimerosal, shows a 20-fold increase in the rate of DCFH oxidation in the presence of external hydrogen peroxide and this rate is not affected by the presence of 250 nM thimerosal in their growth media; n = 6. The three cell lines of the ASD family all show poorer antioxidant defenses than the control and all the members of Family H. The ASD cells of Family B show a 23-fold increase in oxidation rate after addition of 100 µM H_2O_2 but start from a much higher level. Moreover, there is a clear statistically significant difference in the rate of DCFH oxidation in the ASD cells grown in the presence and absence of 250 nM thimerosal ($P = 0.01$). We believe this difference is evidence of an inherent defect of antioxidant defense in the cells derived from this particular ASD individual. The changes induced in the other three cell types of Family B were not statistically significant.

TABLE 2: The DCFH oxidation (nMole $mg^{-1} hr^{-1}$) of cell families B and H after addition of $100 \mu M$ H_2O_2 and $250 nM$ thimerosal. ASD B-cells from family B showed a significant difference (P = 0.01) of DCFH oxidation when exposed to thimerosal. None of the other cells lines in B or H showed any statistical difference. This indicates an inherent defect of antioxidant defense in the ASD population of cells.

Cell ID	DCFH oxidation with $100 \mu M$ H_2O_2	DCFH oxidation with $100 \mu M$ H_2O_2 and $250 nM$ Thimerosal	Difference
ASD-H	49.85 ± 4.34	48.25 ± 2.02	−1.61
Twin-H	49.32 ± 6.19	49.31 ± 2.42	−0.01
Sib-H	48.35 ± 6.7	43.34 ± 2.35	−5.01
Cont-H	47.15 ± 4.8	41.48 ± 5.46	−5.67
ASD-B	83.5 ± 13.76	93.86 ± 13.76	10.396 **
Twin-B	61.32 ± 6.19	60.41 ± 10.69	2.963
Sib-B	62.55 ± 6.7	58.22 ± 10.81	3.816
Cont-B	46.93 ± 4.8	42.03 ± 17.6	4.990

**Indicates statistically significant difference.

10.4 DISCUSSION

In this study we have examined the action of low levels, $\leq 1000 nM$, of thimerosal on immortalized B-cells taken from ASD subjects, their fraternal twins, a sibling, and from an age/sex matched control. We have examined such 11 family groups and identified 4 families, with at least 8 and as many as 10 members of these families, who have a hypersensitivity to thimerosal. The concentration of thimerosal required to inhibit cell proliferation in these individuals is only 40% that required in hyposensitive controls. We have shown that in these hypersensitive cells mitochondria are the target organelle conferring thimerosal sensitivity. Cells that can maintain mitochondrial energy production are robust, showing little effects on growth, on lactate generation, or on cell death levels. Cells that lose mitochondrial function show increased levels of lactate generation and higher death rates.

Recently James et al. [27] examined B-cells derived from ASD individuals drawn from the AGRE collection and compared them to unaffected controls from the Coriell collection. In their study they examined the effect of three hours incubation with thimerosal, 0.156 to 2.5 μM, on endogenous oxidative stress in B-cells. We have independently conducted a similarly designed study but examined the effects that thimerosal, 0.05 to 1 μM, has on cell growth over the course of six days. Cell numbers, measured using the lactate dehydrogenase method [40] modified to read the fluorescence of resorufin generated by NADH/Diaphorase [42], and mitochondrial function, measured by the XTT reduction rate [41, 43], were examined in eleven family groups of B-cell lines from AGRE consisting of an ASD individual, an unaffected fraternal twin (who shared the same in utero environment), an unaffected sibling, and an age/sex/ethnically matched control from a separate population (Coriell). We have also measured the media lactate levels [45] and the levels of protein carbonyls to assess levels of anaerobic respiration. We report that we find that the sensitivity towards thimerosal amongst these cells is bimodal, with ≈18% of the cells (all AGRE) displaying more than 2.5x the sensitivity to thimerosal as the rest of the population.

Thimerosal, Methylmercury, Ethylmercury, and Inorganic Mercury in Baby's Blood and Brains. We used concentrations of thimerosal which reflect the in vivo concentrations in infants and newborns following vaccinations. Stajich and coworkers [10] examined the levels of blood mercury prior to and following a single dose of a thimerosal (12.5 μg) containing vaccine and found that in term infants the concentration rose to an average of 11 nM, but that in preterm infants this was 36.7 ± 24.4 nM SD, indicating that 15% of the infants may have a blood concentration of >60 nM. The estimated blood half-life of mercury after administration of thimerosal in babies is between 5 and 7 days [46]; however, mouse [47] and primate [48] studies indicate that both organic and inorganic mercury levels in brain have a much longer residency (>3 weeks). The concentration of organic/inorganic mercury in brain is typically higher than in blood as organomercury partitions into the lipid rich environment. The partition coefficient into the brain of thimerosal derived organic/inorganic mercury in young primates is 5-6. Thus, blood organic/inorganic mercury concentrations reflect one-sixth of the brain levels [48]. The concentration range that reflects brain organic/inorganic mercury postthimerosal vaccination is in the order of 100 and 500 nM, drawing on the epidemiological data of Ball, Stajich & Burbacher, and coworkers [12, 48, 49].

We find evidence for oxidative stress being a contributing mechanism in hypersensitivity. Cells which are hypersensitive to thimerosal also have higher levels of oxidative stress markers, protein carbonyls, and higher levels of oxidant generation. These same cells also showed compromise of their antioxidant defenses after being grown in the presence of low levels, 250 nM, thimerosal. Our findings are consistent with the only other thimerosal/B-cell study that found mitochondria were thimerosal targets and that antioxidant defenses, especially those linked to glutathione, were intrinsically compromised in ASD cells and were further eroded by exposure to thimerosal [27]. This completely independent study also shows that when an ASD B-cell population is hypersensitive to thimerosal, the twins/siblings have a 50% chance of being the same. The hypersensitivity of twins and siblings was directly dependent on having a familial ASD who was hypersensitive. It implies that there is a genetic component to thimerosal hypersensitivity and this hypersensitivity is only found in a third of the ASD sufferers. This supports a multi-insult model of ASD causation where many individuals have the genetic background that makes them vulnerable to a particular type of insult at a particular time in their brain development; that is, one-third of ASD sufferers couldhave a genetic predisposition to mitochondrial/antioxidant insults [9, 18], one-third a genetic predisposition to in utero testosterone exposure [50], and the final third a genetic predisposition to toxoplasmosis [51].

ASD is a disorder caused by a problem in brain development. If the B-cells from the families in the AGRE collection are at all representative of the neurons in the brains of the cell donors, we can say that a third of them have a sensitivity to thimerosal that would restrict cell proliferation at levels that were/are typically found after vaccination [11, 12, 16, 46–48].

Moreover, we find that hypersensitive populations have poorer antioxidant defenses, elevated markers of oxidative stress, and high lactate levels.

These findings are consistent with a metabolic fingerprint typically found in 20% of ASD individuals, plasma hyperlactacidemia [52].

Although we have established that a third of our ASD subjects have a heightened sensitivity to thimerosal, and this sensitivity is shared by one-third of their twins/siblings, this study does not address etiology. What we suggest is that although standard toxicology studies of thimerosal indicate a LDH-G50 of 1000 nM with a SD of 300 nm, a minority of subjects from a discrete subpopulation have a LDH-G50 of <350 nM with a SD of <100 nm. In our recently published work, we have shown that the mitochondria of normal human astrocytes accumulate the ethylmercury lipophilic cation and that after this primary insult cell death occurs [53]. Here we show that a subpopulation of four individuals with autism, along with some of their siblings, have B-cells exhibiting hypersensitivity toward thimerosal that can be attributed to their mitochondrial phenotype. Thus, certain individuals with a mild mitochondrial defect may be highly susceptible to mitochondrial specific toxins like the vaccine preservative thimerosal.

REFERENCES

1.   CDC, "Autism Spectrum Disorders (ASDs)," in: C.f.D.C.a. Prevention, (Ed.), US Government, 2012.

2.   CDC, "Prevalence of autism spectrum disorders—autism and developmental disabilities monitoring network, 14 sites, United States, 2002," MMWR. Surveillance Summaries: Morbidity and Mortality Weekly Report. Surveillance Summaries, vol. 56, pp. 12–28, 2007.

3.   M. Knapp, R. Romeo, and J. Beecham, "Economic cost of autism in the UK," Autism, vol. 13, no. 3, pp. 317–336, 2009.

4.   M. L. Ganz, "The lifetime distribution of the incremental societal costs of autism," Archives of Pediatrics and Adolescent Medicine, vol. 161, no. 4, pp. 343–349, 2007.

5.   T. T. Shimabukuro, S. D. Grosse, and C. Rice, "Medical expenditures for children with an autism spectrum disorder in a privately insured population," Journal of Autism and Developmental Disorders, vol. 38, no. 3, pp. 546–552, 2008.

6.   D. L. Leslie and A. Martin, "Health care expenditures associated with autism spectrum disorders," Archives of Pediatrics and Adolescent Medicine, vol. 161, no. 4, pp. 350–355, 2007.

7.   USEPA, "TMDL Status by EPA Region," US Government, 2007.

8.   D. A. Geier, L. K. Sykes, and M. R. Geier, "A review of Thimerosal (Merthiolate) and its ethylmercury breakdown product: specific historical considerations regard-

ing safety and effectiveness," Journal of Toxicology and Environmental Health Part B, vol. 10, no. 8, pp. 575–596, 2007.

9. S. Bernard, A. Enayati, L. Redwood, H. Roger, and T. Binstock, "Autism: a novel form of mercury poisoning," Medical Hypotheses, vol. 56, no. 4, pp. 462–471, 2001.

10. G. François, P. Duclos, H. Margolis et al., "Vaccine safety controversies and the future of vaccination programs," Pediatric Infectious Disease Journal, vol. 24, no. 11, pp. 953–961, 2005.

11. M. E. Pichichero, E. Cernichiari, J. Lopreiato, and J. Treanor, "Mercury concentrations and metabolism in infants receiving vaccines containing thiomersal: a descriptive study," The Lancet, vol. 360, no. 9347, pp. 1737–1741, 2002.

12. G. V. Stajich, G. P. Lopez, S. W. Harry, and W. R. Sexson, "Iatrogenic exposure to mercury after hepatitis B vaccination in preterm infants," Journal of Pediatrics, vol. 136, no. 5, pp. 679–681, 2000.

13. C. J. Clements and P. B. McIntyre, "When science is not enough—a risk/benefit profile of thiomersal-containing vaccines," Expert Opinion on Drug Safety, vol. 5, no. 1, pp. 17–29, 2006.

14. C. Gallagher and M. Goodman, "Hepatitis B triple series vaccine and developmental disability in US children aged 1-9 years," Toxicological & Environmental Chemistry, vol. 90, no. 5, pp. 997–1008, 2008.

15. K. M. Madsen, M. B. Lauritsen, C. B. Pedersen et al., "Thimerosal and the occurrence of autism: negative ecological evidence from Danish population-based data," Pediatrics, vol. 112, no. 3, pp. 604–606, 2003.

16. H. A. Young, D. A. Geier, and M. R. Geier, "Thimerosal exposure in infants and neurodevelopmental disorders: an assessment of computerized medical records in the Vaccine Safety Datalink," Journal of the Neurological Sciences, vol. 271, no. 1-2, pp. 110–118, 2008.

17. N. Badawi, G. Dixon, J. F. Felix et al., "Autism following a history of newborn encephalopathy: more than a coincidence?" Developmental Medicine and Child Neurology, vol. 48, no. 2, pp. 85–89, 2006.

18. D. A. Geier and M. R. Geier, "A case series of children with apparent mercury toxic encephalopathies manifesting with clinical symptoms of regressive autistic disorders," Journal of Toxicology and Environmental Health Part A, vol. 70, no. 10, pp. 837–851, 2007.

19. D. Holtzman, "Autistic spectrum disorders and mitochondrial encephalopathies," Acta Paediatrica, International Journal of Paediatrics, vol. 97, no. 7, pp. 859–860, 2008.

20. J. S. Poling, R. E. Frye, J. Shoffner, and A. W. Zimmerman, "Developmental regression and mitochondrial dysfunction in a child with autism," Journal of Child Neurology, vol. 21, no. 2, pp. 170–172, 2006.

21. A. Doja, "Genetics and the myth of vaccine encephalopathy," Paediatrics and Child Health, vol. 13, no. 7, pp. 597–599, 2008.

22. P. A. Offit, "Vaccines and autism revisited—the Hannah poling case," The New England Journal of Medicine, vol. 358, no. 20, pp. 2089–2091, 2008.

23. W. R. McGinnis, "Could oxidative stress from psychosocial stress affect neurodevelopment in autism?" Journal of Autism and Developmental Disorders, vol. 37, no. 5, pp. 993–994, 2007.

24. H. Tsukahara, "Biomarkers for oxidative stress: clinical application in pediatric medicine," Current Medicinal Chemistry, vol. 14, no. 3, pp. 339–351, 2007.

25. A. Chauhan and V. Chauhan, "Oxidative stress in autism," Pathophysiology, vol. 13, no. 3, pp. 171–181, 2006.

26. S. S. Zoroglu, F. Armutcu, S. Ozen et al., "Increased oxidative stress and altered activities of erythrocyte free radical scavenging enzymes in autism," European Archives of Psychiatry and Clinical Neuroscience, vol. 254, no. 3, pp. 143–147, 2004.

27. S. J. James, S. Rose, S. Melnyk et al., "Cellular and mitochondrial glutathione redox imbalance in lymphoblastoid cells derived from children with autism," FASEB Journal, vol. 23, no. 8, pp. 2374–2383, 2009.

28. S. F. Cave, "The history of vaccinations in the light of the autism epidemic," Alternative Therapies in Health and Medicine, vol. 14, no. 6, pp. 54–57, 2008.

29. H. C. Hazlett, M. D. Poe, G. Gerig et al., "Early brain overgrowth in autism associated with an increase in cortical surface area before age 2 years," Archives of General Psychiatry, vol. 68, no. 5, pp. 467–476, 2011.

30. E. R. Whitney, T. L. Kemper, M. L. Bauman, D. L. Rosene, and G. J. Blatt, "Cerebellar Purkinje cells are reduced in a subpopulation of autistic brains: a stereological experiment using calbindin-D28k," Cerebellum, vol. 7, no. 3, pp. 406–416, 2008.

31. J. Wegiel, I. Kuchna, K. Nowicki et al., "The neuropathology of autism: defects of neurogenesis and neuronal migration, and dysplastic changes," Acta Neuropathologica, vol. 119, no. 6, pp. 755–770, 2010.

32. N. M. Kleinhans, T. Richards, L. Sterling et al., "Abnormal functional connectivity in autism spectrum disorders during face processing," Brain, vol. 131, no. 4, pp. 1000–1012, 2008.

33. D. Han, X. Chen, R. Liang, B. Dong, and W. Yin, "Inhibition of proliferation and induction of apoptosis and differentiation of leukemic cell line HL-60 by sodium valproate," Journal of Experimental Hematology, vol. 14, no. 1, pp. 21–24, 2006.

34. A. Hrzenjak, F. Moinfar, M. Kremser et al., "Valproate inhibition of histone deacetylase 2 affects differentiation and decreases proliferation of endometrial stromal sarcoma cells," Molecular Cancer Therapeutics, vol. 5, no. 9, pp. 2203–2210, 2006.

35. M. Miyata, E. Tamura, K. Motoki, K. Nagata, and Y. Yamazoe, "Thalidomide-induced suppression of embryo fibroblast proliferation requires CYP1A1-mediated activation," Drug Metabolism and Disposition, vol. 31, no. 4, pp. 469–475, 2003.

36. C. W. Spraul, C. Kaven, J. Kampmeier, G. K. Lang, and G. E. Lang, "Effect of thalidomide, octreotide, and prednisolone on the migration and proliferation of RPE cells in vitro," Current Eye Research, vol. 19, no. 6, pp. 483–490, 1999.

37. A. L. Moreira, D. R. Friedlander, B. Shif, G. Kaplan, and D. Zagzag, "Thalidomide and a thalidomide analogue inhibit endothelial cell proliferation in vitro," Journal of Neuro-Oncology, vol. 43, no. 2, pp. 109–114, 1999.

38. C. Korzeniewski and D. M. Callewaert, "An enzyme-release assay for natural cytotoxicity," Journal of Immunological Methods, vol. 64, no. 3, pp. 313–320, 1983.

39. T. Decker and M.-L. Lohmann-Matthes, "A quick and simple method for the quantitation of lactate dehydrogenase release in measurements of cellular cytotoxicity and tumor necrosis factor (TNF) activity," Journal of Immunological Methods, vol. 115, no. 1, pp. 61–69, 1988.

40. E. Weidmann, J. Brieger, B. Jahn, D. Hoelzer, L. Bergmann, and P. S. Mitrou, "Lactate dehydrogenase-release assay: a reliable, nonradioactive technique for analysis of cytotoxic lymphocyte-mediated lytic activity against blasts from acute myelocytic leukemia," Annals of Hematology, vol. 70, no. 3, pp. 153–158, 1995.

41. A. H. Cory, T. C. Owen, J. A. Barltrop, and J. G. Cory, "Use of an aqueous soluble tetrazolium/formazan assay for cell growth assays in culture," Cancer Communications, vol. 3, no. 7, pp. 207–212, 1991.

42. T. L. Riss and R. A. Moravec, "Cytotoxicity assay," in: U.P. Office, (Ed.), Promega Corporation, Fitchburg, Wis, USA, 2006.

43. D. A. Scudiero, R. H. Shoemaker, K. D. Paull et al., "Evaluation of a soluble tetrazolium/formazan assay for cell growth and drug sensitivity in culture using human and other tumor cell lines," Cancer Research, vol. 48, no. 17, pp. 4827–4833, 1988.

44. H. Holzmann and S. Vollmer, "A likelihood ratio test for bimodality in two-component mixtures with application to regional income distribution in the EU," AStA Advances in Statistical Analysis, vol. 92, no. 1, pp. 57–69, 2008.

45. B. F. Howell, S. McCune, and R. Schaffer, "Lactate-to-pyruvate or pyruvate-to-lactate assay for lactate dehydrogenase: a re-examination," Clinical Chemistry, vol. 25, no. 2, pp. 269–272, 1979.

46. M. E. Pichichero, A. Gentile, N. Giglio et al., "Mercury levels in premature and low birth weight newborn infants after receipt of thimerosal-containing vaccines," Journal of Pediatrics, vol. 155, no. 4, pp. 495–e2, 2009.

47. G. Zareba, E. Cernichiari, R. Hojo et al., "Thimerosal distribution and metabolism in neonatal mice: comparison with methyl mercury," Journal of Applied Toxicology, vol. 27, no. 5, pp. 511–518, 2007.

48. T. M. Burbacher, D. D. Shen, N. Liberato, K. S. Grant, E. Cernichiari, and T. Clarkson, "Comparison of blood and brain mercury levels in infant monkeys exposed to methylmercury or vaccines containing thimerosal," Environmental Health Perspectives, vol. 113, no. 8, pp. 1015–1021, 2005.

49. L. K. Ball, R. Ball, and R. D. Pratt, "An assessment of thimerosal use in childhood vaccines," Pediatrics, vol. 107, no. 5, pp. 1147–1154, 2001.

50. S. Baron-Cohen, "The extreme male brain theory of autism," Trends in Cognitive Sciences, vol. 6, no. 6, pp. 248–254, 2002.

51. J. Prandota, "Autism spectrum disorders may be due to cerebral toxoplasmosis associated with chronic neuroinflammation causing persistent hypercytokinemia that resulted in an increased lipid peroxidation, oxidative stress, and depressed metabolism of endogenous and exogenous substances," Research in Autism Spectrum Disorders, vol. 4, no. 2, pp. 119–155, 2010.

52. G. Oliveira, L. Diogo, M. Grazina et al., "Mitochondrial dysfunction in autism spectrum disorders: a population-based study," Developmental Medicine and Child Neurology, vol. 47, no. 3, pp. 185–189, 2005.

53. M. A. Sharpe, A. D. Livingston, and D. S. Baskin, "Thimerosal-derived ethylmercury is a mitochondrial toxin in human astrocytes: possible role of fenton chemistry in the oxidation and breakage of mtDNA," Journal of Toxicology, vol. 2012, Article ID 373678, 12 pages, 2012.

PART III

ADHD, LEARNING DISABILITIES, AND OTHER NEURODEVELOPMENTAL DISORDERS

ATTENTION DEFICIT/HYPERACTIVITY DISORDER: A FOCUSED OVERVIEW FOR CHILDREN'S ENVIRONMENTAL HEALTH RESEARCHERS

ANDRÉA AGUIAR, PAUL A. EUBIG, AND SUSAN L. SCHANTZ

In recent years, there has been increasing awareness of the role of environmental factors in neurodevelopmental disorders, including attention deficit/hyperactivity disorder (ADHD) (e.g., Banerjee et al. 2007; Nigg 2006b; Swanson et al. 2007). In this review we provide a focused overview of ADHD for researchers who are interested in the association between environmental exposures and ADHD risk but have little familiarity with the disorder's diagnosis and prevalence, the functional domains that are impaired, or the underlying changes in brain structure and function. A second goal is to summarize behavioral deficits that are hallmarks of ADHD in order to facilitate comparisons with behavioral deficits associated with widely dispersed environmental chemicals—specifically lead and polychlorinated biphenyls (PCBs), which are reviewed in the companion paper by Eubig et al. (2010). At present, there is compelling evidence suggest-

Reproduced with permission from Environmental Health Perspectives. Aguiar A, Eubig PA, and Schantz SL. Attention Deficit/Hyperactivity Disorder: A Focused Overview for Children's Environmental Health Researchers. Environmental Health Perspectives *118 (2010); http://dx.doi.org/10.1289/ ehp.1002326.*

ing that several key brain functions are implicated in ADHD—attention, executive functions, processing of temporal information, and responses to reinforcement (Nigg and Nikolas 2008)—all of which are critical for modulating behavior (Barkley 1997; Nigg and Casey 2005). We review several meta-analyses published since 2004 that compare the performance of children and adolescents diagnosed with ADHD against non-ADHD controls on neuropsychological tasks measuring attention and executive functions. Additionally, we summarize the performance of ADHD children and adolescents on tests of temporal information processing and responses to reinforcement, which have not been evaluated in meta-analyses to date.

Meta-analyses were obtained through searches of PubMed (http://www.ncbi.nlm.nih.gov/pubmed/) using the terms "ADHD," "meta-analysis," "attention," "executive," and "neuropsychological functions," among others. Meta-analytic studies were included if they originated in 2004 or later, included children or adolescents, and measured the effect size of the association between neuropsychological deficits and ADHD in terms of Cohen's d, which is a metric that is discussed ahead. If no meta-analysis was available for a particular neuropsychological function, nonquantitative reviews were included.

11.1 ADHD PREVALENCE AND DIAGNOSTIC CRITERIA

ADHD is characterized by impulsivity and inattention, has an onset in early school age, and can persist into adulthood, although the prevalence lessens with age (Faraone et al. 2006). The pooled worldwide prevalence of ADHD in children and adolescents is 5.29%, with a range of about 5–10% when children are considered alone and about 2.5–4% when adolescents are considered by themselves (Polanczyk et al. 2007). Among adults, the pooled prevalence of ADHD is 2.5% (Simon et al. 2009). Estimates of rates for ADHD persistence into adulthood vary depending on the definition of ADHD persistence. When only those meeting the full criteria for ADHD are considered, persistence rates are lower, around 15% at 25 years of age, whereas when cases of ADHD in partial remission are considered, rates climb to around 65% at 25 years of age (Faraone et al. 2006). Using retrospective self-reports, Kessler et al. (2005) found that ADHD persisted into adulthood in about 36.3% of cases.

One of the challenges with ADHD is the great heterogeneity of symptoms among affected children (Nigg 2006b; Nigg and Nikolas 2008; Nigg et al. 2006). The most common clinical scale for diagnosing ADHD, the scale in the *Diagnostic and Statistical Manual of Mental Disorders,* 4th edition (*DSM-IV*), Text Revision (American Psychiatric Association 2000), consists of 18 behavioral items and distinguishes among three ADHD subtypes (see Appendix). A predominantly inattentive type (ADHD-PI) is diagnosed when at least six items are selected from the inattentive-disorganized dimension; a predominantly hyperactive–impulsive type (ADHD-PH) is diagnosed when at least six items are selected from the hyperactive–impulsive dimension; and a combined type (ADHD-C) is diagnosed when at least six items are selected from each of the two dimensions. Behavioral symptoms listed in the scale are selected only if they occur often, have persisted for the preceding 6 months, and are maladaptive and incongruent with the individual's developmental level. Additionally, an ADHD diagnosis is given only if at least some of the behavioral symptoms were present before 7 years of age, happen in more than one setting, cause clear and significant impairment in social, school, or work functioning, and do not happen in the course of another mental disorder.

Children with ADHD-C make up most clinical referrals, which could explain why some authors have noted that most research has focused on this ADHD subtype (Nigg 2006a; Nigg and Nikolas 2008). ADHD-PI tends to be more prevalent in girls (Nigg and Nikolas 2008), whereas ADHD-C is most frequently diagnosed in boys. Like many other childhood-onset behavioral disorders, ADHD is diagnosed more frequently in boys than in girls (Pastor and Reuben 2002; Polanczyk et al. 2007).

ADHD often co-occurs with one or more other *DSM-IV* disorders. Young (2008) estimates that up to two-thirds of ADHD children have one or more coexisting disorders. The most common disorders co-occurring with ADHD-C in boys in the large, multisite study of ADHD, the Multimodal Treatment Study of Children with ADHD (MTA) (National Institute of Mental Health 1999), were oppositional defiant disorder (> 32%), anxiety (> 22%), and conduct disorder (> 7%). According to Young (2008), anxiety disorders seem to be even more common in girls (~ 33%) than in boys, when ADHD children 6–17 years of age are considered. Depression and bipolar disorders are also common comorbidities among adolescents with ADHD, as are substance use disorders (Spencer 2006; Spencer et al. 2007; Young 2008). Other comorbidities that are less common among ADHD adolescents are eating disorders, sleep disorders, learning disabilities, and certain medical conditions such as tic disorders, epilepsy, and celiac disease (Young 2008). Comorbidity is another challenging factor in interpreting ADHD data and evaluating theoretical claims about underlying mechanisms.

11.2 NEUROPSYCHOLOGICAL FUNCTIONS AFFECTED IN ADHD

Attention. Attention is a multidimensional construct (Stefanatos and Baron 2007) that can be broadly defined as the facilitated processing of one piece of information over others (Nigg and Nikolas 2008). Attention consists of several interrelated processes including alertness and vigilance (Oken et al. 2006; Posner 1995). In psychology and cognitive neuroscience the term "alertness" is described as the ability to obtain an alert state by focusing rapidly on new or unexpected information or stimuli (Nigg and Nikolas 2008). Similarly, vigilance or sustained attention is described as the ability to maintain attention on a task for a period of time once the alert state is entered (Oken et al. 2006).

Research indicates that children with ADHD have problems with alertness as well as with vigilance. These two attentional functions can both be assessed with continuous performance tasks (CPTs), which measure the ability to respond to a rare target (e.g., the letter "X" when it is preceded by the letter "A" but not by other letters) over an extended period of time (usually ≥ 15 min).

Table 1 lists the two attention functions that are impaired in ADHD individuals, the neuropsychological tasks used to assess the functions, the behavioral findings obtained with ADHD individuals, and meta-analyses that estimated the strength of association between deficits in these functions and ADHD based on Cohen's d, which is defined as the difference in means divided by the pooled standard deviation across study populations.

TABLE 1: Attention functions impaired in ADHD: meta-analyses of studies comparing ADHD and control.

Attention function	Task name and description	Behavioral finding[a]	No. of studies in meta-analysis (k)	ADHD subjects summed across studies (n)	Age range[b]	Effect size (Cohen's d)	Reference
Alertness	CPT: Latency to respond to target sequence is the hit RT; its SE indicates the consistency in focusing attention	↑ SE hit RT	13	NA	Children to adult	0.39	Frazier et al. 2004
Vigilance	CPT: Respond rapidly to target sequence; failure counts as omission error	↑ omission errors	33	NA	Children to adult	0.66	Frazier et al. 2004
			30	1,366	Children to teens	0.64	Willcutt et al. 2005

Abbreviations: CPT, continuous performance task; NA, not available; RT, reaction time; SE, standard error. [a] ↑ indicates significant increase associated with ADHD. [b] Age range is for all studies examined in the referenced article; an age breakdown was not given for the individual neuropsychological tasks included in the meta-analyses.

Cohen's d is a standardized measure often used to compare the effects of variables measured on different scales and to estimate effect size across different studies. Cohen (1988) categorizes effect sizes around 0.2 as small, around 0.5 as moderate, and around 0.8 as large. Meta-analyses that focused only on ADHD adults, were published before 2004, or did not measure effect sizes in terms of Cohen's d are not included.

Alertness. Alertness can be measured by the subject's reaction time or how quickly the individual responds to the target stimuli (Posner 1995). Based on a meta-analysis of 13 studies of CPT performance in individuals diagnosed with ADHD, Frazier et al. (2004) reported that those with an ADHD diagnosis were slower than non-ADHD controls in responding to the target, with a small to moderate pooled effect size across studies (d = 0.39) (Table 1). Slower reaction times in ADHD children are not constrained to CPT tasks. For example, a recent study (Albrecht et al. 2008) compared boys diagnosed with ADHD with their unaffected siblings and with non-ADHD controls using a computerized reaction time task in which the stimuli were either congruent or incongruent with a previous target stimulus. ADHD boys were slower in their correct responses on both congruent and incongruent trials than were the non-ADHD controls. Interestingly, the unaffected siblings of the ADHD boys were midway between the two other groups; they did not differ significantly from either their ADHD siblings or the controls.

Vigilance. Vigilance is commonly assessed by errors of omission (misses) on CPTs. Two meta-analyses, one of 30 and the other of 33 studies that were published in 2004 or later, found that on CPTs, ADHD children made more errors of omission than non-ADHD controls did (Frazier et al. 2004; Willcutt et al. 2005). Both meta-analyses reported moderate effect sizes. The two meta-analyses did not employ completely unique data sets. Unfortunately, not enough information was available in Frazier et al. (2004) to ascertain the degree of overlap.

Executive functions. Executive function refers to a set of abilities including working memory, response inhibition, and error correction that are involved in goal-directed problem solving (Marcovitch and Zelazo 2009). Executive function allows an individual to plan a series of steps necessary to achieve a desired goal, keep these steps in mind while acting on the goal, monitor progress through these steps, and have the cognitive flexibility to adjust or change the steps if progress is not being made toward the original goal. Table 2 lists the executive functions that have been identified as impaired in a number of meta-analytic studies of ADHD children and adolescents published since 2004 (Alderson et al. 2007; Frazier et al. 2004; Homack and Riccio 2004; Lansbergen et al. 2007; Lijffijt et al. 2005; Martinussen et al. 2005; Romine et al. 2004; van Mourik et al. 2005; Walshaw et al. 2010; Willcutt et al. 2005). Table 2 includes the neuropsychological tasks commonly used to assess these functions, the behavioral findings obtained with ADHD individuals, and the strength of the association, with the resulting effect sizes expressed as Cohen's d. The inclusion criteria for Table 2 are similar to those for Table 1: The table lists only meta-analyses published since 2004 that reported effect sizes as Cohen's d and that analyzed studies whose samples included children. As in Table 1, there is overlap in the studies included in the various meta-analyses in Table 2.

Working memory. Working memory is the ability to hold something in mind momentarily while doing something else or while using the information to perform an action (Baddeley 1986). Research indicates that there are separate neural circuits for working memory processes that involve verbal information (verbal working memory) versus spatial information (spatial working memory) (Baddeley 1996). Myriad neuropsychological tasks index verbal and spatial working memory function. Since 2004, three meta-analyses (Martinussen et al. 2005; Walshaw et al. 2010; Willcutt et al. 2005) evaluated studies on working memory in ADHD children and adolescents. These studies found moderate effect sizes ranging from 0.55 to 0.63 for impairments in ADHD children and adolescents compared with non-ADHD controls on seven different verbal working memory tasks: Digits Backward, Sentence Span, Color/Digit Span, Children's Memory Scale Numbers Backward, Counting Span, Paced Auditory Serial Addition Task, and Self-Ordered Pointing Task (SOPT)-Objects. Table 2 gives short descriptions of each of these tasks. Larger effect sizes ranging from 0.63 to 1.04 were observed for impairments in children and adolescents diagnosed with ADHD compared with non-ADHD controls in five spatial working memory tasks: spatial span, a spatial working memory task from the Cambridge Neuropsychological Test Automated Battery (CANTAB); Finger Windows Test Backward; SOPT-Abstract; and the Spatial Span

Backward task from the Wechsler Adult Intelligence Scale (WAIS). Table 2 also provides brief descriptions of these spatial working memory tasks.

Response inhibition. Response inhibition refers to the ability to inhibit or interrupt a response during dynamic moment-to-moment behavior (Nigg and Nikolas 2008). Key paradigms that tap this ability and have shown significant deficits in ADHD children are the go/no-go task, the stopping or stop signal time (SST) task (Aron and Poldrack 2005; Winstanley et al. 2006), the fixed interval schedule of reinforcement (Sagvolden et al. 1998), and CPTs. Only meta-analyses of studies of response inhibition in SST and CPT tasks met the criteria for inclusion in Table 2, so this discussion focuses on these two response inhibition measures.

As Huizenga et al. (2009) describe, in the SST task subjects are typically required to make rapid choice responses to "go" signals (e.g., press a button with the right hand if they see an X and a button with the left hand if they see an O). At random and occasional time intervals, a stop signal (e.g., the letter A or a tone) is presented shortly after the go signal, instructing the subject to inhibit the already initiated response activated by the go signal. As listed in Table 2, since 2004, five meta-analyses (Alderson et al. 2007; Frazier et al. 2004; Lijffijt et al. 2005; Walshaw et al. 2010; Willcutt et al. 2005) estimated Cohen's d effect size for SST studies that included or were limited to children. The analyses indicated that, compared with non-ADHD individuals, those diagnosed with ADHD were consistently slower in stopping an ongoing response, suggesting difficulty in response inhibition. Effect sizes for stop signal reaction times in ADHD samples were in the moderate range (d = 0.54–0.63).

Commission errors (or false alarms) in CPTs are also often used as a marker of response inhibition deficits in ADHD children. Since 2004, three meta-analyses (Frazier et al. 2004; Walshaw et al. 2010; Willcutt et al. 2005) have examined the strength of the association between CPT commission errors and ADHD diagnosis in studies that included children and teens and calculated Cohen's d effect sizes (Table 2). As in the SST analyses, the results for CPT commission errors were in the moderate range (d = 0.51–0.56).

Cognitive flexibility. The ability to switch attention from one aspect of an object to another, or to adapt and shift one's response based on situational demands, such as changes in the rules, schedule, or type of reinforcement in a task, is defined as cognitive flexibility or set shifting (Monsell 2003; Stemme et al. 2007). Tests used to assess cognitive flexibility in children include the Wisconsin Card Sorting Test (WCST), the Stroop Color-Word test (Stroop task), and the Trail Making Test Part B (Trails-B).

On the WCST, subjects are asked to sort into two different piles a series of cards with figures that can differ in color, shape, and/or number. Each time a card is sorted, the subject receives feedback as to whether the choice was correct or incorrect, and based on this feedback the subject must infer the correct category (color, shape, or number) for sorting (Romine et al. 2004). After the subject correctly sorts the cards in a series of consecutive trials, the sorting category is changed and the subject must learn the new sorting category by trial and error. An indicator of impairments in cognitive flexibility is the tendency to make perseverative errors or persist in sorting the cards by the previously correct category, even after being told the sorting strategy is incorrect. Four recent meta-analyses (Frazier et al. 2004; Romine et al. 2004; Walshaw et al. 2010; Willcutt et al. 2005) computed small (0.35) to medium (0.52) effect sizes for the differences in mean perseverative errors between ADHD individuals and non-ADHD controls on the WCST (Table 2). ADHD individuals made more perseverative errors on the WCST than did non-ADHD controls, suggesting that ADHD is associated with impaired cognitive flexibility.

In the Stroop task, problems in cognitive flexibility are measured by the degree of difficulty subjects have in naming the color of the ink used to print color words when the two are mismatched (e.g., when the word "green" is printed in blue ink). Interference scores quantify subjects' difficulty in the task, with higher scores indicating greater difficulty. Effect sizes for Stroop interference scores reported in five recent meta-analyses (Frazier et al. 2004; Homack and Riccio 2004; Lansbergen et al. 2007; van Mourik et al. 2005; Walshaw et al. 2010) vary widely from small (0.35) to large (1.11), making it hard to characterize the findings (Table 2). This inconsistency may be at least partially due to variation in the method used to calculate the interference score across studies. [For a description of different ways of deriving interference scores, see Homack and Riccio (2004).]

Another widely used tool for assessing cognitive flexibility is Trails-B, in which subjects are presented with numbers and letters inside circles that are randomly arranged on a sheet of paper. Subjects are asked to connect in ascending order the numbers and letters while alternating between them (e.g., 1–A–2–B–3–C–4); they are asked to do this as quickly as possible (Lezak et al. 2004). Time to complete the task is measured, with longer response times indicative of difficulties in cognitive flexibility. Two meta-analyses (Frazier et al. 2004; Willcutt et al. 2005) have reported medium effect sizes (d = 0.55 and 0.59 respectively, as shown in Table 2) as evidence of reduced cognitive flexibility in ADHD versus control children based on Trails-B scores.

Planning. Some researchers have found that deficits in planning and strategy development discriminate well between children with ADHD and those without (Papadopoulos et al. 2005). ADHD children have been found to perform poorly in four tasks that are commonly used to assess planning ability: Tower of Hanoi (TOH) task and its variant the Tower of London (TOL) task, Porteus Maze, and Rey-Osterrieth Complex Figure Task (ROCF).

Tower tasks such as TOH and TOL are a popular neuropsychological measure of planning (Riccio et al. 2004). The many variations of this task basically involve moving stacked beads or disks of different sizes to new positions that match the model provided. This must be accomplished in a minimum number of moves and while following rules for moving the objects (e.g., only one disk can be moved at a time, no disk can be placed on top of a smaller disk) (Papadopoulos et al. 2005; Riccio et al. 2004). It is assumed that subjects will generate a more efficient solution if they plan a series of moves before actually beginning to move the beads or disks (Riccio et al. 2004).

In the Porteus Maze task, subjects are presented with mazes of increasing difficulty. They must find a solution (i.e., the way out) while following a number of rules (e.g., no entering a dead end, no backtracking) (Levin et al. 2001). Planning the movement through the maze increases the subjects' ability to adhere to the rules. In the ROCF, individuals are asked to copy and later recall a complex figure composed of 64 segments. In both stages the examiner can rate the accuracy of the different lines as well as the level of organization when clustering lines during the copying and recall phases (Sami et al. 2003). Higher levels of organization are indicative of better strategic planning. Three recent meta-analyses (Frazier et al. 2004; Walshaw et al. 2010; Willcutt et al. 2005) indicate effect sizes in the low to medium range (d = 0.24–0.69) (Table 2) for the differences between ADHD individuals and non-ADHD controls in these four planning tasks.

Summary of meta-analytic studies. In summary, meta-analyses indicate that performance is impaired in ADHD individuals on a large number of attention and executive function tasks. Within the attention and executive function domains, larger deficits are found on tasks measuring vigilance, working memory (especially spatial working memory), and response inhibition abilities, whereas smaller but significant deficits are also seen on tasks measuring alertness, cognitive flexibility, and planning abilities. There is overlap in the studies included in some of the meta-analyses discussed herein. Thus, the individual analyses cannot be taken as totally independent indicators of the effect. Also, deficits on any single test of attention or executive function are not sufficient for a diagnosis of ADHD (e.g., Homack and Riccio 2004) or for differentiating ADHD from other mental or learning disorders (e.g., Walshaw et al. 2010). This should not be surprising given the great heterogeneity of symptoms across affected individuals. Finally, meta-analyses to date have lacked in-depth analyses of the associations between patterns of behavioral deficits on the various neuropsychological tasks and the three different ADHD diagnoses (ADHD-C, ADHD-PI, and ADHD-PH), primarily because most ADHD studies, especially older studies, have not evaluated ADHD subtypes.

Temporal information processing and responses to reinforcement. Two other types of deficits related to the processing of temporal information and to responses to the reinforcing properties of rewards have been reported in ADHD children but have not been subjected to meta-analysis. These deficits could contribute to the difficulties ADHD children have in executive function tasks. Recent studies have focused increasingly on temporal information processing, which is believed to be key to the control and modulation of behavior (Barkley 1997; Nigg and Casey 2005). Toplak et al. (2006) reviewed 38 studies that measured temporal information processing in ADHD children. Most of these studies used tasks in which the child was asked to indicate the end of a specific time interval, either by holding down a response key for the specified interval or by responding verbally to indicate the end of the interval. There were no external cues by which the child could estimate the interval. Most studies found poor time estimation in children with ADHD, especially when longer time intervals were employed.

In terms of responses to reinforcement, Luman et al. (2005) reviewed 22 studies comparing the responses of children with and without an ADHD diagnosis to reinforcement contingencies in a variety of tasks. The authors concluded that ADHD is associated with increased weighting of near-term over long-term (but larger) rewards, positive response to high-intensity reinforcement, and a lack of a physiological response, such as heart rate acceleration, to potential rewards. The pattern of results in these studies suggests that ADHD children have difficulty reasoning about rewards and, as a result, do not respond appropriately to reinforcements. Although abnormalities in responses to reinforcement have been studied in the context of motivation, they could be related to impairments in executive functioning, especially in the case of difficulties in weighing near-term versus long-term rewards.

11.3 NEURAL IMAGING STUDIES OF ADHD PATIENTS

The heterogeneity in symptoms and functional deficits observed in ADHD is paralleled by heterogeneity in the results of brain imaging studies. Although many individuals with ADHD do not have abnormal structural magnetic resonance imaging (MRI) results, when the results are considered across individuals in an ADHD sample, a pattern of structural changes becomes evident (Nigg and Nikolas 2008). Overall, there is a reduction of up to 5% in brain volume, with greater reductions in the prefrontal cortex, caudate nucleus, cerebellum, and corpus callosum (Nigg and Nikolas 2008; Valera et al. 2007) (Figure 1A). Smaller brain volume tends to be associated with a greater severity of ADHD symptoms (Krain and Castellanos 2006).

There is strong evidence for altered corticostriatal circuitry in ADHD. This circuit includes the dorsolateral prefrontal and dorsoanterior cingulate cortices, the dorsal striatum (especially the caudate nucleus), and the thalamus, which links to the cerebellum (Sonuga-Barke 2005; Vaidya and Stollstorff 2008). The dorsolateral prefrontal cortex has roles in planning and organizing behavior, working memory, and response inhibition (Nigg and Nikolas 2008). The anterior cingulate cortex has roles in cognition and motor control and is specifically involved in processes underlying the arousal/drive state of the organism (Makris et al. 2009). The dorsal striatum plays an important modulatory role in controlling responses (Nigg and Nikolas 2008), whereas the cerebellum is important for coordinating motor activities as well as timing and shifting attention (Krain and Castellanos 2006).

Bilateral prefrontal cortices, the right caudate, and regions of the cerebellum were all found to be reduced in size in a meta-analysis of structural MRI findings (Valera et al. 2007), whereas the left dorsolateral prefrontal and anterior cingulate cortices, right caudate, and right thalamus were shown to be hypoactive in a meta-analysis of functional MRI data from ADHD individuals performing tests of executive functioning (Dickstein et al. 2006).

A limited number of functional MRI studies suggest alterations in functional connections between components of the corticolimbic circuit (Vaidya and Stollstorff 2008). This circuit includes the orbitofrontal and anterior cingulate cortices, the ventral striatum (especially the nucleus accumbens), the thalamus, and regions of the amygdala (Sonuga-Barke 2005; Vaidya and Stollstorff 2008) (Figure 1). The orbitofrontal cortex integrates sensory and affective information as part of reward processing, whereas the ventral striatum has roles in reward-related emotion and motivation (Fareri et al. 2008).

11.4 NEUROCHEMISTRY OF ADHD

Converging lines of evidence argue that dysfunctional catecholaminergic signaling underlies the cognitive alterations seen with ADHD (Vaidya and Stollstorff 2008). The prefrontal cortex receives both dopaminergic and noradrenergic innervation, whereas the striatum has generous dopaminergic innervation but sparse noradrenergic innervation (Figure 1B,C). In these regions, both of which are implicated in ADHD, catecholaminergic systems modulate glutaminergic and GABAergic (γ-aminobutyric acid) neurotransmitter release (Brennan and Arnsten 2008). Catecholaminergic transporters, including both dopamine and norepinephrine transporters, exert an important influence on dopamine neurotransmission in the prefrontal cortex and striatum.

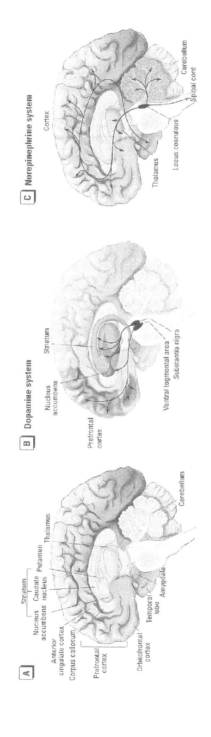

FIGURE 1: Neuroanatomical structures and dopaminergic and noradrenergic neuronal projections that have roles in ADHD. The illustrations are of the medial surface of a hemisected human brain. (A) Reductions in prefrontal cortical, caudate nucleus, corpus callosum, and cerebellar volumes are seen in ADHD. Altered functioning of the anterior cingulate and orbitofrontal cortices, the amygdala, and the nucleus accumbens has also been demonstrated in ADHD. The striatum includes the caudate nucleus, the putamen, and the nucleus accumbens. (B) Dopaminergic neurons that are important in ADHD arise in the ventral tegmental area of the midbrain and project to the frontal cortical and limbic structures, where they serve to modulate neurochemical signaling. Other dopaminergic neurons arise from the substantia nigra and project to the striatum, where they participate in controlling voluntary movement. (C) Noradrenergic neurons arise from the locus coeruleus and project to numerous structures including the prefrontal cortex, the limbic system, the thalamus, and the cerebellum. Adapted from Bear et al. (2001).

Although the exact nature of the neurochemical deficits underlying ADHD is still unknown, there is evidence that hypoactivity of frontostriatal dopamine circuits (reviewed by Swanson et al. 2007) and abnormal noradrenergic signaling (Brennan and Arnsten 2008) play a role. Imaging studies have identified apparent increases of dopamine transporter and dopamine D2 receptor numbers in ADHD patients (Nikolaus et al. 2007), although a recent study in medication-naive ADHD adults found decreases in dopamine transporter and dopamine D2/3 receptors (Volkow et al. 2009). Finally, the improvements in symptoms seen with medications that target catecholaminergic systems indirectly suggest dysfunctional dopaminergic signaling in ADHD. Effective pharmacotherapies for ADHD include stimulant medications, such as methylphenidate and amphetamine, which increase synaptic dopamine release (Madras et al. 2005; Pliszka 2005). Other beneficial medications include the norepinephrine transporter inhibitor atomoxetine, which inhibits the reuptake of dopamine in the prefrontal cortex, and the α2A agonist guanfacine, which increases delay-related firing in the prefrontal cortex (Brennan and Arnsten 2008; Madras et al. 2005; Pliszka 2005).

ADHD cannot be explained by simple deficiencies or excesses of synaptic catecholamines (Pliszka 2005). Alterations in the interactions between neurotransmitter systems are likely to better explain ADHD. Also, the relative levels of monoamines (including serotonin) may be more important than absolute levels (Winstanley et al. 2006). However, these ambiguities should not distract from the large body of evidence that implicates alterations in dopaminergic and noradrenergic signaling as important underlying factors in the pathogenesis of ADHD.

11.5 GENETICS OF ADHD

ADHD is a highly heritable disorder based on findings from family, twin, and adoption studies. The risk of ADHD in parents and siblings of children with ADHD is increased two to eight times (Franke et al. 2009), with heritability estimated at 76% based on pooled data from twin studies (Franke et al. 2009; Smith et al. 2009). Hence, much effort has focused on genetic studies of ADHD.

Candidate gene studies focus on specific genes identified a priori as important in neurotransmitter pathways relevant to ADHD (Brookes et al. 2006; Nigg and Nikolas 2008). Polymorphisms in the dopamine transporter gene (*DAT1, SLC6A3*) and the dopamine 4 (D4) receptor gene (*DRD4*) have been most often associated with ADHD; other candidate genes with significant associations in meta-analyses include the dopamine D5 receptor (*DRD5*), serotonin transporter (*5HTT, SLC6A4*), serotonin receptor 1B (*5HT1B, HTR1B*), and synaptosomal-associated protein 25 (*SNAP25*) (Gizer et al. 2009; Smith et al. 2009). Polymorphisms in the norepinephrine transporter gene (*NET1, SLC6A2*) also have been associated with ADHD (e.g., Brookes et al. 2006; Kim et al. 2008), although meta-analytic findings have not been strong for *NET1*. Overall, the associations from candidate gene studies have been very modest, with no gene accounting for > 3–4% of the total variance in ADHD phenotype (Smith et al. 2009).

Genomewide linkage scans, which are family based, and genome-wide association studies (GWAS), which are population based, differ from candidate gene studies in that the entire genome is analyzed without a priori hypotheses (Franke et al. 2009). These approaches can suggest novel genes that may be involved in the pathogenesis of ADHD. Although genomewide linkage scans have identified chromosome regions that might contain genes associated with ADHD (reviewed by Smith et al. 2009), the findings have not replicated well across studies (Zhou et al. 2008). This may be attributable partly to the fact that linkage studies are best able to identify polymorphisms that account for ≥ 10% of the phenotypic variance of a disorder (Franke et al. 2009). The absence of significant findings from genomewide linkage studies suggests that the effects of DNA risk variants are individually very small despite the high heritability of ADHD (Faraone et al. 2008). In line with this, a recent meta-analysis of seven ADHD genomewide linkage studies identified a significant signal on chromosome 16, whereas none of the individual studies was able to detect a signal at that location (Zhou et al. 2008), suggesting that combining individual studies to increase power may be a valuable approach.

GWAS is a more powerful, unbiased method used to search for risk genes of smaller effect (Psychiatric GWAS Consortium Coordinating Committee et al. 2009). So far, GWAS of ADHD has produced a limited number of significant findings and little overlap between studies (Banaschewski et al. 2010; Franke et al. 2009). However, genes related to cell–cell communication and adhesion, neuronal migration, and potassium-related signaling are commonly found in the top ADHD GWAS rankings, suggesting candidate genes for further study (Banaschewski et al. 2010; Franke et al. 2009). Much remains to be understood about the genetic causes of ADHD. However, GWAS with greater sample size is under way, which, when combined with meta-analytical approaches, holds much promise for further elucidating the genetics of ADHD.

11.6 CONCLUSION

ADHD is a complex disorder with great heterogeneity in the behavioral symptoms presented and brain functions and structures affected. It is clear, however, that several aspects of attention and executive function—particularly vigilance, working memory, and response inhibition—are compromised in ADHD children. Deficits in the processing of temporal information and the processing of rewards are also associated with ADHD and could be either related to or exacerbated by the deficits in executive function.

Although much research has been done on the neuropsychological, neuroanatomical, neurochemical, and genetic bases of ADHD, we are still far from fully understanding its etiology. Given the inability to explain ADHD on a solely genetic basis, interest in the contribution of environmental factors—including exposure to chemical contaminants—has intensified. To date, most of what has been written on this topic focuses on just two contaminants, lead and PCBs, although potential contributions of other chemicals are beginning to be explored. In our companion review (Eubig et al. 2010), we discuss evidence for effects of lead and PCBs on the components of attention and executive function that are impaired in ADHD children. It is our hope that by highlighting the parallels between the neurobehavioral effects of these contaminants and the deficits observed in ADHD children, we will motivate further research on the contribution of environmental chemical exposures to ADHD.

11.A1: APPENDIX I: DIAGNOSTIC CRITERIA FOR ADHD[A]

At least six behavioral symptoms from list A or list B occur often, have persisted for the preceding 6 months, and are maladaptive and inappropriate given the individual's developmental level.

1. Inattentive–Disorganized Dimension:

   - Fails to give close attention to details or makes careless mistakes in schoolwork, work, or other activities
   - Has difficulty sustaining attention in tasks or play activities
   - Does not seem to listen when directly spoken to
   - Fails to follow through on instructions and fails to finish schoolwork, chores, or work duties
   - Has difficulty organizing tasks and activities
   - Avoids, dislikes, or is reluctant about engaging in tasks that require sustained mental effort
   - Loses things necessary for tasks or activities (e.g., toys, school assignments, or tools)
   - Gets easily distracted by extraneous stimuli
   - Is forgetful in daily activities

2. Hyperactivity–Impulsivity Dimension:

   - Fidgets with hands or feet or squirms in seat
   - Leaves seat in classroom or in other situations in which remaining seated is expected
   - Runs about or climbs excessively in situations in which it is inappropriate (in adolescents or adults, may be limited to subjective feelings of restlessness)
   - Has difficulty playing or engaging in leisure activities quietly
   - Is "on the go" or acts as if "driven by a motor"
   - Talks excessively
   - Blurts out answers before questions have been completed
   - Has difficulty awaiting turn
   - Interrupts or intrudes on others (e.g., butts into conversations or games)

3. Some symptoms that cause impairment were present before 7 years of age.
4. Some impairment from the symptoms is present in two or more settings.

5. There is clear evidence of significant impairment in social, school, or work functioning.

6. Symptoms do not happen only during the course of a pervasive developmental disorder, schizophrenia, or other psychotic disorder, and they are not better accounted for by another mental disorder (e.g., mood, anxiety, dissociative, or personality disorder).

Based on criteria I–V, three types of ADHD are identified:

1. Predominantly inattentive (ADHD-PI): if at least six symptoms from list A but not B are present

2. Predominantly hyperactive–impulsive (ADHD-PH): if at least six symptoms from list B but not A are present

3. Combined (ADHD-C): if at least six symptoms from each of the lists, A and B, are present

[a]Adapted from American Psychiatric Association (2000).

REFERENCES

1. Albrecht B, Brandeis D, Uebel H, Heinrich H, Mueller UC, Hasselhorn M, et al. 2008. Action monitoring in boys with attention-deficit/hyperactivity disorder, their nonaffected siblings, and normal control subjects: evidence for an endophenotype. Biol Psychiatry 64(7):615–625.

2. Alderson RM, Rapport MD, Kofler MJ. 2007. Attention-deficit/hyperactivity disorder and behavioral inhibition: a meta-analytic review of the stop-signal paradigm. J Abnorm Child Psychol 35(5):745–758.

3. American Psychiatric Association 2000. Diagnostic and Statistical Manual of Mental Disorders. 4th ed., Text Revision. Washington, DC:American Psychiatric Association.

4. Aron AR, Poldrack RA. 2005. The cognitive neuroscience of response inhibition: relevance for genetic research in attention-deficit/hyperactivity disorder. Biol Psychiatry 57(11):1285–1292.

5. Baddeley A. 1986. Working Memory. New York:Oxford University Press.

6. Baddeley A.. 1996. The fractionation of working memory. Proc Natl Acad Sci U S A 93(24):13468–13472.

7. Banaschewski T, Becker K, Scherag S, Franke B, Coghill D.. 2010. Molecular genetics of attention-deficit/hyperactivity disorder: an overview. Eur Child Adolesc Psychiatry 19(3):237–257.

8. Banerjee TD, Middleton F, Faraone SV. 2007. Environmental risk factors for attention-deficit hyperactivity disorder. Acta Paediatr 96(9):1269–1274.
9. Barkley RA. 1997. Behavioral inhibition, sustained attention, and executive functions: constructing a unifying theory of ADHD. Psychol Bull 121(1):65–94.
10. Bear MF, Connors BW, Paradiso MA. 2001. Neuroscience: Exploring the Brain. 2nd ed. Baltimore, MD:Lippincott Williams & Wilkins.
11. Brennan AR, Arnsten AF. 2008. Neuronal mechanisms underlying attention deficit hyperactivity disorder: the influence of arousal on prefrontal cortical function. Ann NY Acad Sci 1129:236–245.
12. Brookes K, Xu X, Chen W, Zhou K, Neale B, Lowe N, et al. 2006. The analysis of 51 genes in DSM-IV combined type attention deficit hyperactivity disorder: association signals in DRD4, DAT1 and 16 other genes. Mol Psychiatry 11(10):934–953.
13. Cohen J. 1988. Statistical Power Analysis for the Behavioral Sciences. 2nd ed. Hillsdale, NJ:Lawrence Erlbaum Associates.
14. Dickstein SG, Bannon K, Castellanos FX, Milham MP. 2006. The neural correlates of attention deficit hyperactivity disorder: an ALE meta-analysis. J Child Psychol Psychiatry 47(10):1051–1062.
15. Eubig PA, Aguiar A, Schantz SL. 2010. Lead and PCBs as risk factors for attention deficit/hyperactivity disorder. Environ Health Perspect 118:1654–1667.
16. Faraone SV, Biederman J, Mick E. 2006. The age-dependent decline of attention deficit hyperactivity disorder: a meta-analysis of follow-up studies. Psychol Med 36(2):159–165.
17. Faraone SV, Doyle AE, Lasky-Su J, Sklar PB, D'Angelo E, Gonzalez-Heydrich J, et al. 2008. Linkage analysis of attention deficit hyperactivity disorder. Am J Med Genet B Neuropsychiatr Genet 147B(8):1387–1391.
18. Fareri DS, Martin LN, Delgado MR. 2008. Reward-related processing in the human brain: developmental considerations. Dev Psychopathol 20(4):1191–1211.
19. Franke B, Neale BM, Faraone SV. 2009. Genome-wide association studies in ADHD. Hum Genet 126(1):13–50.
20. Frazier TW, Demaree HA, Youngstrom EA. 2004. Meta-analysis of intellectual and neuropsychological test performance in attention-deficit/hyperactivity disorder. Neuropsychology 18(3):543–555.
21. Gizer IR, Ficks C, Waldman ID. 2009. Candidate gene studies of ADHD: a meta-analytic review. Hum Genet 126(1):51–90.
22. Homack S, Riccio CA. 2004. A meta-analysis of the sensitivity and specificity of the Stroop color and word test with children. Arch Clin Neuropsychol 19(6):725–743.
23. Huizenga HM, van Bers BM, Plat J, van den Wildenberg WP, van der Molen MW. 2009. Task complexity enhances response inhibition deficits in childhood and adolescent attention-deficit/hyperactivity disorder: a meta-regression analysis. Biol Psychiatry 65(1):39–45.
24. Kessler RC, Adler LA, Barkley R, Biederman J, Conners CK, Faraone SV, et al. 2005. Patterns and predictors of attention-deficit/hyperactivity disorder persistence into adulthood: results from the national comorbidity survey replication. Biol Psychiatry 57(11):1442–1451.

25. Kim JW, Biederman J, McGrath CL, Doyle AE, Mick E, Fagerness J, et al. 2008. Further evidence of association between two NET single-nucleotide polymorphisms with ADHD. Mol Psychiatry 13(6):624–630.

26. Krain AL, Castellanos FX. 2006. Brain development and ADHD. Clin Psychol Rev 26(4):433–444.

27. Lansbergen MM, Kenemans JL, van Engeland H. 2007. Stroop interference and attention-deficit/hyperactivity disorder: a review and meta-analysis. Neuropsychology 21(2):251–262.

28. Levin HS, Song J, Ewing-Cobbs L, Roberson G. 2001. Porteus maze performance following traumatic brain injury in children. Neuropsychology 15(4):557–567.

29. Lezak MD, Howieson DB, Loring DW. 2004. Neuropsychological Assessment.New York:Oxford University Press.

30. Lijffijt M, Kenemans JL, Verbaten MN, van Engeland H. 2005. A meta-analytic review of stopping performance in attention-deficit/hyperactivity disorder: deficient inhibitory motor control? J Abnorm Psychol 114(2):216–222.

31. Luman M, Oosterlaan J, Sergeant JA. 2005. The impact of reinforcement contingencies on AD/HD: a review and theoretical appraisal. Clin Psychol Rev 25(2):183–213.

32. Madras BK, Miller GM, Fischman AJ. 2005. The dopamine transporter and attention-deficit/hyperactivity disorder. Biol Psychiatry 57(11):1397–1409.

33. Makris N, Biederman J, Monuteaux MC, Seidman LJ. 2009. Towards conceptualizing a neural systems-based anatomy of attention-deficit/hyperactivity disorder. Dev Neurosci 31(1–2):36–49.

34. Marcovitch S, Zelazo PD. 2009. A hierarchical competing systems model of the emergence and early development of executive function. Dev Sci 12(1):1–18.

35. Martinussen R, Hayden J, Hogg-Johnson S, Tannock R.. 2005. A meta-analysis of working memory impairments in children with attention-deficit/hyperactivity disorder. J Am Acad Child Adolesc Psychiatry 44(4):377–384.

36. Monsell S.. 2003. Task switching. Trends Cogn Sci 7(3):134–140.

37. Nigg J, Nikolas M. 2008. Attention-Deficit/Hyperactivity disorder. In: Child and Adolescent Psychopathology (Beauchaine TP, Hinshaw SP, eds). Hoboken, NJ:John Wiley & Sons.

38. Nigg JT. 2006.. Temperament and developmental psychopathology. J Child Psychol Psychiatry 47(3–4):395–422.

39. Nigg JT. 2006b. What Causes ADHD? Understanding What Goes Wrong and Why. New York:Guilford.

40. Nigg JT, Casey BJ. 2005. An integrative theory of attention-deficit/ hyperactivity disorder based on the cognitive and affective neurosciences. Dev Psychopathol 17(3):785–806.

41. Nigg JT, Hinshaw SP, Huang-Pollock C. 2006. Disorders of attention and impulse regulation. In: Developmental Psychopathology (Ciccheti D, Cohen D, eds). New York:Wiley. pp. 358–403.

42. Nikolaus S, Antke C, Kley K, Poeppel TD, Hautzel H, Schmidt D, et al. 2007. Investigating the dopaminergic synapse in vivo. I. Molecular imaging studies in humans. Rev Neurosci 18(6):439–472.

43. National Institute of Mental Health, MTA Cooperative Group. 1999. A 14-month randomized clinical trial of treatment strategies for attention-deficit/hyperactivity

disorder. Multimodal Treatment Study of Children with ADHD. Arch Gen Psychiatry 56(12):1073–1086.

44. Oken BS, Salinsky MC, Elsas SM. 2006. Vigilance, alertness, or sustained attention: physiological basis and measurement. Clin Neurophysiol 117(9):1885–1901.
45. Papadopoulos TC, Panayiotou G, Spanoudis G, Natsopoulos D. 2005. Evidence of poor planning in children with attention deficits. J Abnorm Child Psychol 33(5):611–623.
46. Pastor PN, Reuben CA. 2002. Attention deficit disorder and learning disability: United States, 1997–98. Vital Health Stat 10 ((206):1–12.
47. Pliszka SR. 2005. The neuropsychopharmacology of attention-deficit/hyperactivity disorder. Biol Psychiatry 57(11):1385–1390.
48. Polanczyk G, de Lima MS, Horta BL, Biederman J, Rohde LA. 2007. The worldwide prevalence of ADHD: a systematic review and metaregression analysis. Am J Psychiatry 164(6):942–948.
49. Posner MI. 1995. Attention in cognitive neuroscience: an overview. In: The Cognitive Neurosciences (Gazzaniga MS, ed). Cambridge, MA:MIT Press. pp. 615–624.
50. Psychiatric GWAS Consortium Coordinating Committee, Cichon S, Craddock N, Daly M, Faraone SV, Gejman PV, et al. 2009. Genomewide association studies: history, rationale, and prospects for psychiatric disorders. Am J Psychiatry 166(5):540–556.
51. Riccio CA, Wolfe ME, Romine C, Davis B, Sullivan JR. 2004. The Tower of London and neuropsychological assessment of ADHD in adults. Arch Clin Neuropsychol 19(5):661–671.
52. Romine CB, Lee D, Wolfe ME, Homack S, George C, Riccio CA. 2004. Wisconsin Card Sorting Test with children: a meta-analytic study of sensitivity and specificity. Arch Clin Neuropsychol 19(8):1027–1041.
53. Sagvolden T, Aase H, Zeiner P, Berger D.. 1998. Altered reinforcement mechanisms in attention-deficit/hyperactivity disorder. Behav Brain Res 94(1):61–71.
54. Sami N, Carte ET, Hinshaw SP, Zupan BA. 2003. Performance of girls with ADHD and comparison girls on the Rey-Osterrieth Complex Figure: evidence for executive processing deficits. Child Neuropsychol 9(4):237–254.
55. Simon V, Czobor P, Balint S, Meszaros A, Bitter I.. 2009. Prevalence and correlates of adult attention-deficit hyperactivity disorder: meta-analysis. Br J Psychiatry 194(3):204–211.
56. Smith AK, Mick E, Faraone SV. 2009. Advances in genetic studies of attention-deficit/hyperactivity disorder. Curr Psychiatry Rep 11(2):143–148.
57. Sonuga-Barke EJ. 2005. Causal models of attention-deficit/hyperactivity disorder: from common simple deficits to multiple developmental pathways. Biol Psychiatry 57(11):1231–1238.
58. Spencer TJ. 2006. ADHD and comorbidity in childhood. J Clin Psychiatry 67: suppl 827–31.
59. Spencer TJ, Biederman J, Mick E. 2007. Attention-deficit/hyperactivity disorder: diagnosis, lifespan, comorbidities, and neurobiology. J Pediatr Psychol 32(6):631–642.
60. Stefanatos GA, Baron IS. 2007. Attention-deficit/hyperactivity disorder: a neuropsychological perspective towards DSM-V. Neuropsychol Rev 17(1):5–38.

61. Stemme A, Deco G, Busch A.. 2007. The neuronal dynamics underlying cognitive flexibility in set shifting tasks. J Comput Neurosci 23(3):313–331.

62. Swanson JM, Kinsbourne M, Nigg J, Lanphear B, Stefanatos GA, Volkow N, et al. 2007. Etiologic subtypes of attention-deficit/hyperactivity disorder: brain imaging, molecular genetic and environmental factors and the dopamine hypothesis. Neuropsychol Rev 17(1):39–59.

63. Toplak ME, Dockstader C, Tannock R. 2006. Temporal information processing in ADHD: findings to date and new methods. J Neurosci Methods 151(1):15–29.

64. Vaidya CJ, Stollstorff M. 2008. Cognitive neuroscience of attention deficit hyperactivity disorder: current status and working hypotheses. Dev Disabil Res Rev 14(4):261–267.

65. Valera EM, Faraone SV, Murray KE, Seidman LJ. 2007. Meta-analysis of structural imaging findings in attention-deficit/hyperactivity disorder. Biol Psychiatry 61(12):1361–1369.

66. van Mourik R, Oosterlaan J, Sergeant JA. 2005. The Stroop revisited: a meta-analysis of interference control in AD/HD. J Child Psychol Psychiatry 46(2):150–165.

67. Volkow ND, Wang GJ, Kollins SH, Wigal TL, Newcorn JH, Telang F, et al. 2009. Evaluating dopamine reward pathway in ADHD: clinical implications. JAMA 302(10):1084–1091.

68. Walshaw PD, Alloy LB, Sabb FW. 2010. Executive function in pediatric bipolar disorder and attention-deficit hyperactivity disorder: in search of distinct phenotypic profiles. Neuropsychol Rev 20(1):103–120.

69. Willcutt EG, Doyle AE, Nigg JT, Faraone SV, Pennington BF. 2005. Validity of the executive function theory of attention-deficit/hyperactivity disorder: a meta-analytic review. Biol Psychiatry 57(11):1336–1346.

70. Winstanley CA, Eagle DM, Robbins TW. 2006. Behavioral models of impulsivity in relation to ADHD: translation between clinical and preclinical studies. Clin Psychol Rev 26(4):379–395.

71. Young J.. 2008. Common comorbidities seen in adolescents with attention-deficit/hyperactivity disorder. Adolesc Med State Art Rev 19(2):216–228.

72. Zhou K, Dempfle A, Arcos-Burgos M, Bakker SC, Banaschewski T, Biederman J, et al. 2008. Meta-analysis of genome-wide linkage scans of attention deficit hyperactivity disorder. Am J Med Genet B Neuropsychiatr Genet 147B(8):1392–1398.

There is one table that is not available in this version of the article. To view it, please use the citation on the first page of this chapter.

CHAPTER 12

URINARY POLYCYCLIC AROMATIC HYDROCARBON METABOLITES AND ATTENTION/DEFICIT HYPERACTIVITY DISORDER, LEARNING DISABILITY, AND SPECIAL EDUCATION IN U.S. CHILDREN AGED 6 TO 15

ZAYNAH ABID, ANANYA ROY, JULIE B. HERBSTMAN, AND ADRIENNE S. ETTINGER

12.1 INTRODUCTION

Polycyclic aromatic hydrocarbons (PAHs) are a class of ubiquitous environmental contaminants formed by incomplete combustion of organic material. The main sources of human exposure include occupation, passive and active smoking, food, water, and ambient air pollution [1]. Children may face increased vulnerability to environmental exposures, including PAHs, due to their unique behavior patterns and higher ingestion and inhalation rates given their body size. In a representative sample of the U.S. population, children (aged 6–11 years) had higher levels of PAH urinary

Urinary Polycyclic Aromatic Hydrocarbon Metabolites and Attention/Deficit Hyperactivity Disorder, Learning Disability, and Special Education in U.S. Children Aged 6 to 15. © Abid Z, Roy A, Herbstman JB, and Ettinger AS. Journal of Environmental and Public Health **2014** (2014); http://dx.doi.org/10.1155/2014/628508. *Licensed under Creative Commons Attribution 3.0 Unported License, http://creativecommons.org/licenses/by/3.0/.*

metabolites than adolescents (aged 12–19) and adults (aged ≥20 years) [2]. This is consistent with previous studies of urinary PAH metabolites in children [3, 4] and, also is consistent with children's higher PAH intakes from diet, air, and soil [5, 6].

At least five PAH compounds, including benzo(a)pyrene, are considered by the EPA and IARC to be "probable" or "possible" human carcinogens via a genotoxic mechanism [7]. Animal studies have shown that prenatal PAH exposure may cause adverse neurodevelopment, including learning deficits, memory impairments, and behavioral changes [8–10]. The developing brain is particularly vulnerable to these effects and molecular epidemiological studies found that newborns may be up to 10 times more susceptible to DNA-PAH adduct formation than their mothers [11, 12]. The mechanisms by which PAH exposure affects a child's developing brain are not fully understood, but proposed mechanisms include endocrine disruption [13], oxidative stress [8], binding to placental growth factor receptors [14], induction of P450 enzymes via binding to the human Ah receptor [15], DNA damage resulting in activation of apoptotic pathways [16, 17], or epigenetic effects [18].

Prenatal exposure to PAHs predicted lower mental development index and cognitive developmental delay in the first three years of life [19]; symptoms of anxious/depressed and attention problems at age 5–7 years [20, 21]; decreased language, social, and average developmental quotients in 2-year-old children [22]; and decreased IQ at age of 5 [23, 24]. Higher referral by teachers for clinical assessment of learning and behavioral problems has also been reported [25].

Attention-deficit/hyperactivity disorder (ADHD) is a commonly recognized behavioral disorder characterized by symptoms of inattention and/or impulsivity. ADHD is believed to have genetic origins, but it may interact with the environment such that environmental factors act as a trigger for the disorder [26, 27]. Learning disability (LD) is often associated with ADHD, having been reported in 70% of ADHD patients and their relatives [28]. More than half of children with ADHD are also school-identified as eligible for SE services under the Individuals with Disabilities Education Act (IDEA), with most falling under the categories of LD, emotional disturbance, or other health impairment [28]. A study of elementary school children receiving special education (SE) services revealed that 44% of the children met the diagnostic criteria for ADHD, while only half of those were receiving care for the disorder [29]. Weiland et al. [30] estimated annual costs of preschool SE services for low-income NYC children with PAH-induced developmental delay to be $13.7 million per birth cohort.

There have been no reports of associations between children's PAH exposure and clinically significant neurodevelopmental effects in a nationally representative sample. Here, we assess the cross-sectional relationship between concurrent levels of urinary PAH metabolites and ADHD, LD, and SE in a nationally representative sample of U.S. children aged 6 to 15 years.

12.2 MATERIALS AND METHODS

12.2.1 DATA SOURCE

Data were obtained from the 2001-2002 and 2003-2004 cycles of the National Health and Nutrition Examination Survey (NHANES) for children 6–15 years of age. NHANES is a nationally representative, cross-sectional survey of the noninstitutionalized U.S. civilian population, based on a complex, multistage probability sample. Details of the NHANES protocol are described elsewhere [31, 32]. Briefly, one to two weeks after an initial in-person interview, participants undergo a physical examination in specially designed and equipped Mobile Examination Centers (MECs). The laboratory component involves the collection of biological specimens, including urine for subjects aged 6 years and older.

In 2001–2004, laboratory analysis of urinary biomarkers was performed for one-third of participants aged 6 years and over. Monohydroxy-PAH (OH-PAH) metabolites were measured by an analytical method involving enzymatic hydrolysis of urine, extraction, derivatization, and analysis by capillary gas chromatography combined with isotope-dilution high-resolution mass spectrometry (GC-HRMS) [33].

12.2.2 PAH EXPOSURE

Urinary metabolite concentrations (nanograms per liter (ng/L)) of eight PAHs, available in both the 2001-2002 and 2003-2004 cycles, were identified and selected for the data analysis: 1-pyrene, 1-napthol, 2-napthol, 2-fluorene, 3-fluorene, 1-phenanthrene, 2-phenanthrene, and 3-phenanthrene. Analytes below the limit of detection (LOD) were assigned a value of the LOD divided by the square root of 2.

Five exposure variables were used in this analysis: 1-pyrene, 1-napthol, 2-napthol, fluorine "FLUO" metabolites (2-fluorene + 3-fluorene), and phenanthrene "PHEN" metabolites (1-phenanthrene + 2-phenanthrene + 3-phenanthrene). Urinary 1-pyrene is the most commonly utilized PAH biomarker of exposure and is a useful surrogate of total PAH exposure [2]. The metabolites that arise from the same parent compound were combined, so that our exposure variables would more closely reflect environmental exposure to the parent compound. 1-napthol and 2-napthol were not combined, however, because these metabolites may reflect exposures to different source of naphthalene (personal communication, Dr. Andreas Sjödin, PAH Biomarker Laboratory, CDC). Since the ranges of PAH concentrations were positively skewed, the five exposure variables were log-transformed and treated as continuous variables and, in separate analyses, high/low categorical PAH variables, dichotomized at the median, were used.

12.2.3 OUTCOMES

The primary outcome of interest was parental report of ever-doctor-diagnosed ADHD. The survey question, as asked to participants, was "has a doctor or health professional ever told {you/survey participant (SP)} that {s/he/SP} had attention deficit disorder?" Secondary outcomes were parental report of LD and receipt of special education or early intervention services (abbreviated as "SE" throughout). The survey questions were as follows: "has a representative from a school or a health professional ever told {you/SP} that {s/he/SP} had a learning disability?" and "does {SP} receive special education or early intervention services?"

12.2.4 COVARIATES

A number of covariates and potential confounders identified in the literature were investigated, including age, sex, race/ethnicity (non-Hispanic white, non-Hispanic black, Hispanic and other), and body mass index (BMI) (<25, 25–30, and >30). Because urinary PAH metabolite concentrations vary based on urine dilution, log-transformed creatinine concentration was included as a covariate. The poverty-income ratio (PIR) (<1.00, 1–1.84, 1.85–3, >3), a ratio of family income to the poverty threshold, was used as an indicator of socioeconomic status. Health insurance coverage and having a routine health care provider, both of which have been associated with an increased likelihood of an ADHD diagnosis [34], were also included. Birth and early childhood factors including birthweight (<5.5 and ≥5.5 lbs), maternal age at birth, treatment at a newborn care facility, and preschool attendance were evaluated. Maternal smoking during pregnancy (yes/no) and having any smokers in the household (yes/no) were positively correlated (Spearman correlation coefficient = 0.344, P < 0.001); therefore, the "smokers in the household" variable was chosen for inclusion into the multivariate models to represent postnatal environmental tobacco smoke (ETS) given that we are evaluating the effect of concurrent PAH levels, rather than prenatal PAH levels. Log-transformed fasting time (hours since last meal) was also evaluated as a covariate since recent consumption of dietary PAHs may influence urinary metabolite concentrations.

12.2.5 STATISTICAL ANALYSIS

All analyses were performed using SAS v. 9.3 (SAS Institute Inc. Cary, NC), using SAS SURVEY procedures to account for the complex survey design of the NHANES sample. Variables found to be associated with each dichotomous yes/no outcome of interest based on a Chi-square test (categorical) or t-test (continuous) using a statistical threshold of P < 0.2 in bivariate analyses were included in the multivariate logistic regression analysis. Non-significant covariates (P > 0.05) were removed one at a time (backward elimination) as long as effect estimate between PAH exposure and outcome was not altered by greater than 10% in order to arrive at most parsimonious model. Regardless of statistical significance, the final models included age, sex, race/ethnicity, and creatinine, since PAH levels will vary according to urinary dilution, and urinary dilution varies by age, sex, and race/ethnicity group. To assess potential effect modification by sex, the interaction term sex * PAH for each PAH exposure variable was included in modeling, and subgroup analyses were also performed. Because the initially selected covariates for each outcomes were nested within the larger group of covariates selected in the SE model and the results did not change appreciably (data not shown), the covariates found to be significant in the SE model were also used in the final models for ADHD and LD in order to achieve consistency among the three outcomes. Thus, the final models included adjustment for age, sex, race/ethnicity, creatinine, smokers in the household, PIR, birthweight, and having a routine source of health care. The sample was restricted to participants with no missing data for the PAH measures, covariates, or outcomes of interest.

12.3 RESULTS

Table 1 shows the concentrations of the eight urinary PAH metabolites in the 2001-2002 and 2003-2004 NHANES participants aged 6–15 with no missing covariates or outcomes (N = 1257). Median urinary PAH metabolite concentrations (ng/L) were 1-pyrene, 76.1; 1-napthol, 1290.1; 2-napthol, 2036.6; 2-fluorene, 254.3; 3-fluorene, 102.2; 1-phenanthrene, 128.7; 2-phenanthrene, 49.1; 3-phenanthrene, 106.0. No influential outliers of the continuous covariates were observed and, thus, no observations were excluded prior to analysis.

Prevalences of ADHD, LD, and SE were 7.1%, 13.2%, and 11.4%, respectively, and the Spearman correlation coefficients were for ADHD and LD, $\rho = 0.344$ (P < 0.001); for ADHD and SE, $\rho = 0.301$ (p < 0.001); and for LD and SE, $\rho = 0.679$ (P < 0.001). Spearman correlation coefficients between PAH exposure variables and having any smokers in the household were all statistically significant (P < 0.05) and ranged from $\rho = 0.056$ for log-transformed 1-napthol to $\rho = 0.437$ for high/low FLUO metabolites. The dichotomous high/low exposure variables generally demonstrated a

TABLE 1: Urinary PAH metabolite concentrations (ng/L), NHANES 2001–2004 participants aged 6–15 with no missing covariates or outcomes (N=1257).

PAH metabolite	Percent below LOD[a]	Minimum	Percentiles (95% confidence intervals)						Maximum
			5th	10th	25th	50th	75th	95th	
1-pyrene	0.5	2.1	15.3 (11.6, 18.9)	21.7 (18.6, 24.8)	37.9 (32.9, 42.9)	76.1 (65.0, 87.2)	161.0 (143.4, 178.6)	483.5 (61.6, 357.8)	2216
1-napthol	0.1	33	263.8 (93.5, 334.1)	404.1 (334.7, 473.5)	722.5 (648.2, 796.7)	1290.1 (1140.9, 1439.2)	2969.2 (2572.6, 3365.9)	11165 (9373.5, 12956.1)	567902
2-napthol	0	27	354.5 (269.8, 439.2)	619.3 (527.4, 711.1)	1063.9 (977.8, 1150.0)	2036.6 (1812.7, 2260.5)	3622.8 (3233.3, 4012.3)	9748.2 (7344.2, 12152.1)	345241
FLUO metabolites									
2-fluorene	0	4	52.1 (43.7, 60.4)	81.2 (66.7, 95.8)	141.8 (126.9, 156.8)	254.3 (228.0, 280.6)	395.9 (357.8, 434.0)	875.1 (772.8, 977.3)	7828.6
3-fluorene	0.1	3.5	22.3 (17.2, 27.5)	33.9 (28.1, 39.7)	60.9 (53.5, 68.3)	102.2 (94.7, 109.7)	167.0 (154.7, 179.2)	386.3 (322.8, 449.8)	3462.7
PHEN metabolites									
1-phenanthrene	0.3	2.8	30.0 (24.3, 35.8)	43.0 (36.3, 49.6)	74.8 (66.2, 83.5)	128.7 (116.2, 141.2)	225.1 (201.4, 248.8)	506.5 (407.5, 605.6)	2297
2-phenanthrene	4.1	2.1	5.8 (2.0, 9.6)	12.4 (8.9, 16.0)	24.9 (20.5, 29.3)	49.1 (43.9, 54.4)	82.9 (74.2, 91.7)	226.6 (195.2, 257.9)	2469
3-phenanthrene	0.6	2.8	22.9 (18.3, 27.4)	35.1 (30.3, 40.0)	61.3 (55.6, 66.9)	106.0 (94.0, 118.0)	186.8 (167.7, 205.8)	413.6 (315.1, 512.1)	19643

[a]Limits of detection (LOD) (ng/L) for PAH metabolites, 2001-2002: 1-pyrene: 3.3, 1-napthol: 6.2, 2-napthol: 2.4, 2-fluorene: 3.6, 3-fluorene: 2.0, 1-phenanthrene: 3.5, 2-phenanthrene: 3.2, and 3-phenanthrene: 3.6. 2003-2004: 1-pyrene: 4.9, 1-napthol: 18, 2-napthol: 12, 2-fluorene: 4.5, 3-fluorene: 6.9, 1-phenanthrene: 2.6, 2-phenanthrene: 3.8, and 3-phenanthrene: 2.6.

higher correlation coefficient with the "smokers in the household" variable than did the log-transformed continuous variables.

Bivariate analyses showed significant associations between sex, having smokers in the household, and maternal smoking during pregnancy with ADHD (Table 2). Additionally, race/ethnicity, birthweight, PIR, and fasting time were significant bivariate predictors for LD. All of those variables, as well as age and having a routine source of medical care, were significant bivariate predictors of SE.

TABLE 3: Multivariate associations[a] between PAH metabolites and ADHD, NHANES 2001–2004 (N = 1257).

	All (N = 1257) OR (95% CI)	Male (N = 608) OR (95% CI)	Female (N = 649) OR (95% CI)	P value for interaction[b]
1-Pyrene				
Log-transformed	0.91 (0.69, 1.21)	1.13 (0.88, 1.46)	0.46 (0.23, 0.94)	0.2
High versus low	1.22 (0.65, 2.28)	1.39 (0.76, 2.55)	0.90 (0.28, 2.88)	0.7
1-Napthol				
Log-transformed	1.00 (0.83, 1.21)	1.10 (0.87, 1.38)	0.85 (0.55, 1.31)	0.5
High versus low	1.00 (0.60, 1.69)	1.28 (0.62, 2.61)	0.63 (0.22, 1.81)	0.4
2-Napthol				
Log-transformed	0.75 (0.59, 0.94)	0.76 (0.58, 0.99)	0.78 (0.50, 1.20)	0.8
High versus low	0.59 (0.35, 1.01)	0.75 (0.44, 1.30)	0.39 (0.16, 0.98)	0.5
FLUO metabolites				
Log-transformed	0.93 (0.70, 1.24)	0.98 (0.69, 1.41)	0.84 (0.42, 1.70)	0.7
High versus low	1.40 (0.72, 2.72)	1.50 (0.68, 3.31)	1.22 (0.42, 3.53)	0.6
PHEN metabolites				
Log-transformed	0.93 (0.61, 1.42)	1.07 (0.75, 1.52)	0.68 (0.27, 1.74)	0.9
High versus low	0.71 (0.36, 1.39)	0.64 (0.33, 1.25)	0.87 (0.23, 3.20)	0.9

[a]*Adjusted for age, race/ethnicity, sex, creatinine, smokers in the household, PIR, birthweight, and having a routine source of medical care.* [b]*value for interaction term sex * PAH.*

TABLE 4: Multivariate associations[a] between PAH metabolites and LD, NHANES 2001–2004 (N = 1257).

	All (N =1257) OR (95% CI)	Male (N = 608) OR (95% CI)	Female (N = 649) OR (95% CI)	P value for interaction[b]
1-Pyrene				
Log-transformed	0.85 (0.68, 1.05)	0.99 (0.77, 1.27)	0.58 (0.34, 0.98)	0.8
High versus low	0.87 (0.50, 1.51)	1.28 (0.68, 2.41)	0.42 (0.16, 1.11)	0.4
1-Napthol				
Log-transformed	1.03 (0.85, 1.23)	1.01 (0.75, 1.35)	1.19 (0.84, 1.68)	0.3
High versus low	1.65 (0.96, 2.81)	1.81 (0.83, 3.93)	1.46 (0.64, 3.31)	0.9
2-Napthol				
Log-transformed	0.91 (0.71, 1.17)	1.00 (0.68, 1.46)	0.89 (0.54, 1.45)	0.5
High versus low	0.63 (0.31, 1.28)	0.75 (0.32, 1.76)	0.50 (0.18, 1.41)	0.9
FLUO metabolites				
Log-transformed	0.89 (0.68, 1.17)	0.67 (0.42, 1.08)	1.50 (0.80, 2.81)	0.2
High versus low	1.14 (0.58, 2.23)	0.93 (0.46, 1.89)	1.54 (0.56, 4.24)	0.3
PHEN metabolites				
Log-transformed	0.91 (0.67, 1.24)	0.90 (0.57, 1.42)	1.03 (0.49, 2.13)	0.1
High versus low	0.74 (0.42, 1.32)	0.69 (0.33, 1.44)	0.76 (0.29, 2.005)	0.1

[a]*Adjusted for age, race/ethnicity, sex, creatinine, smokers in the household, PIR, birthweight, and having a routine source of medical care.* [b]*P value for interaction term sex * PAH.*

Multivariate analyses resulted in a significant inverse association between log-transformed (continuous) 2-napthol and ADHD (OR = 0.75; 95% C.I. 0.59, 0.94) (Table 3). Smokers in the household and sex remained significant, independent predictors of ADHD in the final models for each of the continuous and categorical exposure variables (data not shown). In models stratified by sex, a significant inverse association was found between log-transformed 1-pyrene and ADHD (OR = 0.46; 95% C.I. 0.23, 0.94) and between high 2-napthol and ADHD (OR = 0.39; 95% C.I. 0.16, 0.98) among females. The interaction terms of PAH exposure variables with sex were all nonsignificant.

TABLE 5: Multivariate associations[a] between PAH metabolites and SE, NHANES 2001–2004 (N = 1257).

	All (N =1257) OR (95% CI)	Male (N = 608) OR (95% CI)	Female (N = 649) OR (95% CI)	P value for interaction[b]
1-Pyrene				
Log-transformed	1.10 (0.86, 1.42)	1.24 (0.94, 1.63)	0.82 (0.49, 1.38)	0.3
High versus low	1.52 (0.86, 2.68)	1.83 (1.00, 3.34)	1.07 (0.43, 2.66)	0.8
1-Napthol				
Log-transformed	1.05 (0.88, 1.26)	1.02 (0.77, 1.37)	1.17 (0.81, 1.69)	0.1
High versus low	1.32 (0.77, 2.25)	1.55 (0.73, 3.29)	1.01 (0.41, 2.51)	0.3
2-Napthol				
Log-transformed	1.18 (0.89, 1.57)	1.27 (0.88, 1.82)	1.06 (0.71, 1.59)	0.5
High versus low	1.00 (0.53, 1.89)	1.27 (0.62, 2.60)	0.68 (0.27, 1.74)	0.9
FLUO metabolites				
Log-transformed	1.32 (0.92, 1.89)	1.24 (0.88, 1.75)	1.55 (0.79, 3.03)	0.4
High versus low	2.00 (1.05, 3.84)	2.25 (1.24, 4.07)	1.78 (0.59, 5.35)	0.2
PHEN metabolites				
Log-transformed	1.25 (0.89, 1.75)	1.25 (0.87, 1.80)	1.25 (0.67, 2.34)	0.2
High versus low	1.01 (0.61, 1.66)	1.01 (0.53, 1.91)	1.07 (0.44, 2.63)	0.7

[a]*Adjusted for age, race/ethnicity, sex, creatinine, smokers in the household, PIR, birthweight, and having a routine source of medical care.* [b] *P value for interaction term sex * PAH.*

Overall, there were no significant associations between PAH metabolites and LD in multivariate analyses (Table 4). Smokers in the household, birthweight, sex, poverty, and race/ethnicity (higher risk for Hispanics and "other" race compared to whites) remained significant, independent predictors of LD in the final models for each of the continuous and categorical exposure variables (data not shown). However, in models stratified by sex, a significant inverse association was found between log-transformed 1-pyrene and LD (OR = 0.58; 95% C.I. 0.34, 0.98) (Table 4) among females.

Conversely, a marginally significant positive association between high 1-pyrene and SE (OR = 1.83; 95% C.I. 1.00, 3.34) was observed among males in multivariate adjusted models (Table 5). Additionally, high fluorine metabolite levels were significantly and positively associated with SE (OR = 2.00; 95% C.I. 1.05, 3.84). Smokers in the household, birthweight, male sex, poverty, and having a routine source of care remained significant, independent predictors of SE in the final models for each of the continuous and categorical exposure variables (data not shown). In models stratified by sex, a significant positive association between high fluorine and SE remained among males (OR = 2.25; 95% C.I. 1.24, 4.07), but it was not statistically significant among females (OR = 1.78; 95% C.I. 0.59, 5.35).

12.4 DISCUSSION

Previous studies which have examined neurotoxic effects of prenatal PAHs in children were of modest sample size and many were based in New York City [19–21, 24] and China [22] where the results pertaining to highly-exposed populations may not be applicable to the general U.S. population. This study evaluated the association between childhood PAH biomarkers and parental report of ever doctor-diagnosed ADHD, LD, and receipt of SE services in a large, nationally-representative sample of U.S. children.

Significant inverse associations were observed between log-transformed 2-napthol and ADHD. Additionally, sex-stratified analyses indicated significant inverse associations among females between 1-pyrene and both ADHD and LD and between high 2-napthol and ADHD.

Conversely, significant positive associations were observed between high fluorine metabolites and SE. When stratified by sex, this association remained statistically significant for males but not for females. These findings suggest that PAH exposure may increase or decrease the risks of certain developmental disorders depending on the child's sex and the specific compounds to which they are exposed.

A number of limitations in this study must be considered. Unlike previous research on neurotoxic effects of PAHs, NHANES data are collected cross-sectionally thereby limiting our ability to infer causality. Current PAH levels may not reflect past exposures, and if prenatal and early childhood periods alone are the critical windows for susceptibility to the effects of exposure, then the use of current PAH levels as surrogate measures of etiologically-relevant exposures may have biased our results. Despite our findings regarding specific metabolites, it is difficult to attribute health effects to specific PAHs because most exposures are to PAH mixtures and not to individual PAH compounds [7].

Furthermore, use of urinary PAH metabolites, which have half-lives as short as 6–35 hours, will not reflect long-term exposures [35]. PAH-DNA adducts, which do not depend solely on the magnitude of recent dose, are a better measure of chronic exposure. Urinary concentrations are also affected by time of day when spot urine samples are collected—the within-day variance of urinary PAHs contributes 72 to 89% to total variance among individuals—a fluctuation which may be caused by diet, metabolism, or changes in daily routine [36]. Taking urine measurements at multiple time points or over a 24-hour period could help correct for exposure misclassification, although concentrations of urinary PAH metabolites reflect metabolic/detoxification capacity which also will vary among individuals. Our primary outcome is limited by its reliance on parental report of doctor-diagnosed ADHD rather than confirmed diagnosis using the *Diagnostic and Statistical Manual of Mental Disorders*, Fourth Edition (*DSM-IV*) criteria, or the Diagnostic Interview Schedule for Children IV (DISC-IV) used in previous studies. Similarly, diagnosis of LD and receipt of SE, including early intervention services, were both assessed via parental report. However, maternal reports of ADHD have been previously found to have high reliability and accuracy [37]. Nonetheless, any misclassification of the outcome should not be related to PAH exposures and, therefore, would have biased results towards the null.

Adjustment for potential confounders was limited to variables available for both NHANES cycles. Although presence of smokers in the household was included as a measure of ETS exposure, the potential for residual confounding exists. We did not quantitatively adjust for multiple comparisons in our statistical tests, which may have resulted in one or more of the observed effects. Additionally, because our sample size was limited by age restrictions, rarity of outcomes, and the one-third subsample of PAH measurements, we may have had insufficient power to detect some of the independent effects.

It is possible, as we found with some of the exposure variables, that PAH exposure does not increase the risk of ADHD, LD, or receipt of SE services in the general U.S. child population when controlling for other known risk factors. This would be consistent with a recent finding that prenatal exposures to PAHs showed no significant association with DSM-oriented attention deficit/hyperactivity problems at age 6-7 years in the Columbia Center for Children's Environmental Health (CCCEH) cohort [21].

Finally, as we have shown here, the effects of PAH exposure may differ by sex. Our sex-specific findings suggest that males may be at higher risk than females of PAH-induced neurodevelopmental effects. Recent research implicates sex-specific epigenetic marks—triggered by environmental factors—as a potential cause of the sex bias observed in many common diseases [38]. Epigenetic malprogramming caused by environmental factors may occur in a sex-specific manner, thereby leading to dimorphic gene expression and increased sensitivity of males (or females) to environmentally induced adverse health outcomes. PAHs, in particular, have been shown to alter gene expression in hormonal regulatory pathways (that are crucial to early brain development), alter expression of proinflammatory cytokines, upregulate COX-2 (an enzyme involved in inflammation and associated with reactive oxygen species) [39], and, in the CCCEH cohort, to lead to differential methylation in umbilical cord white blood cell DNA of newborns [40]. More research is needed to detect whether these or other epigenetic alterations mediate the neurodevelopmental effects of PAHs and whether these effects are sex-specific.

Nonetheless, this is the first study to examine the relationship between childhood PAH exposure and ADHD, LD, and SE in a nationally representative sample of U.S. children. Our results suggest an association between fluorine metabolites and increased need for SE services among the general U.S. population of school-aged children aged 6–15 years with possible sex-specific effects. Large, nationally representative, prospective studies are needed to fully investigate the neurodevelopmental effects of PAH exposure in children and to disentangle the effects of prenatal and postnatal exposures.

REFERENCES

1. G. Castaño-Vinyals, A. D'Errico, N. Malats, and M. Kogevinas, "Biomarkers of exposure to polycyclic aromatic hydrocarbons from environmental air pollution," Occupational and Environmental Medicine, vol. 61, no. 4, p. e12, 2004.

2. Z. Li, C. D. Sandau, L. C. Romanoff et al., "Concentration and profile of 22 urinary polycyclic aromatic hydrocarbon metabolites in the US population," Environmental Research, vol. 107, no. 3, pp. 320–331, 2008.

3. U. Heudorf and J. Angerer, "Internal exposure to PAHs of children and adults living in homes with parquet flooring containing high levels of PAHs in the parquet glue," International Archives of Occupational and Environmental Health, vol. 74, no. 2, pp. 91–101, 2001.

4. W. Huang, S. P. Caudill, J. Grainger, L. L. Needham, and D. G. Patterson Jr., "Levels of 1-hydroxypyrene and other monohydroxy polycyclic aromatic hydrocarbons in children: a study based on U.S. reference range values," Toxicology Letters, vol. 163, no. 1, pp. 10–19, 2006.

5. G. Falcó, J. L. Domingo, J. M. Llobet, A. Teixidó, C. Casas, and L. Müller, "Polycyclic aromatic hydrocarbons in foods: human exposure through the diet in Catalonia, Spain," Journal of Food Protection, vol. 66, no. 12, pp. 2325–2331, 2003.

6. R. Preuss, J. Angerer, and H. Drexler, "Naphthalene—an environmental and occupational toxicant," International Archives of Occupational and Environmental Health, vol. 76, no. 8, pp. 556–576, 2003.

7. Agency for Toxic Substances and Disease Registry (ATSDR), Polycyclic Aromatic Hydrocarbons (PAHs) What Health Effects Are Associated with PAH Exposure?2006, http://www.atsdr.cdc.gov/csem/csem.asp?csem=13&po=11.

8. C. R. Saunders, S. K. Das, A. Ramesh, D. C. Shockley, and S. Mukherjee, "Benzo(a) pyrene-induced acute neurotoxicity in the F-344 rat: role of oxidative stress," Journal of Applied Toxicology, vol. 26, no. 5, pp. 427–438, 2006.

9. D. D. Wormley, A. Ramesh, and D. B. Hood, "Environmental contaminant-mixture effects on CNS development, plasticity, and behavior," Toxicology and Applied Pharmacology, vol. 197, no. 1, pp. 49–65, 2004.

10. S. Yokota, K. Mizuo, N. Moriya, S. Oshio, I. Sugawara, and K. Takeda, "Effect of prenatal exposure to diesel exhaust on dopaminergic system in mice," Neuroscience Letters, vol. 449, no. 1, pp. 38–41, 2009.

11. F. P. Perera, W. Jedrychowski, V. Rauh, and R. M. Whyatt, "Molecular epidemiologic research on the effects of environmental pollutants on the fetus," Environmental Health Perspectives, vol. 107, supplement 3, pp. 451–460, 1999.

12. F. Perera, D. Tang, R. Whyatt, S. A. Lederman, and W. Jedrychowski, "DNA damage from polycyclic aromatic hydrocarbons measured by benzo[a]pyrene-DNA adducts in mothers and newborns from Northern Manhattan, the World Trade Center Area, Poland, and China," Cancer Epidemiology Biomarkers and Prevention, vol. 14, no. 3, pp. 709–714, 2005.

13. K. Takeda, N. Tsukue, and S. Yoshida, "Endocrine-disrupting activity of chemicals in diesel exhaust and diesel exhaust particles," Environmental science, vol. 11, no. 1, pp. 33–45, 2004.

14. J. Dejmek, I. Solanský, I. Beneš, J. Leníček, and R. J. Šrám, "The impact of polycyclic aromatic hydrocarbons and fine particles on pregnancy outcome," Environmental Health Perspectives, vol. 108, no. 12, pp. 1159–1164, 2000.

15. D. K. Manchester, S. K. Gordon, C. L. Golas, E. A. Roberts, and A. B. Okey, "Ah receptor in human placenta: stabilization by molybdate and characterization of binding of 2,3,7,8-tetrachlorodibenzo-p-dioxin, 3-methylcholanthrene, and benzo(a)pyrene," Cancer Research, vol. 47, no. 18, pp. 4861–4868, 1987.

16. C. J. Nicol, M. L. Harrison, R. R. Laposa, I. L. Gimelshtein, and P. G. Wells, "A teratologic suppressor role for p53 in benzo[a]pyrene-treated transgenic p53-deficient mice," Nature Genetics, vol. 10, no. 2, pp. 181–187, 1995.

17. K. A. Wood and R. J. Youle, "The role of free radicals and p53 in neuron apoptosis in vivo," Journal of Neuroscience, vol. 15, no. 8, pp. 5851–5857, 1995.

18. V. L. Wilson and P. A. Jones, "Inhibition of DNA methylation by chemical carcinogens in vitro," Cell, vol. 32, no. 1, pp. 239–246, 1983.

19. F. P. Perera, V. Rauh, R. M. Whyatt et al., "Effect of prenatal exposure to airborne polycyclic aromatic hydocarbons on neurodevelopment in the first 3 years of life among inner-city children," Environmental Health Perspectives, vol. 114, no. 8, pp. 1287–1292, 2006.

20. F. P. Perera, S. Wang, J. Vishnevetsky et al., "Polycyclic aromatic hydrocarbons-aromatic DNA adducts in cord blood and behavior scores in New York city children," Environmental Health Perspectives, vol. 119, no. 8, pp. 1176–1181, 2011.

21. F. P. Perera, D. Tang, S. Wang et al., "Prenatal polycyclic aromatic hydrocarbon (PAH) exposure and child behavior at age 6-7 years," Environmental Health Perspectives, vol. 120, no. 6, pp. 921–926, 2012.

22. D. Tang, T.-Y. Li, J. J. Liu et al., "Effects of prenatal exposure to coal-burning pollutants on children's development in China," Environmental Health Perspectives, vol. 116, no. 5, pp. 674–679, 2008.

23. S. C. Edwards, W. Jedrychowski, M. Butscher et al., "Prenatal exposure to airborne polycyclic aromatic hydrocarbons and children's intelligence at 5 years of age in a prospective cohort study in Poland," Environmental Health Perspectives, vol. 118, no. 9, pp. 1326–1331, 2010.

24. F. P. Perera, Z. Li, R. Whyatt et al., "Prenatal airborne polycyclic aromatic hydrocarbon exposure and child IQ at age 5 years," Pediatrics, vol. 124, no. 2, pp. e195–e202, 2009.

25. R. J. Šrám, I. Beneš, B. Binková et al., "Teplice Program—the impact of air pollution on human health," Environmental Health Perspectives, vol. 104, no. 4, pp. 699–714, 1996.

26. J. G. Millichap, "Etiologic classification of attention-deficit/hyperactivity disorder," Pediatrics, vol. 121, no. 2, pp. e358–e365, 2008.

27. T. D. Banerjee, F. Middleton, and S. V. Faraone, "Environmental risk factors for attention-deficit hyperactivity disorder," Acta Paediatrica, vol. 96, no. 9, pp. 1269–1274, 2007.

28. C. Schnoes, R. Reid, M. Wagner, and C. Marder, "ADHD among students receiving special education services: a national survey," Exceptional Children, vol. 72, no. 4, pp. 483–496, 2006.

29. R. Bussing, B. T. Zima, A. R. Perwien, T. R. Belin, and M. Widawski, "Children in special education programs: attention deficit hyperactivity disorder, use of services, and unmet needs," American Journal of Public Health, vol. 88, no. 6, pp. 880–886, 1998.

30. K. Weiland, M. Neidell, V. Rauh, and F. Perera, "Cost of developmental delay from prenatal exposure to airborne polycyclic aromatic hydrocarbons," Journal of Health Care for the Poor and Underserved, vol. 22, no. 1, pp. 320–329, 2011.

31. Centers for Disease Control and Prevention (CDC). National Center for Health Statistics (NCHS), National Health and Nutrition Examination Survey Data, U.S. Department of Health and Human Services, Centers for Disease Control and Prevention, Hyattsville, Md, USA, 2001–2004, http://wwwn.cdc.gov/nchs/nhanes/search/nhanes01_02.aspx, http://wwwn.cdc.gov/nchs/nhanes/search/nhanes03_04.aspx.

32. Centers for Disease Control and Prevention (CDC). National Center for Health Statistics (NCHS), National Health and Nutrition Examination Survey Public Data General Release File Documentation, U.S. Department of Health and Human Services, Centers for Disease Control and Prevention, Hyattsville, Md, USA, 2005, http://www.cdc.gov/nchs/data/nhanes/nhanes_01_02/general_data_release_doc.pdf, http://www.cdc.gov/nchs/data/nhanes/nhanes_03_04/general_data_release_doc_03-04.pdf.

33. Centers for Disease Control and Prevention (CDC). National Center for Health Statistics (NCHS), National Health and Nutrition Examination Laboratory Procedure Manual, U.S. Department of Health and Human Services, Centers for Disease Control and Prevention, Hyattsville, Md, USA, 2003-2004, http://www.cdc.gov/nchs/data/nhanes/nhanes_03_04/l31pah_c_met.pdf.

34. J. Stevens, J. S. Harman, and K. J. Kelleher, "Race/ethnicity and insurance status as factors associated with ADHD treatment patterns," Journal of Child and Adolescent Psychopharmacology, vol. 15, no. 1, pp. 88–96, 2005.

35. F. J. Jongeneelen, F. E. van Leeuwen, S. Oosterink et al., "Ambient and biological monitoring of cokeoven workers: determinants of the internal dose of polycyclic aromatic hydrocarbons," British Journal of Industrial Medicine, vol. 47, no. 7, pp. 454–461, 1990.

36. Z. Li, L. C. Romanoff, M. D. Lewin et al., "Variability of urinary concentrations of polycyclic aromatic hydrocarbon metabolite in general population and comparison of spot, first-morning, and 24-h void sampling," Journal of Exposure Science and Environmental Epidemiology, vol. 20, no. 6, pp. 526–535, 2010.

37. S. V. Faraone, J. Biederman, and S. Milberger, "How reliable are maternal reports of their children's psychopathology? One-year recall of psychiatric diagnoses of ADHD children," Journal of the American Academy of Child and Adolescent Psychiatry, vol. 34, no. 8, pp. 1001–1008, 1995.

38. A. Gabory, L. Attig, and C. Junien, "Sexual dimorphism in environmental epigenetic programming," Molecular and Cellular Endocrinology, vol. 304, no. 1-2, pp. 8–18, 2009.

39. F. Perera and J. Herbstman, "Prenatal environmental exposures, epigenetics, and disease," Reproductive Toxicology, vol. 31, no. 3, pp. 363–373, 2011.

40. J. B. Herbstman, D. Tang, D. Zhu et al., "Prenatal exposure to polycyclic aromatic hydrocarbons, benzo[a]pyrene-DNA adducts, and genomic DNA methylation in cord blood," Environmental Health Perspectives, vol. 120, no. 5, pp. 733–738, 2012.

There is one table that is not available in this version of the article. To view it, please use the citation on the first page of this chapter.

CHAPTER 13

SERUM PERFLUORINATED COMPOUND CONCENTRATION AND ATTENTION DEFICIT/ HYPERACTIVITY DISORDER IN CHILDREN 5–18 YEARS OF AGE

CHERYL R. STEIN AND DAVID A. SAVITZ

Perfluorooctanoic acid (PFOA) is a synthetic chemical that has been used in the manufacture of fluoropolymers since the 1950s [U.S. Environmental Protection Agency (EPA) 2009a] and may also result from the breakdown of a related group of chemicals called fluorinated telomers (U.S. EPA 2009b). Fluoropolymers are used in nonstick cookware and clothing made from waterproof, breathable fabric (U.S. EPA 2009b).

PFOA and other perfluorinated compounds (PFCs) with comparable industrial uses—perfluorooctane sulfonate (PFOS), perfluorohexane sulfonate (PFHxS), and perfluorononanoic acid (PFNA)—are persistent environmental pollutants that have been detected worldwide in both wildlife and humans, with higher exposure closer to urbanized and industrialized regions (Houde et al. 2006). In the U.S. general population, PFOA, PFOS,

Reproduced with permission from Environmental Health Perspectives. Stein CR and Savitz DA. Serum Perfluorinated Compound Concentration and Attention Deficit/Hyperactivity Disorder in Children 5–18 Years of Age. Environmental Health Perspectives *119,10 (2011); doi:10.1289/ehp.1003538.*

and PFHxS were detected in all serum samples from the 1999–2000 National Health and Nutrition Examination Survey (NHANES); PFNA was detected in 95% of samples (Calafat et al. 2007a). NHANES 2003–2004 data showed minor reductions in the percentage of samples with detectable levels of PFOA, PFOS, and PFHxS, and the geometric mean concentrations for these three compounds dropped slightly (Calafat et al. 2007b). For PFNA, however, the percentage of serum samples with detectable levels increased, and the geometric mean increased from 0.5 ng/mL to 1.0 ng/mL, between the NHANES waves. PFOA and PFOS, the two most commonly studied PFCs, have been detected in maternal and umbilical cord blood (Inoue et al. 2004; Midasch et al. 2007; Monroy et al. 2008) and breast milk (Kuklenyik et al. 2004; So et al. 2006; Tao et al. 2008a, 2008b; Volkel et al. 2008). The serum elimination half-life for PFOA is estimated at 2.3 years (Bartell et al. 2010) to 4 years (Olsen et al. 2007); for PFOS, 5 years (Olsen et al. 2007); and for PFHxS, 8.5 years (Olsen et al. 2007). A half-life estimate is not available for PFNA.

Toxicology studies highlight the potential for PFCs to affect fetal growth and development (reviewed by Lau et al. 2004, 2007; Olsen et al. 2009). Rat pups prenatally exposed to PFOS show delayed behavioral milestones (Luebker et al. 2005), and delayed task learning has been noted in female pups prenatally exposed to PFOS and maternal restraint (Fuentes et al. 2007). The limited developmental toxicology literature suggests possible adverse effects of PFOA and PFOS on fetal growth and viability and postnatal growth (Butenhoff et al. 2004; Lau et al. 2004).

One epidemiologic study examined developmental milestones in relation to PFC exposure (Fei et al. 2008). In a substudy of the Danish National Birth Cohort (n = 1,400), early pregnancy plasma PFOA and PFOS levels were essentially unrelated to motor or mental development through 18 months of age, although there were weak associations between increased PFOS levels and sitting without assistance or using wordlike sounds to indicate wants (Fei et al. 2008). A single study has examined the association between PFC exposure and attention deficit/hyperactivity disorder (ADHD) among children from the 1999–2000 and 2003–2004 NHANES and reported increased odds of disease with higher serum PFC levels (Hoffman et al. 2010).

ADHD is a relatively common neurodevelopmental disorder with suspected environmental and genetic etiology (reviewed by Aguiar et al. 2010; Banerjee et al. 2007; Swanson et al. 2007). The disorder, generally recognized by early school age, is characterized by developmentally inappropriate levels of inattention, hyperactivity, and impulsivity [Centers for Disease Control and Prevention (CDC) 2010]. In the 2007 U.S. National Survey of Children's Health, the estimate of parent-reported ADHD among children 4–17 years of age was 9.5%; 4.8% reported both diagnosis and medication use (CDC 2010). Although prevalence estimates vary, it is generally accepted that the prevalence of this disorder is rising (Aguiar et al. 2010; CDC 2010; Pastor and Reuben 2008). In contrast, the prevalence of learning disorders among children 6–17 years of age, estimated at 8.7%, has been relatively stable from 1997 to 2006 (Pastor and Reuben 2008). Prenatal exposures to alcohol and cigarettes, as well as childhood exposure to lead, polychlorinated biphenyls (PCBs), and methyl mercury, have all been positively associated with ADHD or ADHD-like behaviors (reviewed by Banerjee et al. 2007; Eubig et al. 2010). PFCs, with their widespread exposure and potential for developmental toxicity, warrant examination as an environmental risk factor for ADHD.

A chemical plant in the Mid-Ohio Valley near Parkersburg, West Virginia, has used PFOA in the manufacture of fluoropolymers since 1951. In 2001, a group of residents from the West Virginia and Ohio communities surrounding the plant filed a class action lawsuit alleging health damage from drinking water supplies drawing on PFOA-contaminated groundwater (Frisbee et al. 2009). Groundwater contamination from the Ohio River and air deposition are believed to be the primary exposure routes for this population (Emmett et al. 2006). The settlement of the class action lawsuit included a baseline survey, the C8 Health Project (C8 is another name for PFOA, denoting its chain of eight carbons) (Frisbee et al. 2009). The C8 Health Project included demographic and health questionnaires and measurement of 10 PFCs in serum. In the present study we used these data to examine the cross-sectional association between serum PFOA, PFOS, PFHxS, and PFNA measurements at C8 Health Project enrollment and report of a diagnosis with ADHD or a learning problem among children 5–18 years of age.

13.1 METHODS

C8 Health Project population. The C8 Health Project enrolled participants between August 2005 and July 2006. The project's purpose was to collect health data from members of the class action lawsuit through questionnaires and blood tests, including measurement of PFCs. This community was highly exposed to PFOA, but exposure to other PFCs reflects typical background levels. Individuals were eligible to participate in the C8 Health Project if they could provide documentation proving they had consumed water for at least 1 year between 1950 and 3 December 2004 in a water district supplied by Little Hocking Water Association of Ohio; City of Belpre, Ohio; Tupper Plains–Chester District of Ohio; Village of Pomeroy, Ohio; Lubeck Public Service District of West Virginia; Mason County Public Service District of West Virginia; or private water sources within areas of documented PFOA contamination. Participants provided informed consent and were compensated $400 for completing the questionnaire and providing blood. At the time of enrollment, participants did not know their individual exposure to PFOA. The C8 Health Project collected data on 69,030 people. The total number of people eligible to join the class action lawsuit is unknown. Participation rates based on U.S. Census counts of current residents of the eligible water districts are estimated at around 80% and in some ZIP codes within eligible water districts appear close to 100% (Frisbee et al. 2009). The overall participation rate is likely < 80% because former residents were also eligible to participate. In this population, the strongest predictor of PFOA serum level was current residence in a contaminated water district, with distance to the plant directly affecting PFOA levels (Steenland et al. 2009). Because plant emissions varied over the 50-year contamination period, the relative PFOA exposure levels of the water districts remained the same, such that high-exposure water districts were always more exposed than low-exposure water districts, regardless of the absolute exposure levels. Exposure to other PFCs is not determined by residence in a PFOA-contaminated water district and reflects typical background levels, which likely occur through dietary and consumer product exposures (Vestergren and Cousins 2009). Of the 69,030 C8 Health

Project participants, 12,016 were 5–18 years of age at enrollment. Of these children, 11,046 (92%) had serum PFC measurements.

Measures. Laboratory analysis (Exygen Research Inc., State College, PA) of PFCs used automated solid-phase extraction combined with reverse-phase high-performance liquid chromatography (Kuklenyik et al. 2004). Four PFCs were detectable in 100% of samples (PFOA, PFOS, PFHxS, PFNA); we included these four in our analyses. We examined the association between PFCs and ADHD using restricted cubic splines (Desquilbet and Mariotti 2010) and determined that quartiles of exposure best captured the nonlinear nature of the PFC–outcome associations. All analyses categorized PFCs into quartiles.

We examined the relation between PFC serum concentrations and a diagnosis of ADHD as reported in the C8 Health Project questionnaire. Participants were asked "Has a doctor or health professional ever told you that you have/had 'Attention Deficit Disorder' (ADD or ADHD)?" We additionally constructed a second, more sensitive ADHD definition by combining report of ADHD diagnosis with current use of a medication commonly used to treat ADHD (Braun et al. 2006). Participants were asked to list all current prescription and over-the-counter medications they were currently taking for any reason. Based on guidance from clinical experts, medications considered treatment for ADHD were methylphenidate, dextroamphetamine, mixed amphetamine salts, lisdexamfetamine, dexmethylphenidate, atomoxetine, clonidine, guanfacine, imipramine, nortriptyline, bupropion, and carbamazepine. We included several medications that are prescribed off-label for complicated and recalcitrant cases of ADHD. This decision yielded 23 children who reported a diagnosis with ADHD and use of off-label medications only that would not have been included in the analysis of ADHD with medication had we restricted the category solely to those taking licensed drugs. These children tended to be older and male. Finally, we examined report of learning problems based on the question "Has a representative from a school or a health professional ever told you that you have/had a learning problem?" Among the 60% of the C8 Health Project population that gave permission to use identifying information allowing us to determine precisely who completed the questionnaire, 10.7% of children reported completing the questionnaires for themselves.

Parents or legal guardians accounted for 98.2% of nonchild responders. As a sensitivity analysis, among the 60% of children where the respondent was identified, we compared the results for all children versus children where the parent or legal guardian completed the survey. Restriction to the subset with the parent/guardian as the named respondent had no effect on the pattern of results. The vast majority of the 682 children responding for themselves were old enough to be in high school and were likely adequate reporters of whether they had been diagnosed with ADHD. It is also possible that these children provided the preliminary information on the questionnaire themselves (name, birth date, address, and identification of who was completing the survey) and then passed the survey to a parent to answer the more involved questions on health outcomes. This change in respondent would not have been noted on the questionnaire.

Other covariates available for analysis included age (modeled as quintiles), sex, race/ethnicity (non-Hispanic white vs. other), body mass index (BMI) z-score based on the 2000 CDC growth charts of BMI for age (CDC 2009), and average household income ($\leq$ \$30,000 vs. > \$30,000). Institutional review board approval was granted from the Mount Sinai Program for the Protection of Human Subjects.

Statistical analysis. Analysis was performed using SAS software (version 9.2; SAS Institute Inc., Cary, NC). Given the concern that PFCs may be hormonally active (White et al. 2011), we first examined the potential for sex to modify the association between exposure and outcome by comparing the effect estimates of stratified and unstratified models and by examining the p-value for the PFC–sex interaction term (Rothman and Greenland 1998). There was little evidence that sex modified the exposure–outcome association, although for PFOA there was a modest, imprecise, suggestion of a stronger association among females; we report unstratified models. We assessed the potential for age, sex, race/ethnicity, BMI z-score, and average household income to act as confounders by looking for associations between these covariates and the exposure, and these covariates and the outcome (Rothman and Greenland 1998). Neither BMI z-score nor race/ethnicity met the criteria for confounding, although we restricted analyses to 10,546 non-Hispanic white children (95.0%) to facilitate comparisons with other studies requiring adjustment for race/ethnicity. Because average household income was missing for 21.3% of participants, we compared odds ratios (ORs) adjusted for age, sex, and income with ORs adjusted for age and sex only. There was a < 10% change in ORs between the fully and partially adjusted models, so we excluded average household income from analysis, allowing us to retain a larger study population. We ran logistic regression models adjusted for age and sex to calculate the OR and 95% confidence intervals (CIs) for each PFC–outcome combination.

We also performed several secondary analyses: a) For all 10,546 children, we ran each model, simultaneously adjusting all PFCs for one another to account for confounding. For instance, in the model for PFOA, we adjusted for age, sex, PFOS, PFHxS, and PFNA. b) Among the 6,523 children permitting use of identifying information, we restricted analysis to the 2,437 children who lived in the same PFOA-exposed water district their entire life. Because PFOA exposure is directly related to residential location, this residential restriction is more likely to maintain the same relative ranking of PFOA exposure distribution over time, potentially reducing exposure misclassification, particularly if there is an early-life critical developmental window of susceptibility to PFOA. c) To facilitate comparisons with the NHANES population (Hoffman et al. 2010), we ran two additional analyses. We restricted analysis to the 3,571 children 12–15 years of age so that our age range was comparable to that of NHANES. We also examined the 5,262 children with PFOA exposures below the median (range, 0.6 ng/mL to < 28.2 ng/mL) to align our exposure range more closely to that of NHANES.

13.2 RESULTS

Of the 10,546 non-Hispanic white children 5–18 years of age in the C8 Health Project, 12.4% reported a diagnosis of ADHD and 12.1% a learning problem (Table 1). Using the stricter definition of ADHD diagnosis plus medication, 5.1% of children were counted as cases. Mean ± SD serum PFOA was 66.3 ± 106.1 ng/mL, and the median value was 28.2 ng/mL [interquartile range (IQR), 13.0–65.3 ng/mL], considerably higher than the NHANES 2003–2004 geometric mean of 3.9 ng/mL. Serum PFOS concentration was comparable to that of NHANES, whereas PFHxS and

PFNA concentrations were higher in the C8 Health Project population. The correlation among all PFCs ranged from the weakest Spearman $\rho = 0.11$ ($p < 0.001$) between PFOA and PFNA to the strongest $\rho = 0.54$ ($p < 0.001$) between PFOS and PFHxS. The mean $\pm$ SD age in the population was 13.1 ± 3.8 years, and 51.6% were male. Of the 6,532 children in the subset where residential history was available, 2,437 (37.4%) lived their entire life in a single PFOA-exposed water district.

The association between serum PFOA and ADHD followed an inverted J. We observed a small increase in prevalence for the second quartile of exposure compared with the lowest, and a somewhat larger decrease for the highest versus lowest quartile (Table 2). For PFOS, we observed a small increase in prevalence of ADHD with medication for all quartiles that was most pronounced for the highest exposure group but less apparent for ADHD alone (without consideration of medication use). The strongest association between exposure and outcome was for PFHxS, with elevated ORs for quartiles 2–4 compared with the lowest quartile, ranging from 1.44 to 1.59. We found no discernable pattern for PFNA, with no association for ADHD alone and only a slightly elevated OR for the highest exposure quartile for ADHD with medication. Overall, the associations for ADHD both with and without medication use were similar, with the patterns more pronounced for the more stringent criteria, albeit with less precise CIs.

We observed small reductions in ORs comparing quartiles 2–4 with the lowest quartile for PFOA, PFOS, and PFNA and reported learning problems, but no dose–response gradient (Table 2). The prevalence of a self-reported learning problem was increased for quartiles 2–4 of PFHxS exposure compared with the lowest quartile. The strongest OR compared the highest versus lowest quartiles (OR = 1.19; 95% CI, 1.00–1.41).

Simultaneous adjustment for all PFCs tended to weaken positive ORs and strengthen negative ORs for ADHD. The exception was for PFHxS, where simultaneous adjustment for all PFCs strengthened all of the observed positive associations. For instance, for ADHD with medication, the OR comparing the highest and lowest exposure groups was 1.67 (95% CI, 1.23–2.26) with simultaneous adjustment for all PFCs, compared with 1.59 (95% CI, 1.21–2.08) without the additional adjustment. Overall, the changes to the results with adjustment for all PFCs were minor and did not alter interpretation of the estimates (data not shown).

TABLE 1: Univariate characteristics of non-Hispanic white children 5–18 years of age, C8 Health Project, Mid-Ohio Valley, 2005–2006 (n = 10,546).

Characteristic	Measure
ADHD diagnosis	
Yes	1,303 (12.4)
No	9,243 (87.6)
ADHD diagnosis + medication	
Yes	542 (5.1)
No	10,004 (94.9)
Learning problema	
Yes	1,281 (12.1)
No	9,265 (87.9)
Serum PFOA (ng/mL)	66.3 ± 106.1
Quartile 1: 0.6 to < 13.0	2,643 (25.1)
Quartile 2: 13.0 to < 28.2	2,634 (25.0)
Quartile 3: 28.2 to < 65.3	2,643 (25.1)
Quartile 4: 65.3 to 2070.6	2,626 (24.9)
Serum PFOS (ng/mL)	22.9 ± 12.5,
Quartile 1: 0.25 to < 14.8	2,597 (24.6)
Quartile 2: 14.8 to < 20.2	2,655 (25.2)
Quartile 3: 20.2 to < 27.9	2,632 (25.0)
Quartile 4: 27.8 to 202.1	2,662 (25.2)
Serum PFHxS (ng/mL)	9.3 ± 13.7
Quartile 1: 0.25 to < 2.9	2,716 (25.7)
Quartile 2: 2.9 to < 5.2	2,500 (23.7)
Quartile 3: 5.2 to < 10.1	2,689 (25.5)
Quartile 4: 10.1 to 276.4	2,641 (25.0)
Serum PFNA (ng/mL)	1.7 ± 1.0
Quartile 1: 0.25 to < 1.2	2,552 (24.2)
Quartile 2: 1.2 to < 1.5	2,387 (22.6)
Quartile 3: 1.5 to < 2.0	2,880 (27.3)
Quartile 4: 2.0 to 24.1	2,727 (25.9)
Sex	
Male	5,446 (51.6)
Female	5,100 (48.4)
Age (years)	13.1 ± 3.8

TABLE 1: *Cont.*

Characteristic	Measure
Quintile 1: 5.0 to < 9.3	2,092 (19.8)
Quintile 2: 9.3 to < 12.3	2,099 (19.9)
Quintile 3: 12.3 to < 14.7	2,116 (20.1)
Quintile 4: 14.7 to < 16.8	2,129 (20.2)
Quintile 5: 16.8 to < 19.0	2,110 (20.0)
Average household income	
≤ $30,000	3,968 (47.8)
> $30,000	4,335 (52.2)
BMI (kg/m^2)	21.9 ± 5.5
BMI z-score	0.5 ± 1.3
BMI percentile	
Underweight (< 5th)	440 (4.4)
Healthy weight (5th to < 85th)	5,801 (58.6)
Overweight (85th to < 95th)	1,686 (17.0)
Obese (> 95th)	1,973 (19.9)
Single water districtb	
Yes	2,437 (37.4)
No	4,086 (62.6)

Data are presented as n (%) or mean ± SD. [a]Learning problem denotes a positive response to the question "Has a representative from a school or a health professional ever told you that you have/had a learning problem?" [b]Available for identified subset only (n = 6,523).

TABLE 2: Crude and adjusted[a] associations between serum PFC exposure and ADHD or learning problems[b] among children 5–18 years of age, C8 Health Project, Mid-Ohio Valley, 2005–2006 (n = 10,546).

Serum PFC (ng/mL)	ADHD diagnosis			ADHD diagnosis + medication			Learning problem[b]		
	No. of cases	Crude OR CI)a	Adjusted OR (95% CI)a	No. of cases	Crude OR CI)a	Adjusted OR (95% CI)a	No. of cases	Crude OR	Adjusted OR (95% CI)a
PFOA									
Quartile 1: 0.6 to <13.0	327	1.00	1.00	129	1.00	1.00	326	1.00	1.00
Quartile 2: 13.0 to <28.2	364	1.14	1.10 (0.94–1.30)	159	1.25	1.20 (0.94–1.53)	318	0.98	0.95 (0.81–1.12)
Quartile 3: 28.2 to <65.3	337	1.04	0.98 (0.83–1.15)	146	1.14	1.04 (0.81–1.32)	330	1.01	0.98 (0.83–1.15)
Quartile 4: 65.3 to 2070.6	275	0.83	0.76 (0.64–0.90)	108	0.84	0.72 (0.55–0.94)	307	0.94	0.90 (0.76–1.06)
PFOS									
Quartile 1: 0.25 to <14.8	299	1.00	1.00	107	1.00	1.00	347	1.00	1.00
Quartile 2: 14.8 to <20.2	321	1.06	0.99 (0.83–1.17)	134	1.24	1.15 (0.89–1.50)	317	0.88	0.83 (0.70–0.98)
Quartile 3: 20.2 to <27.9	318	1.06	0.96 (0.81–1.14)	137	1.28	1.14 (0.87–1.48)	288	0.80	0.74 (0.62–0.87)
Quartile 4: 27.9 to 202.1	365	1.22	1.09 (0.93–1.29)	164	1.53	1.27 (0.99–1.64)	329	0.91	0.85 (0.72–1.00)
PFHxS									
Quartile 1: 0.25 to <2.9	258	1.00	1.00	89	1.00	1.00	300	1.00	1.00

TABLE 2: Cont.

Serum PFC (ng/mL)	ADHD diagnosis			ADHD diagnosis + medication			Learning problem[b]		
	No. of cases	Crude OR	Adjusted OR (95% CI)a	No. of cases	Crude OR	Adjusted OR (95% CI)a	No. of cases	Crude OR	Adjusted OR (95% CI)a
Quartile 2: 2.9 to <5.2	304	1.32	1.27 (1.06–1.52)	128	1.59	1.44 (1.09–1.90)	313	1.15	1.13 (0.95–1.34)
Quartile 3: 5.2 to <10.1	364	1.49	1.43 (1.21–1.70)	157	1.83	1.55 (1.19–2.04)	332	1.13	1.12 (0.95–1.33)
Quartile 4: 10.1 to 276.4	377	1.59	1.53 (1.29–1.83)	168	2.01	1.59 (1.21–2.08)	336	1.17	1.19 (1.00–1.41)
PFNA									
Quartile 1: 0.25 to <1.2	311	1.00	1.00	112	1.00	1.00	352	1.00	1.00
Quartile 2: 1.2 to <1.5	302	1.04	1.00 (0.84–1.19)	117	1.12	1.02 (0.78–1.34)	299	0.89	0.87 (0.74–1.03)
Quartile 3: 1.5 to <2.0	349	0.99	0.94 (0.79–1.11)	151	1.21	1.06 (0.82–1.36)	340	0.84	0.81 (0.69–0.95)
Quartile 4: 2.0 to 24.1	341	1.03	0.99 (0.84–1.18)	162	1.38	1.16 (0.90–1.49)	290	0.74	0.74 (0.62–0.87)

[a]Adjusted for age and sex. [b]Learning problem denotes a positive response to the question "Has a representative from a school or a health professional ever told you that you have/had a learning problem?"

TABLE 3: Adjusted[a] associations [OR (95% CI)] between serum PFC exposure and ADHD or learning problems[b] among children 12–15 years of age, C8 Health Project, Mid-Ohio Valley, 2005–2006 (n = 3,571).

Serum PFC (ng/mL)	ADHD diagnosis	ADHD diagnosis + medication	Learning problem[b]
PFOA			
Quartile 1: 0.6 to < 13.0	1.00	1.00	1.00
Quartile 2: 13.0 to < 28.2	1.18 (0.91–1.53)	1.39 (0.95–2.04)	1.13 (0.86–1.47)
Quartile 3: 28.2 to < 65.3	0.93 (0.71–1.21)	1.25 (0.85–1.83)	0.93 (0.71–1.21)
Quartile 4: 65.3 to 2070.6	0.79 (0.60–1.04)	0.87 (0.58–1.32)	0.96 (0.73–1.26)
PFOS			
Quartile 1: 0.25 to < 14.8	1.00	1.00	1.00
Quartile 2:14.8 to < 20.2	0.91 (0.70–1.19)	1.40 (0.94–2.08)	0.78 (0.60–1.01)
Quartile 3: 20.2 to < 27.9	0.92 (0.71–1.21)	1.38 (0.92–2.06)	0.68 (0.52–0.89)
Quartile 4: 27.8 to 202.1	0.99 (0.76–1.30)	1.32 (0.88–1.99)	0.71 (0.54–0.93)
PFHxS			
Quartile 1: 0.25 to < 2.9	1.00	1.00	1.00
Quartile 2: 2.9 to < 5.2	1.46 (1.10–1.93)	1.32 (0.87–1.99)	1.31 (1.00–1.71)
Quartile 3: 5.2 to < 10.1	1.45 (1.10–1.91)	1.32 (0.88–1.97)	1.08 (0.82–1.43)
Quartile 4: 10.1 to 276.4	1.53 (1.15–2.04)	1.42 (0.94–2.13)	1.05 (0.79–1.40)
PFNA			
Quartile 1: 0.25 to < 1.2	1.00	1.00	1.00
Quartile 2: 1.2 to < 1.5	1.16 (0.89–1.51)	1.12 (0.76–1.64)	0.97 (0.74–1.25)
Quartile 3: 1.5 to < 2.0	0.96 (0.74–1.24)	0.99 (0.67–1.45)	0.86 (0.66–1.11)
Quartile 4: 2.0 to 24.1	1.00 (0.75–1.32)	1.15 (0.78–1.71)	0.73 (0.55–0.98)

[a]*Adjusted for age (continuous) and sex.* [b]*Learning problem denotes a positive response to the question "Has a representative from a school or a health professional ever told you that you have/had a learning problem?"*

Among the children living in a single PFOA-exposed water district where presumably the current level of exposure reflects long-term patterns (n = 2,437), the association between PFOA and ADHD was attenuated (data not shown). For ADHD with medication, the modest increased prevalence in quartile 2 remained the same while the reduced prevalence in quartile 4 relative to the first quartile was eliminated (OR = 1.02; 95% CI, 0.60–1.73).

Among the 12- to 15-year-olds (n = 3,571), the patterns of association for ADHD alone and learning problems remained the same as for the full age range (Table 3). For ADHD with medication, the positive ORs were strengthened for PFOA and PFOS and weakened for PFHxS, and we observed no appreciable change for PFNA. Overall, the pattern of associations observed in the full data set was not materially altered by restriction to ages 12–15 years.

When restricting the analysis to children with PFOA exposures below the median (n = 5,262), for ADHD alone all ORs were near the null value and CIs were wide (data not shown). For ADHD with medication, we observed no reduction in prevalence for quartile 4 as we observed in the full population. Rather, the increase in prevalence observed when moving from the lowest quartile to quartile 2 (OR = 1.23; 95% CI, 0.85–1.76) remained consistent for quartile 3 (OR = 1.33; 95% CI, 0.93–1.93) and quartile 4 (OR = 1.35; 95% CI, 0.94–1.93).

13.3 DISCUSSION

Our sporadic positive associations between PFCs and ADHD contrast somewhat with the findings of Hoffman et al. (2010), even when we restricted to the same age range. In a sample of 571 children 12–15 years of age, the prevalence of ADHD was 8.4% (3.6% with medication use) in the Hoffman et al. (2010) population, compared with 14.3% (6.2% with medication use) in our population of 3,571 children 12–15 years of age. In addition to lower ADHD prevalence, the NHANES study also had lower median exposure levels for PFHxS and PFNA and, of course, dramatically lower exposures for PFOA. The median PFOS values were comparable between NHANES and the C8 Health Project. It is not surprising that PFNA exposure was higher in our sample (2005–2006) than in the NHANES samples (1999–2000 and 2003–2004), because PFNA exposure appears to be increasing (Calafat et al. 2007b) and we collected our data subsequent to NHANES. Additionally, we are studying a non-Hispanic white population, which also tends to have higher PFC levels than do non-Hispanic black and Mexican-American populations (Calafat et al. 2007b). Even with lower exposure and disease prevalence estimates, Hoffman et al. (2010) reported increased prevalence of ADHD with increased exposure to all PFCs, ranging from 1.15 (95% CI, 0.93–1.42) for the IQR effect for PFNA to 1.60 (95% CI, 1.10–2.31) for the IQR effect for PFOS. Although the results from these two studies are not directly comparable because we analyzed our exposure by quartiles to best characterize the observed nonlinear association, among our population of 12- to 15-year-olds the only positive association for ADHD alone was with PFHxS (e.g., highest vs. lowest quartile: OR = 1.53; 95% CI, 1.15–2.04). In NHANES, a 2.9-ng/mL (IQR) increase in PFHxS was associated with an OR of 1.19 (95% CI, 1.05–1.34). When examining ADHD with medication, however, our study also yielded a positive association for PFOS. In the subset of children with PFOA exposure below the median, an exposure range more comparable to that in NHANES, PFOA results were null for ADHD alone, but we observed a sustained positive association for ADHD with medication for quartiles 2–4 compared with the lowest quartile.

The pattern of results for PFOA and ADHD in our full population, with a small increase then more notable decrease in prevalence, is unlikely to be causal and may reflect some unmeasured correlate of PFOA exposure. The diagnosis of ADHD requires that behavioral symptoms be present in two or more settings, such as at home and at school (American Psychiatric Association 2000). If the geographic boundaries of water district (the strongest predictor of PFOA exposure) and school district (which may affect the likelihood of being diagnosed with ADHD) overlap, the characteristics of school districts may contribute to this finding. For instance, it is possible that children living in the water districts most highly exposed to PFOA may also be living in the school districts least likely to diagnose ADHD. Alternatively, children living in the less exposed water districts may attend schools that are more likely to diagnose ADHD. Prevalence of ADHD can vary by school district (Daley et al. 1998) as well as characteristics of teacher, school (Schneider and Eisenberg 2006), and clinical provider (Fulton et al. 2009). In addition to the potential for confounding by regional geography, another explanation for the inverted J-shaped association between PFOA and ADHD in this cross-sectional study is that a correlate of the disorder may affect measured exposure. If ADHD or its treatment is related to drinking less tap water, for example, which is a major influence on exposure, a spurious association might result. Additionally, the observed association could also occur if the condition or its treatment affected the uptake, metabolism, or excretion of PFOA. Without additional data, we are unable to more thoroughly examine any of these scenarios.

We found support for a small, positive association between PFC exposure and report of learning problems only for PFHxS. Serum PFNA levels were associated with a modest decrease in the prevalence of a self-reported learning problem. However, this outcome was defined nonspecifically and may indicate disabilities in listening, speaking, basic reading skills, reading comprehension, written expression, mathematical calculation, or mathematical reasoning (Pastor and Reuben 2008). Future investigations should differentiate among specific types of learning disabilities.

A major limitation of this cross-sectional investigation is the reliance on parent or self-report for measurement of the outcome, although we also included the more stringent case definition of ADHD report with medication use (Braun et al. 2006). One study found 83% agreement between parent report and physician records for accessing services for ADHD, and a kappa of 0.94 for agreement on medication use (Bussing et al. 2003). Parent report of ADHD is commonly used in research studies and national surveys. Furthermore, there is little reason to expect that report of ADHD would be differential by PFC exposure level, which would be needed to bias our findings away from the null. The laboratory-determined exposure measurement does not suffer from the same quality issues as do reported ADHD and learning problems. However, the simultaneous measurement of the exposure and reporting of the outcome allows for confounding by behaviors or physiologic changes associated with ADHD, such as moving to a different water district or altering tap water consumption after diagnosis, which would affect measured PFOA serum level and, additionally, preclude examining potential critical windows of developmental effects.

To assess a potential causal role of PFCs in ADHD or learning problems, a prospective study is required. School-level information on this population may be needed to more adequately understand the pattern of association between PFOA and report of ADHD diagnosis. Additionally, data on other health and environmental risk factors, such as prenatal exposures to nicotine or alcohol, gestational age at birth, childhood exposures to toxicants such as lead and PCBs, and better socioeconomic information, would have enriched these analyses.

13.4 CONCLUSION

With only two studies, each with its own limitations, research on the developmental health effects of PFCs is at a very early stage. The suggestive findings of these cross-sectional studies examining PFCs as risk factors for ADHD call for a more thorough evaluation of the association.

REFERENCES

1. Aguiar A, Eubig PA, Schantz SL. Attention deficit/hyperactivity disorder: a focused overview for children's environmental health researchers. Environ Health Perspect. 2010;118:1646–1653.
2. American Psychiatric Association. Washington, DC: American Psychiatric Association; 2000. Diagnostic and Statistical Manual of Mental Disorders: DSM-IV-TR. 4th ed., text revision.
3. Banerjee TD, Middleton F, Faraone SV. Environmental risk factors for attention-deficit hyperactivity disorder. Acta Paediatr. 2007;96:1269–1274.
4. Bartell SM, Calafat AM, Lyu C, Kato K, Ryan PB, Steenland K. Rate of decline in serum PFOA concentrations after granular activated carbon filtration at two public water systems in Ohio and West Virginia. Environ Health Perspect. 2010;118:222–228.
5. Braun JM, Kahn RS, Froehlich T, Auinger P, Lanphear BP. Exposures to environmental toxicants and attention deficit hyperactivity disorder in U.S. children. Environ Health Perspect. 2006;114:1904–1909.
6. Bussing R, Mason DM, Leon CE, Sinha K. Agreement between CASA parent reports and provider records of children's ADHD services. J Behav Health Serv Res. 2003;30:462–469.
7. Butenhoff JL, Kennedy GL, Jr, Frame SR, O'Connor JC, York RG. The reproductive toxicology of ammonium perfluorooctanoate (APFO) in the rat. Toxicology. 2004;196:95–116.

8. Calafat AM, Kuklenyik Z, Reidy JA, Caudill SP, Tully JS, Needham LL. Serum concentrations of 11 polyfluoroalkyl compounds in the U.S. population: data from the National Health and Nutrition Examination Survey (NHANES). Environ Sci Technol. 2007a;41:2237–2242.

9. Calafat AM, Wong LY, Kuklenyik Z, Reidy JA, Needham LL. Polyfluoroalkyl chemicals in the U.S. population: data from the National Health and Nutrition Examination Survey (NHANES) 2003–2004 and comparisons with NHANES 1999–2000. Environ Health Perspect. 2007b;115:1596–1602.

10. CDC (Centers for Disease Control and Prevention) A SAS Program for the CDC Growth Charts. 2009. Available: http://www.cdc.gov/nccdphp/dnpao/growthcharts/resources/sas.htm [accessed 20 October 2010]

11. CDC (Centers for Disease Control and Prevention). Increasing prevalence of parent-reported attention-deficit/hyperactivity disorder among children—United States, 2003 and 2007. MMWR Morb Mortal Wkly Rep. 2010;59:1439–1443.

12. Daley CE, Onwuegbuzie AJ, Griffin H. Attention-deficit/hyperactivity disorder: relations between prevalence rate and school district size, diagnostic method, and referral process. Psychol Rep. 1998;83:593–594.

13. Desquilbet L, Mariotti F. 2010. Dose-response analyses using restricted cubic spline functions in public health research. Stat Med; doi:[Online 19 January 2010]10.1002/sim.3841

14. Emmett EA, Shofer FS, Zhang H, Freeman D, Desai C, Shaw LM. Community exposure to perfluorooctanoate: relationships between serum concentrations and exposure sources. J Occup Environ Med. 2006;48:759–770.

15. Eubig PA, Aguiar A, Schantz SL. Lead and PCBs as risk factors for attention deficit/hyperactivity disorder. Environ Health Perspect. 2010;118:1654–1667.

16. Fei C, McLaughlin JK, Lipworth L, Olsen J. Prenatal exposure to perfluorooctanoate (PFOA) and perfluorooctanesulfonate (PFOS) and maternally reported developmental milestones in infancy. Environ Health Perspect. 2008;116:1391–1395.

17. Frisbee SJ, Brooks AP, Jr, Maher A, Flensborg P, Arnold S, Fletcher T, et al. The C8 health project: design, methods, and participants. Environ Health Perspect. 2009;117:1873–1882.

18. Fuentes S, Colomina MT, Vicens P, Domingo JL. Influence of maternal restraint stress on the long-lasting effects induced by prenatal exposure to perfluorooctane sulfonate (PFOS) in mice. Toxicol Lett. 2007;171:162–170.

19. Fulton BD, Scheffler RM, Hinshaw SP, Levine P, Stone S, Brown TT, et al. National variation of ADHD diagnostic prevalence and medication use: health care providers and education policies. Psychiatr Serv. 2009;60:1075–1083.

20. Hoffman K, Webster TF, Weisskopf MG, Weinberg J, Vieira VM. Exposure to polyfluoroalkyl chemicals and attention deficit/hyperactivity disorder in U.S. children 12–15 years of age. Environ Health Perspect. 2010;118:1762–1767.

21. Houde M, Martin JW, Letcher RJ, Solomon KR, Muir DC. Biological monitoring of polyfluoroalkyl substances: a review. Environ Sci Technol. 2006;40:3463–3473.

22. Inoue K, Okada F, Ito R, Kato S, Sasaki S, Nakajima S, et al. Perfluorooctane sulfonate (PFOS) and related perfluorinated compounds in human maternal and cord blood samples: assessment of PFOS exposure in a susceptible population during pregnancy. Environ Health Perspect. 2004;112:1204–1207.

23. Kuklenyik Z, Reich JA, Tully JS, Needham LL, Calafat AM. Automated solid-phase extraction and measurement of perfluorinated organic acids and amides in human serum and milk. Environ Sci Technol. 2004;38:3698–3704.

24. Lau C, Anitole K, Hodes C, Lai D, Pfahles-Hutchens A, Seed J. Perfluoroalkyl acids: a review of monitoring and toxicological findings. Toxicol Sci. 2007;99:366–394.

25. Lau C, Butenhoff JL, Rogers JM. The developmental toxicity of perfluoroalkyl acids and their derivatives. Toxicol Appl Pharmacol. 2004;198:231–241.

26. Luebker DJ, Case MT, York RG, Moore JA, Hansen KJ, Butenhoff JL. Two-generation reproduction and cross-foster studies of perfluorooctanesulfonate (PFOS) in rats. Toxicology. 2005;215:126–148.

27. Midasch O, Drexler H, Hart N, Beckmann MW, Angerer J. Transplacental exposure of neonates to perfluorooctanesulfonate and perfluorooctanoate: a pilot study. Int Arch Occup Environ Health. 2007;80:643–648.

28. Monroy R, Morrison K, Teo K, Atkinson S, Kubwabo C, Stewart B, et al. Serum levels of perfluoroalkyl compounds in human maternal and umbilical cord blood samples. Environ Res. 2008;108:56–62.

29. Olsen GW, Burris JM, Ehresman DJ, Froehlich JW, Seacat AM, Butenhoff JL, et al. Half-life of serum elimination of perfluorooctanesulfonate, perfluorohexanesulfonate, and perfluorooctanoate in retired fluorochemical production workers. Environ Health Perspect. 2007;115:1298–1305.

30. Olsen GW, Butenhoff JL, Zobel LR. Perfluoroalkyl chemicals and human fetal development: an epidemiologic review with clinical and toxicological perspectives. Reprod Toxicol. 2009;27:212–230.

31. Pastor PN, Reuben CA. Diagnosed attention deficit hyperactivity disorder and learning disability: United States, 2004–2006. Vital Health Stat 10. 2008:1–14.

32. Rothman KJ, Greenland S. Philadelphia: Lippincott-Raven; 1998. Modern Epidemiology. 2nd ed.

33. Schneider H, Eisenberg D. Who receives a diagnosis of attention-deficit/ hyperactivity disorder in the United States elementary school population? Pediatrics. 2006;117:e601–e609.

34. So MK, Yamashita N, Taniyasu S, Jiang Q, Giesy JP, Chen K, et al. Health risks in infants associated with exposure to perfluorinated compounds in human breast milk from Zhoushan, China. Environ Sci Technol. 2006;40:2924–2929.

35. Steenland K, Jin C, MacNeil J, Lally C, Ducatman A, Vieira V, et al. Predictors of PFOA levels in a community surrounding a chemical plant. Environ Health Perspect. 2009;117:1083–1088.

36. Swanson JM, Kinsbourne M, Nigg J, Lanphear B, Stefanatos GA, Volkow N, et al. Etiologic subtypes of attention-deficit/hyperactivity disorder: brain imaging, molecular genetic and environmental factors and the dopamine hypothesis. Neuropsychol Rev. 2007;17:39–59.

37. Tao L, Kannan K, Wong CM, Arcaro KF, Butenhoff JL. Perfluorinated compounds in human milk from Massachusetts, U.S.A. Environ Sci Technol. 2008a;42:3096–3101.

38. Tao L, Ma J, Kunisue T, Libelo EL, Tanabe S, Kannan K. Perfluorinated compounds in human breast milk from several Asian countries, and in infant formula and dairy milk from the United States. Environ Sci Technol. 2008b;42:8597–8602.

39. U.S. EPA (U.S. Environmental Protection Agency) Perfluorooctanoic Acid (PFOA) and Fluorinated Telomers. 2009a. Available: http://www.epa.gov/oppt/pfoa/index. html [accessed 21 January 2009]

40. U.S. EPA (U.S. Environmental Protection Agency) Perfluorooctanoic Acid (PFOA) and Fluorinated Telomers Basic Information. 2009b. Available: http://www.epa.gov/ oppt/pfoa/pubs/pfoainfo.html [accessed 21 January 2009]

41. Vestergren R, Cousins IT. Tracking the pathways of human exposure to perfluoro-carboxylates. Environ Sci Technol. 2009;43:5565–5575.

42. Volkel W, Genzel-Boroviczeny O, Demmelmair H, Gebauer C, Koletzko B, Twardella D, et al. Perfluorooctane sulphonate (PFOS) and perfluorooctanoic acid (PFOA) in human breast milk: results of a pilot study. Int J Hyg Environ Health. 2008;211:440–446.

43. White SS, Fenton SE, Hines EP. 2011. Endocrine disrupting properties of perfluo-rooctanoic acid. J Steroid Biochem Mol Biol; doi:[Online 11 March 2011]10.1016/j. jsbmb.2011.03.011

IN UTERO AND CHILDHOOD POLYBROMINATED DIPHENYL ETHER (PBDE) EXPOSURES AND NEURODEVELOPMENT IN THE CHAMACOS STUDY

BRENDA ESKENAZI, JONATHAN CHEVRIER,
STEPHEN A. RAUCH, KATHERINE KOGUT, KIM G. HARLEY,
CAROLINE JOHNSON, CELINA TRUJILLO, ANDREAS SJÖDIN,
AND ASA BRADMAN

Polybrominated diphenyl ether (PBDEs) flame retardant chemicals, used in the manufacture of furniture, infant products, and electronics, are ubiquitous in U.S. households (Sjödin et al. 2008). An unintended consequence of California's Technical Bulletin 117 (TB 117)—a fire safety law promulgated in the 1970s which requires that furniture, baby, and other household products resist open flame (California Department of Consumer Affairs 2000; Zota et al. 2008)—is that PBDE concentrations in California children are now among the highest measured worldwide (Eskenazi et al. 2011). Until 2005, the predominant chemical flame retardant used to comply with TB 117 was pentaBDE (comprising congeners BDEs 47, 99, 100,

Reproduced with permission from Environmental Health Perspectives. Eskenazi B, Chevrier J, Rauch SA, Kogut K, Harley KG, Johnson C, Trujillo C, Sjödin A, and Bradman A. Nitrate Leaching From Intensive Organic Farms to Groundwater. Environmental Health Perspectives 121,2 (2013); DOI:10.1289/ehp.1205597.

and 153). Although pentaBDE was banned in California and phased out by the manufacturer in 2004, pentaBDEs continue to leach from older household items. Exposure is also perpetuated by decaBDEs, still used in many electronic products, which can break down into lower-brominated congeners (Noyes et al. 2011). Because PBDEs are semivolatile and not chemically bound to substrates, they migrate into house dust, placing young children, who crawl on the floor and exhibit frequent hand-to-mouth behaviors, at risk of higher exposures (Stapleton et al. 2008).

PBDEs are endocrine-disrupting compounds with half-lives in humans ranging from 2 to 12 years (Geyer et al. 2004). Recent research suggests that PBDE exposures are associated with altered thyroid hormone levels in pregnant women (Chevrier et al. 2010) and infants (Herbstman et al. 2008), and negatively associated with birth weight (Harley et al. 2011). Research also suggests possible neurotoxic effects of in utero and early childhood exposure to PBDEs (Chao et al. 2007; Gascon et al. 2011, 2012; Herbstman et al. 2010; Hoffman et al. 2012; Roze et al. 2009). Herbstman et al. (2010) reported significant decrements in motor and mental development at ages 1–6 years associated with in utero PBDE exposures in New York children (n = 100). In a study of 62 5- to 6-year-old Dutch children, Roze et al. (2009) reported that in utero exposure levels were negatively associated with fine motor coordination and sustained attention, although improved coordination and visual perception and fewer internalizing and externalizing behaviors. Recently, Gascon et al. (2011) reported that 4-year-old Spanish children with detectable blood concentrations of BDE-47 were significantly more likely to demonstrate attention symptoms [*DSM-IV* (*Diagnostic and Statistical Manual of Mental Disorders, 4th ed.*) (American Psychiatric Association 1994) scores > 80th percentile] than less-exposed peers, but not motor or cognitive deficits. Cord blood BDE-47 concentrations were not associated with any neurobehavioral parameters at 4 years of age. Hoffman et al. (2012) found a positive association between breast milk levels of BDEs 47, 99, and 100 and externalizing behaviors, specifically activity/impulsivity behaviors in 220 30-month-olds.

In this analysis, we examined the relationship of prenatal maternal and child PBDE concentrations with attention, cognition, and motor development in California children at 5 and 7 years of age.

14.1 METHODS

The Center for the Health Assessment of Mothers and Children of Salinas (CHAMACOS) is a longitudinal birth cohort study of predominantly Mexican-American families in California's Salinas Valley. Detailed methods for CHAMACOS are published elsewhere (Eskenazi et al. 2004, 2006). Eligible pregnant women ($\geq$ 18 years old, < 20 weeks gestation, Spanish- or English-speaking, qualifying for low-income health insurance, and planning to deliver at the public hospital) were recruited between October 1999 and October 2000 from community clinics. The cohort included 601 women, 526 of whom delivered live-born singletons.

Women were interviewed twice during pregnancy (at ~ 13 and 26 weeks gestation), after delivery, and when children were 6 months old, and 1, 2, 3.5, 5, and 7 years old. Mothers completed the Peabody Picture Vocabulary Test (PPVT) or Test de Vocabulario en Imágenes Peabody (TVIP) of verbal intelligence (Dunn and Dunn 1981) at the 6-month visit and the Center for Epidemiologic Studies Depression Scale (CES-D) (Radloff 1977) at the 1-year visit. Age-appropriate versions of the HOME (Home Observation for Measurement of the Environment) survey were completed at most postdelivery visits (Caldwell and Bradley 1984). Birth weight and gestational duration were abstracted from medical records.

Neurobehavioral assessments were performed by bilingual psychometricians, and children were assessed in their dominant language. A total of 310 children were assessed at 5 years (mean = 60.0 ± 2.6 months) and 323 at 7 years (85.2 ± 2.9 months). The present analysis excludes four children with autism, Down syndrome, cerebral palsy/hydrocephalus, or deafness and 63 children who lacked PBDE measurements.

Compared with children in the cohort who were not followed, children included in the present analyses were more likely to be female and born full term, with mothers who were older, breastfed longer, and were less likely to smoke or drink during pregnancy (data not shown). They did not differ according to other sociodemographic characteristics or by their maternal prenatal PBDE levels [median = 24.9 ng/g lipid; interquartile range (IQR) 14.0–42.1] for those followed versus 23.8 ng/g lipid (IQR = 14.9–41.3) for those not followed].

Mothers provided written informed consent at both visits, and children provided verbal assent at 7 years of age. Study activities were approved by the University of California at Berkeley (UC) Committee for the Protection of Human Subjects. A technical assistance agreement was established between the Division of Laboratory Sciences at the National Center for Environmental Health, Centers for Disease Control and Prevention (CDC), and UC Berkeley.

Attention. At the 5-year visit, mothers completed the Child Behavior Checklist (CBCL)/1.5–5 (CBCL) (Achenbach and Rescorla 2000). We analyzed two subscales as continuous raw scores: the Attention Problems scale and the DSM-IV–oriented Attention Deficit/Hyperactivity Disorder (ADHD) Problems scale. We also analyzed a "borderline clinical range" ($\geq$ 93rd percentile in the standardization sample) indicator variable for each scale (Achenbach and Rescorla 2000). In addition, children were assessed on the Conners' Kiddie Continuous Performance Test (K-CPT) (Conners and Staff 2001), a 7-min computerized vigilance task that assesses reaction time, accuracy, and impulse control. We determined continuous T-scores (standardized to a nonclinical population) for errors of commission, errors of omission, and hit reaction time (Conners and Staff 2001). We also examined the continuous ADHD Confidence Index score, which indicates the probability that children are correctly classified as having clinical ADHD, and a binary variable indicating a Confidence Index score $\geq$ 70th percentile.

At child's age 7 years, mothers and teachers completed the Conners' ADHD/DSM-IV Scales (CADS) (Conners 2001) and the Behavior Assessment System for Children, 2nd edition (BASC) (Reynolds and Kamphaus 2004). CADS data from four subscales (Conners ADHD index score, and DSM-IV–based Inattentive, Hyperactive/Impulsive, and Total ADHD scores) were analyzed both as continuous, standardized scores (T-scores; mean $\pm$ SD = 50 $\pm$ 10) and as a binary variable indicating scores in the "Moderately" or "Markedly Atypical" range (T-score $\geq$ 65) (Conners 2001). BASC data from Hyperactivity and Attention Problems subscales were analyzed as standardized T-scores and as a binary "at-risk" or "clinically significant" variable (T-score $\geq$ 60) (Reynolds and Kamphaus 2004).

Motor function. At ages 5 and 7 years, children's gross motor skills were assessed using select subscales of the McCarthy Scales of

Children's Abilities (McCarthy 1972). Their fine motor dexterity was assessed with a pegboard test (Wide Range Assessment of Visual Motor Ability; WRAVMA) (Adams and Sheslow 1995) (age-standardized mean = 100 ± 15) and with a finger-tapping task [at 5 years: Behavioral Assessment and Research System (BARS) (Rohlman et al. 2003); and at 7 years: Reitan Neuropsychology Laboratory (Tucson, AZ)]. We standardized McCarthy gross motor and finger tap scores within our study population (z-scores, mean = 0 ± 1).

Cognitive functioning. At 5 years of age, children completed tests of receptive verbal intelligence in both English and Spanish using the PPVT and TVIP, respectively (Dunn and Dunn 1981). We analyzed children's continuous standardized scores (mean = 100 ± 15) in their language of best performance. We assessed children's performance intelligence (PIQ) with the Wechsler Preschool and Primary Scale of Intelligence, 3rd edition (WPPSI-III) (mean = 100 ± 15).

At age 7 years, children were assessed on four subdomains of the Wechsler Intelligence Scale for Children–Fourth Edition (WISC-IV) (Wechsler 2003): Verbal Comprehension, Perceptual Reasoning, Working Memory, and Processing Speed. A Full-Scale IQ was also calculated (mean = 100 ± 15 for the Full-Scale IQ and all components).

Other questions. Mothers were also asked "Has a doctor, nurse, psychologist or teacher ever told you that your child might have 1) attention problems? or 2) learning problems?" Teachers were asked "Do you have any specific concerns about this student (in terms of) 1) emotional problems, 2) behavioral problems, or 3) learning problems?"

PBDE exposure assessment. Blood samples were collected by venipuncture from mothers during pregnancy (mean = 26.7 ± 2.6 weeks gestation, n = 219) or at delivery (n = 60), and from children at the 7-year visit (n = 272). PBDE serum levels in women with data at both time points were very strongly correlated (Pearson $r \geq 0.98$, $p < 0.001$)]. Samples were immediately processed and stored at −80oC until shipment on dry ice to the CDC (Atlanta, GA). Samples were analyzed at CDC for 10 congeners (BDEs 17, 28, 47, 66, 85, 99, 100, 153, 154, and 183) using gas chromatography isotope dilution high-resolution mass spectrometry (Sjödin et al. 2004). PBDE concentrations are expressed on a serum lipid basis (nanograms per gram lipids). Total serum lipid concentrations were determined based on the measurement of triglycerides and total cholesterol using standard enzymatic methods (Roche Chemicals, Indianapolis, IN) (Phillips et al. 1989). The limits of detection (LODs) for BDE-47 ranged from 0.3 to 2.6 ng/g lipids for maternal samples, and 0.4 to 0.8 ng/g lipids for child samples. For all other congeners, LODs ranged between 0.2 and 0.7 ng/g lipids for maternal and 0.3 and 5.6 ng/g lipids for child samples, respectively. Quality control samples (blanks and spikes) were included in each run.

We used the sum of BDEs 47, 99, 100, and 153 congeners as our primary exposure measure. Values < LOD were assigned the machine-read value if a signal was detected. If not, all concentration levels < LOD were imputed at random based on a log-normal probability distribution using maximum likelihood estimation (Lubin et al. 2004).

We assessed maternal exposure to organophosphate (OP) insecticides as measured by dialkyl phosphate (DAP) metabolites in maternal urine (at 13 and 26 weeks gestation), using an isotope dilution gas chromatography-tandem mass spectrometry method (Bradman et al. 2005; Bravo et al. 2002); lead in maternal prenatal and cord blood samples, using graphite furnace atomic absorption spectrophotometry; polychlorinated biphenyls (PCBs) in maternal serum using high-resolution gas chromatography/high-resolution mass spectrometry with isotope dilution quantification (Barr et al. 2003); and maternal thyroid stimulating hormone (TSH; using immunochemiluminometric assay) and free thyroxine (T4; using direct equilibrium dialysis followed by radioimmunoassay) (Bayer ADVIA Centaur system; Siemens Healthcare Diagnostics, Deerfield, IL) at 26 weeks gestation (Chevrier et al. 2010; Nelson and Tomei 1988).

Data analysis. PBDE levels were expressed on the $\log_{10}$ scale. To determine the shape of the dose–response function, we ran generalized additive models using cubic splines. If nonlinearity was detected ($p < 0.10$), additional models were run with categorized PBDE concentrations (quartiles). We re-ran all final models with PBDE concentrations expressed on a serum basis (picograms per gram serum) with total serum lipids as a covariate. We also ran models with the sum of all 10 PBDE congeners; individually for each of the four primary congeners (47, 99, 100, and 153); and excluding outliers (defined as being ≥ 3.5 SD away from the mean for $\log_{10}$ PBDEs or the outcome).

Variables were identified as potential confounders based on their re-lationship to neurodevelopment. We examined the following [see Sup-plemental Material, Table S3 for categories (http://dx.doi.org/10.1289/ehp.1205597)]: maternal age, education, years in the United States, mari-tal status, work outside the home, use of alcohol and tobacco during preg-nancy, depression (CES-D), parity, and PPVT or TVIP score; housing density, household poverty, pregnancy exposure to environmental tobacco smoke, number of children in the home, father's presence in the home, and HOME score at 6 months and 7 years; preschool and out-of-home child care attendance; psychometrician, location, and language of assessment; and child sex, birth weight, preterm delivery status, and handedness (mo-tor outcomes only). Missing values (< 10%) for covariates were imputed by randomly selecting a value from the dataset.

We built separate models for attention, cognition, and motor outcomes, and used the same model for all outcomes within a category. In addition to child's sex and months of age (continuous), final models included all covariates that changed the coefficient for the main exposure and any out-come within the group by > 10%. The covariates maintained in the models are listed in the footnote of the respective tables.

For sensitivity analyses, we adjusted for birth weight, gestational age at birth, maternal thyroid hormone (TSH and free T4), DAPs, lead, and PCBs in separate models (Chevrier et al. 2010; Harley et al. 2011). We evaluated effect modification by child sex. In addition, we included mater-nal and child PBDE levels in the same models, although doing so reduced the sample size (n = 214).

Main effects were considered statistically significant with $p < 0.05$ based on two-tailed tests, and interactions were considered significant if p < 0.10. All analyses were conducted with STATA version 10.1 (StataCorp, College Station, TX).

14.2 RESULTS

For both mothers and children, BDE congeners 47, 99, 100, and 153 had detection frequencies > 97% and dominated the total measure of concen-tration, with BDE-47 in the highest concentration [for maternal and child measures, see Supplemental Material, Tables S1 and S2, respectively (http://dx.doi.org/10.1289/ehp.1205597)]. Children's PBDE levels were more than three times higher than the mothers' for the sum of four congeners, and detection frequencies for most other congeners were also substantially higher in children (Bradman et al. 2012; Castorina et al. 2011; Eskenazi et al. 2011). The correlation between maternal and child ΣPBDE levels was 0.27 (p < 0.001); the correlation for individual congeners ranged from 0.21 for BDE-99 to 0.30 for BDE-153. Supplemental Material, Table S3, presents the distribution of demographic characteristics for children in the study sample and the geometric means (GM) of maternal and child ΣPBDE concentrations by covariates. Supplemental Material, Table S4, summarizes neurobehavioral scores for the study population.

Correlations between reports by teachers and parents concerning attention at 7 years of age, and between measures of attention, cognition, and motor skills, were moderate. For example, correlations between maternal and teacher report on the CADS ranged from $r = 0.2$–0.3 ($p < 0.01$). Similar measures of attention on the BASC and CADS within a reporter (mother/teacher) were more strongly correlated—for example, $r = 0.5$ to 0.8, $p < 0.001$ for maternal report and $r = 0.7$ to 0.8, $p < 0.001$ for teacher report. Maternal and teacher CADS scores were negatively correlated with WISC Full-Scale IQ scores ($r = -0.2$ to -0.3, $p < 0.001$). Motor skills outcomes tended to be positively correlated with IQ scores ($r = 0.1$ to 0.4, several $p < 0.001$) and negatively correlated with attention outcomes ($r = -0.05$ to -0.2, several $p < 0.01$) (data not shown).

Attention. At child age 5 years, maternal prenatal ΣPBDE concentrations (for the 4 main congeners) were marginally associated ($p < 0.10$) with maternally reported CBCL scores above the 93rd percentile for attention problems [adjusted odds ratio (aOR) for a 10-fold increase in ΣPBDE = 4.6; 95%CI: 0.9, 24.5] [see Supplemental Material, Table S5 (http://dx.doi.org/10.1289/ehp.1205597)], and strongly associated with both errors of omission scores and ADHD Confidence Index scores on the K-CPT (Table 1). Quartile categorization suggested that both errors of omission and the ADHD Confidence Index were primarily elevated in children with mothers in the highest quartile of ΣPBDE exposure (> 42 ng/g) (Figure 1).

TABLE 1: Adjusted linear models for attention-related outcome scores in CHAMACOS children at 5 and 7 years of age, per 10-fold increase in maternal prenatal and child $\sum$PBDE concentration (ng/g, lipid-adjusted).

Outcome		Maternal $\sum$PBDE[a,c]		Child $\sum$PBDE[b,c]	
		n	β (95% CI)	n	β (95% CI)
Assessment of 5-year-olds					
CBCL (raw score)	Attention problems	249	0.1 (−0.4, 0.6)		
	ADHD	249	0.4 (−0.5, 1.2)		
K-CPT (T-score)	Errors of omission	246	5.8 (1.5, 10.1)**,#		
	Errors of commission	246	−0.5 (−3.7, 2.7)		
	ADHD Confidence Index	233	7.0 (1.6, 12.4)**,#		
Assessment of 7-year-olds					
Conner's rating scale (CADS)–maternal report (T-score)	ADHD index	266	2.9 (0.7, 5.2)**	270	1.0 (−1.9, 3.9)
	DSM-IV total scale	266	2.6 (0.2, 5.0)**,#	270	1.4 (−1.5, 4.4)
	Inattentive subscale	266	2.2 (0.0, 4.5)**,#	270	0.7 (−2.1, 3.5)#
	Hyperactive/Impulsive subscale	266	1.6 (−0.8, 4.1)	270	1.9 (−1.1, 5.0)
BASC-2–maternal report (T-score)	Hyperactivity scale	257	1.0 (−1.5, 3.6)	269	0.5 (−2.6, 3.5)
	Attention Problems scale	257	0.5 (−1.2, 2.1)	269	−0.1 (−2.1, 1.9)
Conner's rating scale (CADS)–teacher report (T-score)	ADHD index	213	2.4 (−1.4, 6.1)	219	4.6 (−0.4, 9.6)*
	DSM-IV total scale	212	1.8 (−1.4, 5.0)	217	4.0 (−0.3, 8.3)*
	Inattentive subscale	216	1.2 (−1.6, 3.9)	221	3.7 (0.1, 7.4)**
	Hyperactive/Impulsive subscale	216	1.7 (−1.7, 5.0)	221	3.5 (−1.1, 8.0)
BASC-2–teacher report (T-score)	Hyperactivity scale	217	1.8 (−1.3, 4.9)	222	4.8 (0.5, 9.0)**
	Attention Problems scale	257	0.7 (−1.3, 2.7)	222	2.9 (0.4, 5.5)**

[a]*Maternal PBDE models control for child's age at assessment, sex, maternal education, number of children in the home, and psychometrician (5-year assessments only).* [b]*Child PBDE models control for child's age at assessment, sex, and parity.* [c]*Sum of four PBDE congeners: BDEs 47, 99, 100, and 153.* **p < 0.1. **p ≤ 0.05. #Digression from linearity at p < 0.10.*

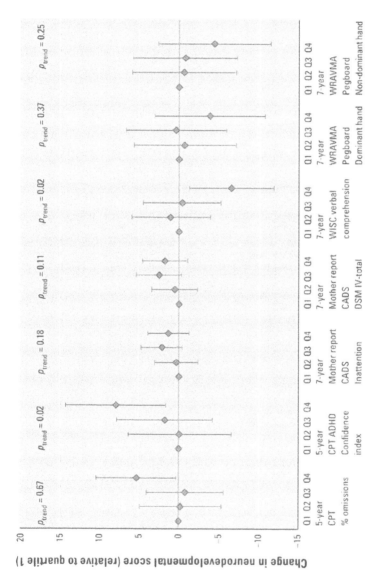

FIGURE 1: The point estimate and 95% CI for each quartile (Q) of maternal $\sum$PBDE concentration for outcomes that showed overall associations and evidence of nonlinearity (at $p < 0.1$). The quartile ranges for maternal PBDEs were ≤ 14.4, 14.5–24.78, 24.8–41.97, and $\geq$ 42 ng/g lipid. Tests for trend come from models using PBDE quartile (1–4) as a continuous variable.

TABLE 2: Adjusted linear models for motor function in CHAMACOS children at 5 and 7 years of age, per 10-fold increase in maternal prenatal and child $\sum$PBDE concentration (ng/g, lipid-adjusted).

Outcome		Maternal $\sum$PBDE[a,b]		Child $\sum$PBDE[b,c]	
		n	β (95% CI)	n	β (95% CI)
Assessment of 5-year-olds					
WRAVMA pegboard (standard score)	Dominant hand	254	−4.3 (−9.6, 1.0)		
	Nondominant hand	252	−5.6 (−10.8, −0.4)**,##		
Finger tap (BARS z-score)	Dominant hand	234	−0.4 (−0.7, 0.0)**		
	Nondominant hand	234	−0.2 (−0.5, 0.1)		
McCarthy (z-score)	Gross motor leg	241	0.0 (−0.3, 0.4)#		
	Bean bag catch	249	−0.1 (−0.4, 0.2)#		
Assessment of 7-year-olds					
WRAVMA pegboard (standard score)	Dominant hand	258	−5.4 (−11.1, 0.3)*,#,##	269	−5.4 (−12.0, 1.2)
	Nondominant hand	258	−6.5 (−12.3, −0.7)**,#	268	−6.1 (−12.7, 0.4)*
Finger tap (BARS z-score)	Dominant hand	258	−0.1 (−0.4, 0.2)#	269	−0.2 (−0.6, 0.2)
	Nondominant hand	258	−0.1 (−0.4, 0.2)#	268	−0.1 (−0.5, 0.2)
McCarthy (z-score)	Gross motor leg	255	−0.1 (−0.4, 0.1)#	266	−0.1 (−0.4, 0.2)#
	Bean bag catch	258	0.0 (−0.3, 0.4)	268	0.0 (−0.4, 0.3)

[a]*Maternal PBDE models control for child's age, sex, home score at 6-month visit, father living with family, handedness, location of testing, whether the child attended preschool, maternal years in United States before giving birth, and psychometrician (5-year assessment only).* [b]*Sum of four PBDE congeners: BDEs 47, 99, 100, and 153.* [c]*Child PBDE models control for child's age, sex, home score at 7-year visit, and location of testing.* *p < 0.1. **p ≤ 0.05. #Digression from linearity at p < 0.10. ##Interaction with child sex at p < 0.10.*

At child age 7 years, maternal $\sum$PBDE exposure was associated with maternally reported ADHD Index scores on the CADS (β = 2.9; 95% CI: 0.7, 5.2), DSM-IV Total scores (β = 2.6; 95% CI: 0.2, 5.0), and DSM-IV

Inattention scale scores ($\beta = 2.2$; 95% CI: 0.0, 4.5) (Table 1). Although there was evidence of nonlinearity for the DSM measures, quartile categorization showed no clear trends (Figure 1). Maternal exposure was also related to somewhat higher odds of a mother having been told that her child had attention problems (aOR = 2.3; 95% CI: 0.9, 5.8), and to teacher reports of child behavior problems (aOR = 2.5; 95% CI: 1.1, 6.0) [see Supplemental Material, Table S5 (http://dx.doi.org/10.1289/ehp.1205597)]. However, there were no associations between maternal ΣPBDE and teacher ratings on the CADS or BASC, or maternal ratings on the BASC, for continuous or dichotomous outcomes.

By contrast, child PBDE concentrations were associated with reports of attention problems from teachers, but not from mothers. Specifically, child ΣPBDEs were associated with more adverse teacher reports on CADS ADHD Index, CADS DSM-IV Total, CADS DSM-IV Inattentive, BASC Hyperactivity, and BASC Attention Problems scales [Table 1; see also Supplemental Material, Table S5 (http://dx.doi.org/10.1289/ehp.1205597)]. Associations were particularly pronounced for some of the dichotomous outcomes: Every 10-fold increase in child ΣPBDE level was associated with 4.5 and 5.5 times higher odds of the child being rated by the teacher as being in the "moderately or markedly atypical" range on CADS DSM-IV Hyperactive/Impulsive subscale (95% CI: 1.2, 16.6) and DSM-IV Total subscale (95% CI: 1.5, 20.3), respectively (see Supplemental Material, Table S5).

Motor function. We observed little evidence of association between either maternal or child ΣPBDE serum concentrations and gross motor performance on McCarthy scales (Table 2). However, maternal ΣPBDEs were related to poorer performance on the WRAVMA pegboard at both 5 and 7 years, particularly for the nondominant hand. For the 5-year-olds, this relationship was observed primarily for the nondominant hand among boys (boys: $\beta = -12.1$; 95% CI: $-19.4, -4.7$; girls: $\beta = 0.8$; 95% CI: -6.8, 8.5; $p_{interaction} = 0.09$), whereas at age 7, it was seen mainly in the dominant hand in girls (boys: $\beta = -2.7$; 95% CI: -10.8, 5.4; girls $\beta = -8.1$; 95% CI: -16.3, 0.1; $p_{interaction} = 0.08$). Associations between maternal ΣPBDEs and pegboard performance at 7 years showed evidence of nonlinearity, with nonsignificantly poorer performance in children of mothers in the highest quartile of exposure (Figure 1). At 5 but not 7 years of age, maternal

ΣPBDEs were also inversely associated with dominant-hand finger taps (Table 2).

Child ΣPBDEs were marginally related to nondominant hand pegboard performance at age 7 years, but not with other motor outcomes.

Cognitive functioning. We observed no associations between maternal ΣPBDE concentrations and child PPVT/TVIP or WPPSI Performance IQ scores at age 5 years (Table 3). However, at age 7 years, maternal ΣPBDEs were associated with significant decrements in WISC Verbal Comprehension IQ, contributing to a somewhat lowered Full-Scale IQ. Quartile analysis indicated that the association was primarily driven by a Verbal Comprehension IQ decrement in the highest quartile ($\beta = -6.0$; 95% CI: $-11.3, -0.7$; see Figure 1).

TABLE 3: Adjusted linear models for measures of cognition at 5 and 7 years of age (standard score), per 10-fold increase in maternal prenatal and child ΣPBDE concentration (ng/g, lipid-adjusted).

Outcome	Maternal ΣPBDE[a,b]		Child ΣPBDE[b,c]	
	n	β (95% CI)	n	β (95% CI)
Assessment of 5-year-olds				
PPVT	252	0.4 (–5.1, 5.9)		
Performance IQ	256	0.9 (–3.5, 5.3)		
Assessment of 7-year-olds				
Full-Scale IQ	231	–4.7 (–9.4, 0.1)*	248	–5.6 (–10.8, –0.3)**
Verbal Comprehension IQ	258	–5.5 (–10.0, –1.0)**,#	269	–4.3 (–9.4, 0.8)*
Perceptual Reasoning IQ	258	–2.4 (–7.6, 2.9)	269	–5.2 (–11.1, 0.7)*
Working Memory IQ	231	–2.4 (–7.2, 2.3)#	249	–2.3 (–7.4, 2.8)
Processing Speed IQ	232	–2.3 (–6.8, 2.3)	249	–6.6 (–11.4, –1.8)**

[a]*Maternal PBDE models control for child's age, sex, home score at 6-month visit, language of assessment, and maternal years living in United States before giving birth.* [b]*Sum of four PBDE congeners: BDEs 47, 99, 100, and 153.* [c]*Child PBDE models control for child's age, sex, home score at 7-year visit, maternal PPVT, language of examination, maternal years living in the United States before giving birth, parity, and prenatal exposure to environmental tobacco smoke.* *p < 0.1. **p ≤ 0.05. #Digression from linearity at p < 0.10.*

Children's ΣPBDE concentrations were also related to Full-Scale IQ at age 7 years (β = –5.6; 95% CI: –10.8, –0.3), particularly with the Perceptual Reasoning IQ, Processing Speed IQ, and Verbal Comprehension IQ subscales (Table 3).

Sensitivity analyses. The above relationships were not confounded by maternal lead, PCB, or OP pesticide exposures, or substantially altered when controlled (in separate models) for birth weight, gestational age, or prenatal thyroid hormones. Overall, associations with individual PBDE congeners or the sum of all 10 congeners [see Supplemental Maternal, Table S6 (http://dx.doi.org/10.1289/ehp.1205597)] were generally consistent with results for the sum of the four major congeners. Depending on the outcome, there were between 0 and 4 outliers with respect to either ΣPBDE concentrations or outcomes; excluding them did not substantively affect the results (data not shown). Except where noted, we did not find evidence of effect modification by child sex.

When both maternal and child ΣPBDE levels were entered into the same model (n = 214), associations were attenuated (data not shown) but child ΣPBDE levels were still associated with a borderline increase in teacher-reported scores for inattention on the BASC (β = 2.8; 95% CI: –0.2, 5.7) and maternal ΣPBDE levels were still associated with maternally-reported CADS DSM-IV Total scale scores (β = 2.6; 95% CI: –0.3, 5.5), decreased Verbal Comprehension IQ (β = –5.2; 95% CI: –10.4, 0.1) and Full-Scale IQ (β = –5.2; 95% CI: –10.6, 0.1), and lower nondominant hand pegboard scores (β = –6.5; 95% CI: –13.4, 0.3).

14.3 DISCUSSION

In the present study, we report associations between mothers' prenatal serum concentrations of PBDEs and evidence of deficits in attention, fine motor coordination, and cognitive functioning (particularly verbal comprehension) in their children at ages 5 and/or 7 years. Despite only weak correlations between PBDE concentrations in maternal prenatal and child age 7 years blood, we found associations between cognition, motor function and attention with both maternal and child PBDE exposures. The observed results appeared to be independent of associations previously reported in this cohort between maternal PB-DEs and maternal thyroid hormone (Chevrier et al. 2010) or child birth weight (Harley et al. 2011) and between maternal organophosphate pesticide exposure and child neurobehavioral development (Bouchard et al. 2011; Eskenazi et al. 2007; Marks et al. 2010). In addition, associations were not confounded by maternal lead or PCB levels, which were at low background levels.

This is the largest study to date on the potential neurodevelopmental impacts of PBDE exposures, and largely supports findings from three smaller studies, including those with substantially lower PBDE serum levels (Gascon et al. 2011; Herbstman et al. 2010; Hoffman et al. 2012; Roze et al. 2009). Our results are also similar to those reported between prenatal exposure to PCBs, which are chemically similar to PBDEs, and poorer attention and cognition or mental development in children (Grandjean et al. 2001; Jacobson and Jacobson 2003; Koopman-Esseboom et al. 1996; Rogan and Gladen 1991; Sagiv et al. 2012).

A notable finding of our study is that, in addition to in utero exposures, childhood PBDE concentrations were also associated with neurodevelopmental deficits. Although we hypothesized a priori that prenatal exposure would be more influential than postnatal exposure, the 7-year-olds' average PBDE concentrations were much higher than those in their mothers during pregnancy; we attribute this difference in part to the lifetime residence of the children in California compared with mothers, many of whom were recent immigrants to California when their levels were measured (Eskenazi et al. 2011).

In animal studies, PBDE exposure has been associated with increased death of cerebellar granule cells, alterations in neuronal arachidonic acid release, and disruption of calcium homeostasis (Birnbaum and Staskal 2004). Other potential mechanisms include perturbations of the cholinergic neurotransmitter system, interference with cellular signaling (Viberg et al. 2002a, 2002b, 2003), and, because of PBDEs' structural similarity to T4, effects on maternal thyroid hormone necessary for normal infant brain development (Darnerud et al. 2007; Richardson et al. 2008; Zhou et al. 2002). However, maternal thyroid hormone did not appear to explain the associations observed in our study population, as adding it to models did not measurably change the results.

Important strengths of the current study include its longitudinal design and use of comprehensive neurobehavioral assessments, which incorporate input from multiple informants. Limitations of this study are that we did not observe consistency in associations with PBDEs across informants for measures of attention (although their responses were moderately correlated), and we constructed numerous statistical models (although performance across domains was also moderately correlated), which increased the possibility of a chance finding. We also did not measure some higher-brominated compounds (e.g., BDE-209), which are present in decaBDE. Another study, however, indicates that BDE-209 represents a very small fraction of total serum PBDE concentrations in a different population of California children (Rose et al. 2010).

14.4 CONCLUSIONS

This study's finding of significant associations of both maternal prenatal and childhood PBDE exposures with poorer attention, fine motor coordination, and cognition in early school-age children contributes to the growing evidence of adverse associations between PBDE exposure and children's neurobehavioral development. Although these results are of particular concern for California children, they are also relevant to other locations, many of which contain products manufactured to meet California's standards. With the phaseout of pentaBDE, other flame retardants have been used to achieve compliance with TB 117. Additional research is needed to determine the potential child health consequences of these new chemical flame retardants.

REFERENCES

1. Achenbach T, Rescorla L. 2000. Manual for the ASEBA Preschool Forms & Profiles. Burlington, VT:University of Vermont, Research Center for Children, Youth, and Families.
2. Adams W, Sheslow D. 1995. Wide Range Assessment of Visual Motor Abilities (WRAVMA). Wilmington, DE:Wide Range, Inc.

3. American Psychiatric Association. 1994. Diagnostic and Statistical Manual of Mental Disorders, 4th ed. Washington, DC:American Psychiatric Association.
4. Barr JR, Maggio VL, Barr DB, Turner WE, Sjödin A, Sandau CD, et al. 2003. New high-resolution mass spectrometric approach for the measurement of polychlorinated biphenyls and organochlorine pesticides in human serum. J Chromatogr B Analyt Technol Biomed Life Sci 794(1):137–148.
5. Birnbaum LS, Staskal DF. 2004. Brominated flame retardants: cause for concern? Environ Health Perspect 112:9–17.
6. Bouchard MF, Chevrier J, Harley KG, Kogut K, Vedar M, Calderon N, et al. 2011. Prenatal exposure to organophosphate pesticides and IQ in 7-year-old children. Environ Health Perspect 119:1189–1195.
7. Bradman A, Castorina R, Sjödin A, Fenster L, Jones RS, Harley KG, et al. 2012. Factors associated with serum polybrominated diphenyl ether (PBDE) levels among school-age children in the CHAMACOS cohort. Environ Sci Technol 46(13):7373–7381.
8. Bradman A, Eskenazi B, Barr D, Bravo R, Castorina R, Chevrier J, et al. 2005. Organophosphate urinary metabolite levels during pregnancy and after delivery in women living in an agricultural community. Environ Health Perspect 113:1802–1807.
9. Bravo R, Driskell WJ, Whitehead RD Jr, Needham LL, Barr DB. 2002. Quantitation of dialkyl phosphate metabolites of organophosphate pesticides in human urine using GC-MS-MS with isotopic internal standards. J Anal Toxicol 26(5):245–252.
10. Caldwell B, Bradley R. 1984. Home Observation for Measurement of The Environment. Little Rock, AR:University of Arkansas.
11. California Department of Consumer Affairs. 2000. Technical Bulletin 117: Requirements, Test Procedure and Apparatus for Testing the Flame Retardance of Resilient Filling Materials Used in Upholstered Furniture. Available: http://www.bhfti.ca.gov/industry/117.pdf [accessed 23 June 2010].
12. Castorina R, Bradman A, Sjödin A, Fenster L, Jones RS, Harley KG, et al. 2011. Determinants of serum polybrominated diphenyl ether (PBDE) levels among pregnant women in the CHAMACOS cohort. Environ Sci Technol 45(15):6553–6560.
13. Chao HR, Wang SL, Lee WJ, Wang YF, Papke O. 2007. Levels of polybrominated diphenyl ethers (PBDEs) in breast milk from central Taiwan and their relation to infant birth outcome and maternal menstruation effects. Environ Int 33(2):239–245.
14. Chevrier J, Harley KG, Bradman A, Gharbi M, Sjödin A, Eskenazi B. 2010. Polybrominated diphenyl ether (PBDE) flame retardants and thyroid hormone during pregnancy. Environ Health Perspect 118:1444–1449.
15. Conners CK. 2001. Conner's Rating Scales–Revised (CSR-R) Technical Manual (includes auxilliary scales: CADS-P and CADS-T). North Tonawanda, NY:Multi-Health Systems Inc.
16. Conners CK, Staff M. 2001. Conners' Kiddie Continuous Performance Test (K-CPT): Computer Program for Windows Technical Guide and Software Manual. Toronto, ON, Canada:Multi-Health Systems Inc.
17. Darnerud PO, Aune M, Larsson L, Hallgren S. 2007. Plasma PBDE and thyroxine levels in rats exposed to Bromkal or BDE-47. Chemosphere 67(9):S386–S392.

18. Dunn L, Dunn L. 1981. Peabody Picture Vocabulary Test, Revised. Circle Pines, MN:American Guidance Service.
19. Eskenazi B, Fenster L, Castorina R, Marks AR, Sjödin A, Rosas LG, et al. 2011. A comparison of PBDE serum concentrations in Mexican and Mexican-American children living in California. Environ Health Perspect 119:1442–1448.
20. Eskenazi B, Harley K, Bradman A, Weltzien E, Jewell NP, Barr DB, et al. 2004. Association of in utero organophosphate pesticide exposure and fetal growth and length of gestation in an agricultural population. Environ Health Perspect 112:1116–1124.
21. Eskenazi B, Marks AR, Bradman A, Fenster L, Johnson C, Barr DB, et al. 2006. In utero exposure to dichlorodiphenyltrichloroethane (DDT) and dichlorodiphenyl-dichloroethylene (DDE) and neurodevelopment among young Mexican American children. Pediatrics 118(1):233–241.
22. Eskenazi B, Marks AR, Bradman A, Harley K, Barr DB, Johnson C, et al. 2007. Organophosphate pesticide exposure and neurodevelopment in young Mexican-American children. Environ Health Perspect 115:792–798.
23. Gascon M, Fort M, Martinez D, Carsin AE, Forns J, Grimalt JO, et al. 2012. Polybrominated diphenyl ethers (PBDEs) in breast milk and neuropsychological development in infants. Environ Health Perspect 120:1760–1765.
24. Gascon M, Vrijheid M, Martinez D, Forns J, Grimalt JO, Torrent M, et al. 2011. Effects of pre and postnatal exposure to low levels of polybromodiphenyl ethers on neurodevelopment and thyroid hormone levels at 4 years of age. Environ Int 37(3):605–611.
25. Geyer HJ, Schramm K-W, Darnerud PO, Aune M, Feicht A, Fried KW. 2004. Terminal elimination half-lives of the brominated flame retardants TBBPA, HBCD, and lower brominated PBDEs in humans. Organohalogen Compounds 66:3867–3872.
26. Grandjean P, Weihe P, Burse VW, Needham LL, Storr-Hansen E, Heinzow B, et al. 2001. Neurobehavioral deficits associated with PCB in 7-year-old children prenatally exposed to seafood neurotoxicants. Neurotoxicol Teratol 23(4):305–317.
27. Harley KG, Chevrier J, Schall RA, Sjödin A, Bradman A, Eskenazi B. 2011. Association of prenatal exposure to polybrominated diphenyl ethers and infant birth weight. Am J Epidemiol 174(8):885–892.
28. Herbstman JB, Sjödin A, Apelberg BJ, Witter FR, Halden RU, Patterson DG, et al. 2008. Birth delivery mode modifies the associations between prenatal polychlorinated biphenyl (PCB) and polybrominated diphenyl ether (PBDE) and neonatal thyroid hormone levels. Environ Health Perspect 116:1376–1382.
29. Herbstman JB, Sjödin A, Kurzon M, Lederman SA, Jones RS, Rauh V, et al. 2010. Prenatal exposure to PBDEs and neurodevelopment. Environ Health Perspect 118:712–719.
30. Hoffman K, Adgent M, Goldman BD, Sjödin A, Daniels JL. 2012. Lactational exposure to polybrominated diphenyl ethers and its relation to social and emotional development among toddlers. Environ Health Perspect 120:1438–1442.
31. Jacobson JL, Jacobson SW. 2003. Prenatal exposure to polychlorinated biphenyls and attention at school age. J Pediatr 143(6):780–788.
32. Koopman-Esseboom C, Weisglas-Kuperus N, de Ridder MA, Van der Paauw CG, Tuinstra LG, Sauer PJ. 1996. Effects of polychlorinated biphenyl/dioxin exposure

and feeding type on infants' mental and psychomotor development. Pediatrics 97(5):700–706.

33. Lubin JH, Colt JS, Camann D, Davis S, Cerhan JR, Severson RK, et al. 2004. Epidemiologic evaluation of measurement data in the presence of detection limits. Environ Health Perspect 112:1691–1696.

34. Marks AR, Harley K, Bradman A, Kogut K, Barr DB, Johnson C, et al. 2010. Organophosphate pesticide exposure and attention in young Mexican-American children: the CHAMACOS study. Environ Health Perspect 118:1768–1774.

35. McCarthy D. 1972. McCarthy Scales of Children's Abilities. New York:Psychological Corporation.

36. Nelson JC, Tomei RT. 1988. Direct determination of free thyroxin in undiluted serum by equilibrium dialysis/radioimmunoassay. Clin Chem 34(9):1737–1744.

37. Noyes PD, Hinton DE, Stapleton HM. 2011. Accumulation and debromination of decabromodiphenyl ether (BDE-209) in juvenile fathead minnows (Pimephales promelas) induces thyroid disruption and liver alterations. Toxicol Sci 122(2):265–274.

38. Phillips DL, Pirkle JL, Burse VW, Bernert JT Jr, Henderson LO, Needham LL. 1989. Chlorinated hydrocarbon levels in human serum: effects of fasting and feeding. Arch Environ Contam Toxicol 18(4):495–500.

39. Radloff L. 1977. The CES-D Scale: a self-report depression scale for research in the general population. Appl Psychol Meas 1(3):385–401.

40. Reynolds CR, Kamphaus RW. 2004. BASC-2: Behaviour Assessment System for Children, Second Edition Manual. Circle Pines, MN:AGS Publishing.

41. Richardson VM, Staskal DF, Ross DG, Diliberto JJ, DeVito MJ, Birnbaum LS. 2008. Possible mechanisms of thyroid hormone disruption in mice by BDE 47, a major polybrominated diphenyl ether congener. Toxicol Appl Pharmacol 226(3):244–250.

42. Rogan W, Gladen B. 1991. PCBs, DDE, and child development at 18 and 24 months. Ann Epidemiol 1(5):407–413.

43. Rohlman DS, Gimenes LS, Eckerman DA, Kang SK, Farahat FM, Anger WK. 2003. Development of the Behavioral Assessment and Research System (BARS) to detect and characterize neurotoxicity in humans. Neurotoxicology 24(4–5):523–531.

44. Rose M, Bennett DH, Bergman A, Fangstrom B, Pessah IN, Hertz-Picciotto I. 2010. PBDEs in 2–5 year-old children from California and associations with diet and indoor environment. Environ Sci Technol 44(7):2648–2653.

45. Roze E, Meijer L, Bakker A, Van Braeckel KN, Sauer PJ, Bos AF. 2009. Prenatal exposure to organohalogens, including brominated flame retardants, influences motor, cognitive, and behavioral performance at school age. Environ Health Perspect 117:1953–1958.

46. Sagiv SK, Thurston SW, Bellinger DC, Altshul LM, Korrick SA. 2012. Neuropsychological measures of attention and impulse control among 8-year-old children exposed prenatally to organochlorines. Environ Health Perspect 120:904–909.

47. Sjödin A, Jones RS, Lapeza CR, Focant JF, McGahee EE III, Patterson DG Jr. 2004. Semiautomated high-throughput extraction and cleanup method for the measurement of polybrominated diphenyl ethers, polybrominated biphenyls, and polychlorinated biphenyls in human serum. Anal Chem 76(7):1921–1927.

48. Sjödin A, Papke O, McGahee E, Focant JF, Jones RS, Pless-Mulloli T, et al. 2008. Concentration of polybrominated diphenyl ethers (PBDEs) in household dust from various countries. Chemosphere 73(1 suppl):S131–S136.

49. Stapleton HM, Kelly SM, Allen JG, McClean MD, Webster TF. 2008. Measurement of polybrominated diphenyl ethers on hand wipes: estimating exposure from hand-to-mouth contact. Environ Sci Technol 42(9):3329–3334.

50. Viberg H, Fredriksson A, Eriksson P. 2002a. Neonatal exposure to the brominated flame retardant 2,2',4,4',5-pentabromodiphenyl ether causes altered susceptibility in the cholinergic transmitter system in the adult mouse. Toxicol Sci 67(1):104–107.

51. Viberg H, Fredriksson A, Eriksson P. 2002b. Neonatal exposure to a brominated flame retardant, 2,2',4,4',5,5'-hexabromodiphenyl ether (PBDE 153) affects behaviour and cholinergic nicotinic receptors in brain of adult mice [Abstract 643]. In: The Toxicologist: Proceedings of the 41st Annual Meeting of the Society of Toxicology, 17–21 March 2002, Nashville, TNReston, VA:Society of Toxicology, 132.

52. Viberg H, Fredriksson A, Eriksson P. 2003. Neonatal exposure to polybrominated diphenyl ether (PBDE 153) disrupts spontaneous behaviour, impairs learning and memory, and decreases hippocampal cholinergic receptors in adult mice. Toxicol Appl Pharmacol 192(2):95–106.

53. Wechsler D. 2003. Wechsler Intelligence Scale for Children–Fourth Edition (WISC-IV) Administration and Scoring Manual. San Antonio, TX:Harcourt Assessment Incorporated.

54. Zhou T, Taylor MM, DeVito MJ, Crofton KM. 2002. Developmental exposure to brominated diphenyl ethers results in thyroid hormone disruption. Toxicol Sci 66(1):105–116.

55. Zota AR, Rudel RA, Morello-Frosch RA, Brody JG. 2008. Elevated house dust and serum concentrations of PBDEs in California: unintended consequences of furniture flammability standards? Environ Sci Technol 42(21):8158–8164.

There are several supplemental files that are not available in this version of the article. To view this additional information, please use the citation on the first page of this chapter.

PART IV

CONCLUSION

CHAPTER 15

TAKING ACTION ON DEVELOPMENTAL TOXICITY: SCIENTISTS' DUTIES TO PROTECT CHILDREN

KRISTIN SHRADER-FRECHETTE

15.1 BACKGROUND

In Spring 2012, organizers of PPTOX III—a conference focused on integrating "the role of environmental exposures and nutrients during development on subsequent diseases/dysfunctions later in life"— issued a white paper. So far, nearly 100 physicians/scientists throughout the world have co-signed it. Reviewing classic scientific research on how developmental exposures to environmental chemicals can cause later disease/dysfunction, the white paper draws two main conclusions. One is that children's in-utero and early-postnatal-developmental periods are "particularly sensitive to developmental disruption by nutritional factors or environmental-chemical exposures, with potentially adverse consequences for health later in life." A second conclusion is that children's heightened developmental sensitivity requires a new "policy and public health response" of "both research and disease-prevention strategies" [1].

15.1.1 DEVELOPMENTAL TOXICITY (DT)

While the white paper provides the scientific basis for special child-developmental protection against environmental chemicals, this paper provides a preliminary ethical basis for protection. It argues that, to varying degrees and for slightly different reasons, citizens, physicians, and scientists each have justice-based, sometimes overlapping, duties to help stop developmental toxicity or DT.

DT refers to the fact that "many of the major diseases—and dysfunctions—that have increased substantially in prevalence over the last 40 years seem to be related in part to developmental factors associated with...exposures to environmental chemicals" [1]. Scientists confirm that, despite the need for much more research to reduce various scientific uncertainties, the concept of the "developmental origins of [much] health and disease... is sufficiently robust and repeatable across species, including humans" [1], that toxin-induced "epigenetic modifications can be passed from one cell generation to the next and, in some cases, when germ cells are targeted, can be transgenerationally transmitted" [2]. These adverse effects, however, "may not be apparent during a latent period which may last from months to years or decades," and they can result from "a combination of developmental stressors...[that] cause effects jointly with similar or other exposures." These harms—manifested as "increased incidence,...earlier onset, or an increased severity" of disease or dysfunction—include "obesity, diabetes, hypertension, cardiovascular disease, asthma and allergy, immune and autoimmune diseases, neurodevelopmental and neurodegenerative diseases, precocious puberty, infertility, some cancer types, osteoporosis, depression, schizophrenia, and sarcopenia" [1].

Although all environmental exposures likely causing DT have not been fully confirmed, low-dose environmental chemicals known to cause DT include "especially endocrine disrupting chemicals" or EDCs. "Examples of EDCs known to alter disease susceptibility as a result of developmental exposures in animal models include bisphenol A (from polycarbonate plastics), phthalates (a softener in plastics), some organophosphate and organochlorine pesticides, nicotine (tobacco smoking), air pollution, per-fluorooctane compounds (stain and water repellents), and polybrominated diphenyl ethers (flame retardants) – all chemicals that are found in detectable concentrations in blood or urine samples from most people" [1].

15.1.2 USING A THOUGHT EXPERIMENT TO HELP DECIDE HOW TO RESPOND TO DT

The preceding list of developmental toxins, however, is not complete. Also, because much DT testing remains to be done, some scientists are uncertain about DT and its potential epigenetic effects. How should scientists/society respond, given such unknowns?

When it is impossible or impractical for scientists to rapidly conduct real-world experiments on some question, they often use thought experiments—apriori, rather than empirical, assessments using only reason and imagination. Richard Feynman famously described thought experiments as more elegant than physical ones. Galileo's "tower" thought experiment showed that, contrary to Aristotle, objects of different masses fall at the same acceleration. Maxwell's "demon" showed that, contrary to the second law of thermodynamics, entropy could be decreased. Einstein used Schrödinger's "cat" to show that, contrary to Copenhagen interpretations of quantum mechanics, observation does not break quantum-state superposition.

Ethicists also use thought experiments. Judith Thomson's "transplant surgeon" showed that, contrary to some utilitarians, one cannot deliberately kill an innocent person to save more lives. Philippa Foot's "trolley" showed that, contrary to some egalitarians, one could allow one death in order to save more people, provided the victim was not used as a means to this end.

Would a thought experiment also help clarify how scientists/society ought to respond to DT—to environmental-chemical exposures that may put children at risk of later disease and dysfunction? To answer this question, consider a thought experiment about another potential harm to children.

Suppose you are on vacation in Brazil, taking an early-morning walk. Crying, a tiny boy's well-dressed "aunt" approaches you, saying she is late for work. She apologizes for bothering you, is clearly distraught, and says she fears losing her job because of her lateness, unless someone takes her visiting "nephew" to his mother. The "aunt" pleads for help, gives you the child and his "address," then offers you money for taking him "home." Should you help the "aunt," take the child to the address, but refuse the money? Or should you take the child to the police?

On one hand, the Brazilian "aunt" may be telling the truth and may need a Good Samaritan. On the other hand, the child may be at risk of organ trafficking. Given the shortage of available organs for transplant, and the millions of "street children" in nations like Brazil, the World Health Organization estimates that organ trafficking accounts for up to 10 percent of all organ transplants. Part of a trillion-dollar annual global-economic output in illicit trade, organ trafficking annually causes thousands of murders among many of those whose organs are harvested for resale [3,4].

What you ought to do about the Brazilian child may illuminate what scientists/society ought to do about DT. After all, although organ transplants and industrial/agricultural chemicals serve important goods, both pose at least 7 serious—and similar—risks. Both involve potential harm, uncertainty, innocent victims, lack of child consent, and high stakes—only "one chance" to possibly avoid organ-harvester murderers or to "develop a brain" [5]. Both also involve questions such as whether to minimize false-negative risks (to children) or false-positive risks (to the aunt/chemical-industry), and whether to make health-economics tradeoffs.

Most informed people probably would find it easier to decide what to do in the Brazilian-child case than in the DT situation, partly because of organ-trafficking publicity. They likely would not give an innocent child to possible traffickers. Yet this commentary argues that—according to all major ethical theories—the answer regarding whether citizens/physicians/ scientists should allow avoidable DT is almost as clear as whether to deliver the Brazilian child to his "home." In both cases, justice and the vulnerability of children argue for their protection.

15.1.3 SCIENTIFIC UNCERTAINTY
ABOUT ORGAN TRAFFICKING AND DT

Why does it seem more difficult to decide the DT, than the Brazilian-child question? One reason, already noted, is that the relevant science is still unfolding. A second reason is that organ trafficking involves threats to specific individuals, while scientists typically can document subtle DT harm mainly to populations, although individuals are affected. Third, human studies reveal organ trafficking, whereas mainly animal studies reveal DT. Fourth, organ trafficking is more obvious to laypeople than is DT. Fifth, because of this obviousness, citizens might claim that in the organ-trafficking case, it is better to risk false positives (false assertions of child harm) than false negatives, whereas in the DT case, scientists might claim it is better to risk false negatives (false assertions of no DT harm to children), than false positives, because scientists typically have more aversion to false positives [6,7]. Sixth, although organ traffickers obviously have no rights to economic gain from their activities, industries (that seriously harm no one) do have such rights. If these industries are unjustly accused, they could face economic harm from DT regulation, but if possible DT victims are not protected, innocent, non-consenting children (and future generations, if epigenetic change is heritable) could face health harm—a possible stealth DT pandemic. Yet, given global recession and government-research-funding cutbacks, arguments for increasing DT funding, so as to reduce all these DT-associated uncertainties, face an uphill battle. The result?

Needed DT-related science is not getting done, and many uncertainties about DT remain. This is partly because of the "Matthew Effect" [8], that most scientific studies—of substances on the US Environmental Protection Agency's (EPA's) risk-based-priority ranking of high-production-volume (HPV) chemicals—focus on the top 10–20 chemicals. Already-overstudied chemicals are studied more, whereas risky chemicals, ranked 50th or 90th among roughly 80,000, are rarely studied [8]. A second cause of DT uncertainty is that only 7 percent of HPV chemicals have ever been assessed for developmental effects or toxicity to children [9]. Third, under the innocent-until-proved-guilty assumption, at least 1000 new chemicals enter the market annually, giving scientists little time to study them before they may cause serious harm [10].

A fourth reason for uncertainty about DT is scientists' disagreement over causal inferences. British statistician Austin Bradford Hill [11] introduced 9 causal-inference guidelines: strength of the mathematical association, biological plausibility (underlying mechanisms), coherence, consistency with other results, specificity of results (one-to-one relationships), temporality (causes' preceding effects), biological gradients (dose–response curves), experimental evidence, and analogies with causal precedents.

So-called "black-box epidemiologists" (the majority camp) emphasize Hill's first guideline and use mathematical/statistical measures like relative risk to assess cause-effect relationships, whereas so-called "eco-epidemiologists" (the minority camp) are methodological pluralists who emphasize the second guideline and often seek cause-effect mechanisms. Although black-box epidemiologists emphasize statistical evidence, even for purely-observational data, are more eager to avoid false positives, and focus on disease treatment—eco-epidemiologists avoid using only statistical tests of observational data, are more eager to false negatives, and focus more on disease prevention. Unsurprisingly, these camps often disagree about harm from specific chemical exposures [12].

15.1.4 FIRST OF FOUR ARGUMENTS: DOMINANT ETHICAL THEORIES DISALLOW DT

Despite some disananogies between organ trafficking and DT exposure, and despite some scientific uncertainties about DT, the ethics is reasonably clear. Any one of at least four different ethical arguments, given in subsequent pages, is alone sufficient to show that it is prima-facie unethical to allow avoidable DT. (To call something prima-facie unethical means (i) that a general ethical principle affirms it is unethical; (ii) that the burden of proof is on anyone wishing to justify a case-specific override of this prima-facie principle; and (iii) that anyone who disagrees (with a case-specific application of the principle) must provide precise, compelling, ultima-facie (all-things-considered) arguments to the contrary [13,14]. Such ultima-facie arguments might be, for instance, that allowing DT, given a specific chemical compound/case/ time/set of circumstances, would cause less human death/disease/dysfunction than not allowing it).

Why do the four arguments (given in subsequent pages) establish merely prima-facie principles against allowing DT? Because ethical principles must be applicable to a wide variety of situations, by definition they do not take into account the millions of case-specific or conflict-specific factual and moral considerations—ultima-facie considerations—that might override them and cause exceptions. Instead, moral principles establish merely prima-facie claims that put the burden of proof on violators.

The four different ethical arguments, each sufficient to show that allowing avoidable DT is prima-facie unethical—focus, respectively, on (1) ethical theory, (2) just political theory, (3) DT causality, and (4) DT benefits. (1) The ethical-theory argument has four parts and argues that no major ethics codes (Aristotelian, Thomistic, utilitarian, egalitarian) allow avoidable DT because, even if epigenetic change is not heritable, DT unjustifiably harms individual human flourishing, life, equality, and good. (2) The just-political-theory argument is that no major political codes allow unequal "takings" from the biological commons, as would occur if DT-induced epigenetic change is heritable. (3) The DT-causality argument is that—even if epigenetic change is not heritable—all citizens, and scientists/physicians in particular, have justice-based duties to take action on avoidable DT because they helped cause it. (4) The DT-benefits argument is that—even if epigenetic change is not heritable—all citizens, and scientists/physicians in particular, have justice-based duties to take action on avoidable DT because they benefit from it. After presenting these four basic arguments, the paper shows that all major objections to them are logically/ethically/scientifically flawed.

To assess argument (1) above, consider four main ethical codes—classical Aristotelian virtue theory, medieval Thomistic natural-law theory, modern/contemporary Millian utilitarianism, and modern/contemporary Rawlsian egalitarianism. A very quick, simple survey reveals that all these ethical theories would mandate that allowing avoidable DT is prima-facie indefensible.

15.1.4.1 ARISTOTELIAN ETHICS

For Aristotelians, the purpose, meaning, goal, or telos of life is human flourishing or eudaimonia, the desired end of all human actions. For Aristotelians, humans achieve this end or telos of flourishing by having a virtuous character. And they attain a virtuous character through practicing the virtues—such as justice and courage. Because DT threatens the fundamental telos or end of human flourishing or eudaimonia—given its increasing disease susceptibility, adverse neurological/other effects, epigenomic disruption, and possible transgenerational effects [2,15-18]—consistent Aristotelians would not allow DT. Moreover, in the Aristotelian world, where the virtue of courage is a key means to flourishing or eudaimonia, those who lack the courage to protect others, such as innocent children, will themselves not attain eudaimonia. Therefore those lacking courage behave unethically, apart from the indefensible harm they allow to children.

Suppose someone objected that allowing DT-inducing environmental toxins promoted overall economic welfare, therefore human flourishing? Consistent Aristotelians would reject this objection because they believe money is merely a medium of exchange, something able to corrupt people and natural exchanges, hence something unable to capture fundamentally incommensurable and superior values—like human flourishing. Aristotelians believe the fundamental ethical end, telos, or eudaimonia is not captured through cost-benefit calculations. Therefore, to show that allowing DT is ethical, for Aristotelians, would require showing that DT promoted greater virtue and eudaimonia or flourishing. Yet there is no reason to believe that allowing DT would lead to greater virtue and flourishing, given the harms it causes [19].

15.1.4.2 NATURAL-LAW ETHICS
AND ALLEGED "FREE-MARKET" OBJECTIONS

A second major class of ethical theorists, consistent followers of Thomas Aquinas' natural-law ethics, likewise must reject avoidable DT. For them, universal law—written on human hearts, discoverable by human reason—binds people/government to act in accord with it, especially its fundamental tenet to preserve human life and authentic happiness [20]. Because DT threatens life and happiness—just as it threatens Aristotelian flourishing—natural-law theorists cannot allow avoidable DT.

Of course, anti-regulatory political theorists—like attorney Cass Sunstein, current (2012) administrator of the US Office of Information and Regulatory Affairs, whose research has been funded by right-wing think tanks, like the American Enterprise Institute—reject this ethics. He and other alleged "free-market" environmentalists would likely claim that allowing DT contributes to preserving human life. Sunstein's argues that (1) monies spent on regulations "produce less employment and more poverty," (2) "wealth buys longevity," and therefore health-related regulations cost money, "increase risk," thus kill people [21].

However, Sunstein's alleged-free-market objection to stopping DT in invalid because it commits three logical fallacies of false cause in premises (1–2) above. The first fallacy consists of assuming in premise (1) that regulations reduce employment. Yet health-related regulations are neither necessary nor sufficient conditions for reduced overall employment. Instead, health-related regulations typically increase overall employment or shift it from one sector/industry to another, with no net job loss. For instance, workers often move from old/dirty to new/clean technologies, with no overall job loss, partly because many clean technologies such as solar/wind are more labor intensive, per kilowatt of electricity produced. Cleaner technologies also often save lives and therefore jobs [22,23].

A second false-cause fallacy in Sunstein's premise (1) is the assumption that industrial profits are always spent to increase employment, an assumption falsified by the last half-century of US economic history. A third false-cause fallacy occurs in premise (2), that "wealth buys longevity." On the contrary, research shows mortality is very strongly associated with societal income-inequality, not with either per-capita or median income [24].

These three false-cause fallacies arise partly because alleged "free-market" environmentalists ignore relevant facts/norms, such as that higher employment has little value for people increasingly made ill by DT, or that higher employment does not excuse injustice to innocent children. It did, one could justify employing many people as "pushers" to children. This supposed free-market argument likewise is invalid for a fourth reason: It begs the question that cost-benefit analysis is the sole test for regulations. A simple counter example shows it is not: Law requires expensive trials and possible prosecution/incarceration/death for accused murderers. Yet, criminologists agree these requirements are rarely cost-effective because most murders are not serial offenders, hence pose no future threat to society. Instead, society tries them because justice requires it. If so, justice trumps cost-effectiveness and therefore alleged "free-market" environmentalism.

Apart from its four logical fallacies, the alleged "free market" objection to avoiding/preventing DT also fails scientifically. Why? Adam Smith and virtually all economists and ethicists agree that economically-efficient (and ethical) market transactions require full information and fully voluntary exchanges. Without them, Coase's famous theorem is inapplicable. (Coase's theorem—a key basis for economic analysis of government regulation—is that, regardless of how property rights are initially apportioned, if there are no transaction costs, and if people can trade in an externality, then bargaining will lead to an economically-efficient outcome.) Yet obviously consumer-market behavior regarding pollutants is neither fully informed nor fully voluntary, partly because polluters often mislead about harm, fight labeling and right-to-know requirements, and resist government/consumer information-gathering [25-28]. If so, supposed "free-market" proponents apply their views to precisely the cases (DT cases without fully informed, voluntary exchanges) that, economists agree, generate no economically-efficient outcomes. Indeed, poor or poorly educated consumers often have neither equal bargaining power nor ability to correct disinformation and skewed market forces. If not, misapplied free-market objections really offer a wolf's argument in sheep's clothing. The sheep is market reasoning; the wolf is "might makes right," defending conclusions that allow harm to poor/innocent people on false grounds that harming them increases overall wealth/employment. Given alleged "free-market" environmentalism's scientific/ethical flaws, it is unsurprising that consistent free-market economists reject claims that regulations kill people [29]. Thus, supposed "free-market" objections to avoiding/preventing DT are invalid. They fail on logical, scientific, and ethical grounds.

15.1.4.3 UTILITARIAN ETHICS

A third major group of ethicists, modern/contemporary utilitarians, maintains ethical actions are those that achieve the greatest good for the greatest number of people, as measured by preferences. They likewise cannot consistently defend allowing avoidable DT because DT death/disease, and people's uncertainty/anxiety regarding whether their loved ones will be DT victims, both harm the greater good. Why? Harms to minorities, like children, hurt the majority. This why utilitarian John Stuart Mill [30] rejected "the tyranny of the majority."

However, an objector might claim that societal inequities from DT do not reduce overall welfare because health-related regulations cause unemployment, thus kill people. Yet, as the previous criticisms of objections to natural-law arguments for avoiding/preventing DT reveal, the alleged "free-market" objection fails to justify allowing avoidable DT because its premises are factually false, and its inferences are invalid.

15.1.4.4 EGALITARIAN ETHICS

A fourth main group of ethicists, modern/contemporary egalitarians, likewise would reject avoidable DT. Egalitarians, like the late Harvard ethicist John Rawls [31], say that because equal opportunity and liberty are primary ethical goals, unavoidable societal inequalities should be arranged so as to benefit the least-well-off, the most vulnerable. Consequently they would reject avoidable DT because it thwarts liberty and equal opportunity, especially among least-well-off victims, like children.

Nevertheless, objectors might counter egalitarianism by appeal to the alleged "free-market" objection, already considered/rejected. Yet the free-market objection relies on rejecting equal opportunity for the sake of alleged economic benefits. Rawls, however, argues no one would sanction equal-opportunity violations unless she were certain not to be a victim, a fact demonstrating the self-interested bias—and invalid arguments—of those who reject egalitarian ethics.

As the preceding considerations reveal, all main ethical theories (based on virtue, equality, overall preferences, and equality) reject allowing avoidable DT, but on different grounds and with different degrees of stringency. Aristotelian virtue ethicists, Thomistic natural-law theorists, and Rawlsian egalitarians would all reject avoidable DT because of its harms to basic goods, respectively, flourishing, life, and equality. Millian utilitarians are a bit less stringent (in disallowing avoidable DT) than are ethicists in the other three groups, because utilitarians in principle allow money/harm tradeoffs. However, even utilitarians would find it nearly impossible to show that most people's preferences would trade DT harm to their children for money.

5.1.5 SECOND ARGUMENT: MAJOR POLITICAL THEORIES DISALLOW DT

Besides all four major ethical theories, dominant political theories—if they are consistent—must disallow avoidable DT. Whether socialist, Marxist, libertarian, capitalist, or anarchist, virtually all political theorists accept John Locke's account of property rights and his labor theory of value. That is, they all maintain human labor/merit/effort creates property rights in things, and that one cannot have full property rights over anything one's labor has not created—although different groups may disagree over what constitutes labor/merit/effort, and how far property rights extend. Because human labor did not create common natural/biological resources (such as land and genes), full property right to them are impossible and, instead, Lockeans argue one can use natural/biological resources only under the constraint of an equal-opportunity criterion—provided "as much and as good" is left for all other people, including future generations. While political theorists may disagree over precisely what is "as much and as good" for future people, they all agree with this Lockean account of property rights and its equal-opportunity criterion for natural/biological resources [32]. Otherwise, despots could illegitimately claim full rights to resources needed for others' survival. Because avoidable DT harms resources (like genomic stability)—possibly for future generations, if epigenetic changes are heritable—avoidable DT harms are never permissible. One never has rights to "take" that over which (like biological resources) one has no property rights.

But doesn't society recognize civil property rights/patents over natural resources like land and genes? While social/civil convention accepts such legal rights as a matter of convenience, even conservative ethical/legal theorists (including William Blackstone) agree that no rational grounds (only grounds of "might makes right") exist for claiming property rights over things not created by labor. Instead, they admit property "rights" to biological resources often originated from fraud, violence, theft, bullying, or colonialism—then were "transferred" through the ages. Thus, virtually all "transfers" have been problematic because original "owners" often had the equivalent of stolen goods, violating Locke's as-much-and-as-good proviso. If so, many current conventional property rights (to biological-commons resources) are as ethically indefensible as conventions of racism, sexism, or homophobia. But if property rights to natural biological resources—such as genomic stability/health—are impossible, and if those who threaten genetic integrity (because of the heritability of epigenetic change) therefore have no rights to do so, then avoidable DT is ethically impermissible [33], and citizens/scientists should not allow it.

5.1.6 THIRD ARGUMENT: HELPING CAUSE DT CREATES GREATER DT DUTIES

Apart from ethical theory, justice-based reasons also show that citizens, and especially physicians/scientists, should not allow avoidable DT. The DT-causality argument is that—even if epigenetic change is not heritable—all citizens, and scientists/physicians in particular, have justice-based duties to take action on avoidable DT because they helped cause this harm to children. How so? Virtually everyone contributes to air pollution, and virtually everyone uses/purchases products containing bisphenol A, phthalates, organophosphate and organochlorine pesticides, nicotine, perfluorooctane compounds, and polybrominated diphenyl ethers—all chemicals known to cause DT [1]. Because everyone contributes to DT through pollution and product use, everyone has duties to help stop this harm they cause. The ethics is basic: if you broke it, you should fix it.

Moreover, because democracy is not a spectator sport, and because all citizens in a democracy are responsible for being politically active, so as to help stop public harms, all citizens have duties to help stop avoidable DT. Those who have never even attempted to help stop avoidable DT have special duties to do so, precisely because they bear a greater responsibility for helping cause DT because of their inaction and their failure to exercise the duties of citizenship. Thus, although everyone who helps cause DT has prima facie duties to help stop it, those duties differ, ultima facie and individual to individual, as a function of factors such as one's fractional contribution to DT, one's knowledge, profession, time, expertise, etc. [34].

5.1.6.1 SCIENTISTS'/PHYSICIANS' GREATER ABILITIES GENERATE GREATER DUTIES

Although scientists/physicians share duties with other citizens to help stop DT because of helping cause it, they have special duties, all other things being equal, because they have greater ability/expertise/intellectual-professional resources (than laypeople) to help stop DT. As all professional ethics codes note, all other things being equal, greater ability to prevent some harm generates greater responsibilities to do so [35]. The American Medical Association, for instance, says that because of their "skills and competency," physicians should "educate the public and policy about present and future threats to the health of humanity" and "advocate for social, economic, educational, and political changes that ameliorate suffering and contribute to human well-being" [36].

5.1.6.2 SCIENTISTS' PHYSICIANS' UNEARNED ADVANTAGES GENERATE GREATER DUTIES

All citizens have duties to help alleviate avoidable DT not merely proportional to their skills and abilities, but also proportional to their unearned advantages from society. All other things being equal, the greater a citizen's wealth, intelligence, freedom, health, etc.—the greater her unearned advantages—the greater her responsibility to help alleviate avoidable DT.

In particular, because scientists/physicians have received increased, unequal, partially unearned, societal advantages, as compared to many other people, they have increased responsibilities to "give back," to help promote equal opportunity/protection from harm, as virtually all professional-ethics codes recognize, e.g., [37]. Scientists'/physicians' increased advantages include government-funded education, research grants, societal protection/licensing for professional careers, and "corners on the market" providing scientific/medical services. These increased advantages arise because of scientists'/physicians' largely-unearned higher intelligence and resulting higher incomes. Granted, most scientists/physicians have worked hard, but without largely-unearned advantages like high intelligence, good parenting, and educational opportunities, their privileges would have been unachievable. Given such privileges, scientists/physicians and others with such increased advantages have greater responsibilities (than most people) to protect society from harm, especially in areas related to their expertise [35]. To the degree that citizens, including scientists/physicians, do not accept any heightened responsibility—which varies, individual to individual, on the basis of unearned advantages like intelligence, education, etc.—their inaction helps cause avoidable DT, for which they are responsible.

5.1.7 FOURTH ARGUMENT: DT BENEFITS CREATE DT DUTIES

Citizens, and especially wealthier citizens like scientists/physicians, also bear justice-based responsibilities to help stop DT because, according to the DT-benefits argument, even if epigenetic change is not heritable—all citizens, and scientists/physicians in particular, have justice-based duties to take action on avoidable DT because they benefit from it. How do they benefit? Just as many people have saved money by purchasing sweatshop-produced goods, and just as wealthier people likely purchase more sweatshop goods and therefore have greater responsibility for the harms they cause, something similar holds for DT harms. To see how all citizens, especially wealthier citizens such as scientists/physicians benefit from DT, consider three examples: fossil-fueled automobiles and electricity, pesticide-laden food, and waste incinerators.

5.1.7.1 DT HARMS DESPITE FOSSIL-FUEL BENEFITS

At least in Europe and the US, fossil-fueled vehicles cause DT risks because they are responsible for roughly half of all ozone and particulates, neither of which has a safe dose, both of which are especially harmful to children [38,39]. Although asthma is a complex disease with multi-factorial, multi-level origins, particulates alone cause at least $2 billion annually in environmentally-attributable asthma harms to US children, apart from possible developmental decrements. Particulates are at least part of the reason that US pediatric-asthma rates have doubled in the last 10 years [39]. Yet, drivers of fossil-fueled vehicles never compensate their child victims for harms they cause.

Something similar holds for recipients of fossil-fuel-generated electricity. Although coal-fired plants produce roughly 45 percent of US, and 41 percent of global, electricity—-and are the largest US source of SO2/mercury/air toxins and major NOX/ozone/particulates sources—virtually all citizens benefit unfairly from this pollution. Why? Coal-generated-electricity users impose developmental risks from pollutants such as mercury, yet they never compensate victims, like US newborns who suffer $9 billion/year in IQ and discounted-lifetime-earnings (DLE) losses from coal-plant-mercury pollution [40]. Instead, fossil-fueled vehicles and electricity plants impose many of their health/economic costs—unpaid by users—on society's most vulnerable members, children.

5.1.7.2 SCIENTISTS'/PHYSICIANS' GREATER FOSSIL-FUEL BENEFITS GENERATE GREATER DT DUTIES

Even worse, uncompensated economic benefits that wealthier people—like scientists/physicians—receive from fossil-fueled vehicles and electricity may dwarf benefits to others and explain the greater responsibilities of wealthier people to address DT. Why? Scientists/physicians tend to have higher incomes, and those in the highest-income decile appear to cause about 25 times more fossil-fuel pollutants than those in the lowest-income decile [41]. If so, wealthier people like scientists/physicians may (unintentionally) be responsible for disproportionate injustice from un-compensated DT harms, such as asthma.

In his classic UK-government report, British economist Nicholas Stern [42] estimated that each person in the developed world causes an average of 11 tons/year of carbon-equivalent emissions—roughly $ 935/year in fossil-fuel, climate-only (droughts, floods) effects that kill about 150,000 people/year. Yet global annual outdoor-air-pollution-related deaths, mostly from fossil fuels, are about 1.3 million/year—roughly 10 times greater than climate-related deaths [43]. But if each person in the developed world causes about $900/year climate-related deaths/harms, and if pollution-related fossil-fuel deaths are up to 10 times greater, then developed-world citizen could cause up to (10 x $900) or $9,000/year in fossil-pollution deaths/harms. If so, wealthier people—like physicians/scientists—each might cause up to (25 x $9000) or $225,000 /year in fossil-fuel-pollution damages, including DT [41], mainly to poor people and children, for which they never compensate anyone.

5.1.7.3 GREATER PESTICIDE AND INCINERATION BENEFITS GENERATE GREATER DUTIES TO STOP DT

Besides DT caused by fossil-fueled electricity and vehicles, pesticides are widely acknowledged neuro-developmental toxins that constitute a third example of how most people profit unfairly from DT because they buy non-organic food. Although pesticides save consumers money, they impose inequitable DT harms on infants/children, especially farmworker children. Moreover, pesticide-related income losses, alone, are substantial—perhaps $61 billion/year, just from organophosphate-pesticide-induced IQ and DLE losses in children aged 0–5. Once organochlorines and carbamates are included, pesticides harms may rise higher. Why? Data show that for a population of 25.5 million children, aged 0–5, organophosphate pesticides cause losses of about 3,400,000 IQ points/year [44]. Yet the monetary value (DLE) of a one-point IQ loss is about $18,000—if one takes the average of a US EPA estimate of about $11,240 [45]; a Harvard estimate of about $16,500 [46]; a US Centers for Disease Control estimate of about $20,000 [47]; and a Mount Sinai School of Medicine estimate of about \$22,300 [40]. Thus \$18,000 x 3,400,000=about \$61 billion/year DLE losses caused by organophosphate-exposed young children—if one counts only the 50-percent-highest-exposed children. (This \$61 billion/year loss may be an underestimate, given the substantial fraction of overall IQ losses that may be contributed by children with exposures at the lower end of the distribution, and given the relative ubiquity of organophosphate exposures). Although adult food consumers—including scientists/physicians—partly benefit from these losses, they never compensate victims. Yet fairness dictates that consumers pay full costs for their activities/goods, not impose them on innocent children [34].

Incinerator emissions, like lead, constitute another example of how many citizens (unintentionally) gain economic and health benefits from imposing DT risks on children. At least some DT occurs because most citizens (who create garbage) fail to cover full waste-management costs/controls. Because most consumers pay only small household-garbage-pickup fees, the waste is often incinerated in poor neighborhoods—where lead and other emissions impose uncompensated IQ and DLE losses on residents, especially poor/minority children [48].

By benefitting from fossil fuels, pesticide-laden foods, and waste incineration, most citizens are at least partial, unintentional "free riders" who save money and health by imposing their DT risks on poor children [34]. Moreover, because their unfair fossil-fuel, pesticide, incinerator, and other DT-related benefits typically are proportional to their consumption and thus wealth, higher-income groups—like physicians/scientists—achieve greater undeserved gains, and thus bear greater responsibility, for DT-associated harms.

5.1.8 ALL MAJOR OBJECTIONS FAIL

In response to previous arguments showing that all citizens—and especially scientists/physicians, because of their greater abilities, training, wealth, etc.—have justice-based duties to help avoid DT, at least 7 questions/objections may arise. These might be called the avoidability, intention, neutrality, economics, excuse, uncertainty, and unfairness objections.

5.1.8.1 THE AVOIDABILITY OBJECTION

The avoidability question is "how is it possible to determine which DT agents are avoidable?". This question can be answered only on a case-by-case basis, depending on whether some DT agent is irreplaceable for human needs, e.g., medicines. Moreover, this question's answer depends in part on the state of science/engineering—including what is known about various chemicals, their DT potential, and possible alternatives to them—and on the ethical theory employed. For instance, all other things being equal, Rawlsian egalitarians would be more likely than Millian utilitarians to say some DT exposure was avoidable, if a much more expensive alternative (to the DT chemical) were available. Why? Rawlsians (more than Millians) require protecting vulnerable minorities, and take less account of the economic costs of protection. Thus, there is no algorithm to answer the avoidability question. As noted earlier, the main (Kantian) point is that "ought implies can." Therefore, if one cannot avoid some DT exposure, one is not obligated to do so. However, whether an exposure is avoidable requires case-specific, science-specific, ethics-specific assessment.

5.1.8.2 THE INTENTION OBJECTION

What about the intention objection: If I don't intend to cause harm, how can I be responsible for DT? This objection fails because, as Aristotle [19] noted, people are responsible when their intended acts, culpable ignorance, or inaction causes harm. Why? People are responsible for what should know and who they allow themselves to become. Asking why people failed to stop Hitler (just as we might ask why people have failed to stop avoidable DT, when many people at the time denied Hitler's atrocities, just as many today deny DT harms), Karl Jaspers [49] and Jean-Paul Sartre [50] charged humankind with "metaphysical guilt." For what? For not creating themselves, through their attitudes/choices/acts, as the sorts of people who would be help avoid societal harms. To the degree that people's own inaction/insensitivity has allowed them to become passive, compassionless, or weak—to live in "bad faith"—they are culpable for inaction in the face of great harms, whether Hitler or DT. Hence, to varying degrees (proportional to individual ability, training, profession, income, etc., as argued), everyone has duties to help prevent avoidable DT [49].

5.1.8.3 THE NEUTRALITY OBJECTION

Scientists/physicians, however, might have a neutrality, objection. If scientists are supposed to be neutral, value-free, and objective, how can they become activists against DT?

The neutrality objection fails on several logical grounds. First, it relies on the false assumption that objectivity is neutrality; it is not. Objectivity is even-handedness, lack of bias. Otherwise, scientists would have to remain neutral about whether the earth is flat, whether evolution is a fact, or whether anthropogenic climate change exists. Second, if scientists remained neutral, instead of speaking out against DT, they also would err through inconsistency. Why? No good scientists are neutral about poor science. Instead, they use rational debate to help resolve scientific controversies. If so, consistency demands scientists' using rational debate to assess possible advocacy in areas related to their scientific expertise. Besides, even in doing science, scientists are forced to make hundreds of value-laden, methodological judgments, about everything from proper sample sizes, measurement errors, and possible model biases, to data interpretations [34]. If they did not make methodological value judgments, they could not do science.

Scientists/physicians also must make ethical value judgments—for instance, about allowing avoidable DT—or they violate principles of virtually all codes of professional (scientific) ethics. These codes bind scientists to be unbiased/objective and to promote human welfare/protection. Thus, the American Association for the Advancement of Science (AAAS) emphasizes the "added responsibility of members of the scientific community, individually and through their formal organizations, to speak out" whenever public health or safety is at risk [34,36,37,51]. Besides, if physicians/scientists do not speak out and instead remain neutral, they cannot fulfill their duties of citizenship, duties to help ensure others' equal protection. Yet no one ought avoid the duties of citizenship. Physicians/scientists therefore do not cease being citizens, just because they are scientists. Indeed, as argued earlier, virtually all ethics codes agree that physicians/ scientists' heightened abilities/training/education arguably give them increased (not reduced) duties as citizens [36,37]. Besides, if physicians/ scientists did not have duties to speak out, especially in areas related to their special expertise, worse harms could occur. As Burke put it: All that is necessary for the triumph of evil is that good people do nothing.

Scientists'/physicians' neutrality on important issues, like DT, also would generate harmful consequences for science itself. Why? The AAAS notes that roughly 75% of US science is funded by industry, 25% by government; that more than half of US-government-funded science is military; and that for every $100 that environmental-health industries spend on their science, government spends about $1 [52]. Consequently, the medical-scientific "playing field" is not level, but often politicized. Declining government science/education funding, and increased special-interest funding, further tilt this playing field, as illustrated by fossil-fuel-industry-funded "science" challenging anthropogenic climate change. The result? Half of Americans believe scientists disagree about whether anthropogenic climate change exists; yet, at least since 1993, no climate scientists publishing in basic-research journals have challenged climate change [53]. Such special-interest "science" helps explains why, even in top medical journals, pharmaceutical-industry-funded studies rarely attribute harmful effects to their drugs, while independent researchers often do so [54], and why chemical-industry-funded studies rarely attribute health damage to their pollutants, while independent researchers often do so [27,55]. Private-interest-science influence also helps explain why university scientists, like Herbert Needleman, were harassed by the lead/gas industry, why the smelting industry harassed Mary Amdur, why the fossil-fuel industry harassed Mike Mann, why the asbestos industry harassed Irving Selikoff, why the beryllium industry harassed Adam Finkel, etc. [34].

Special-interest science also explains why at least 50 percent of environmental epidemiologists—mostly in universities—report polluter harassment after publishing environmental-health research [28]. Given such tilted scientific playing fields, unbiased physicians/scientists who remain neutral serve the status quo, not objectivity. Neutrality allows biased conclusions to become more dominant, science and scientists to be harmed.

Because even-handed inquiry (not neutrality) serves objectivity, unbiased scientists need not fear they lack objectivity, if they take action on DT. The opposite is probably true.

5.1.8.4 THE ECONOMICS OBJECTION

What about a third, or economics, objection. Would preventing avoidable DT cause economic harm? The obvious response is "for whom?" Polluters or innocent children?

The main ethical/logical problem with the economics objection is its begging the questions whether those who seriously harm health should be out of business, whether they have the rights to profit from causing harm. Making this objection is thus a bit like an accused murderer's claiming (correctly, as already noted) that prosecuting him is not cost-effective. Yet the key issue is justice, not cost. After all, no reasonable person asks whether enforcing basic human rights is economical.

The economics objection also errs factually. As already noted, many scientists have shown that costs of preventing serious health harms——such as DT—are likely less than those caused by allowing them. For instance, French researchers examined economic benefits of lead-abatement/prevention. They discovered lead abatement/prevention costs were far less than health/social costs of addressing lead exposure through screening, special-education expenditures, crime, suffering, and reduced DLE. Although France's population is one-fifth that of the US, lead-induced IQ losses cause French children's DLE losses of about 22 Euros/year or $30 billion/year, and French crime losses of 62 Euros/year or $81 billion/year [56]. Similarly, the health, IQ, DLE, etc. losses of US children's mercury exposures are up to $8 billion/year [46]. More generally, US costs of environmentally-attributable (caused) children's lead exposure, asthma, cancer, and neurobehavioral problems are up to $55 billion/year [40]. If lead-pollution costs are analogous to those for other developmental toxins, every $1, spent on lead (or other toxin) controls, causes $17-221 in benefits [57]. If so, the economics objection may have little scientific/factual merit.

5.1.8.5 THE EXCUSE OBJECTION

But suppose scientists/physicians have a fourth, or excuse, objection. Do people who do many good things with their lives—raising children, healing patients, serving the poor, doing important research—have rights not to spend time taking action on DT?

While reasonable, the excuse objection errs in ignoring the fact, already argued, that people who cause DT and benefit from it thereby have justice-based duties to compensate for this injustice. Hence they cannot rationally claim excuses for not taking action, any more than robbers can claim ethical excuses for not compensating their victims. Why not? Justice violations require justice-based restitution [58]. Because taking action on DT is a matter of justice, not charity, it is not optional. If not, scientists/physicians—as citizens—have justice-based duties of democratic responsibility, especially if their failure to be politically active in their areas of expertise contributes to DT. Of course, different people's duties to help address DT differ, depending on their income, health, abilities, etc. Nevertheless, no excuses completely exonerate offenders from justice-based duties to rectify injustice. Otherwise, justice would not exist. Also, it is unreasonable, practically speaking, to offer excuses for completely relinquishing justice-based duties to take action. If such excuses applied to all duties, they would generate question-begging, self-fulfilling prophecies that caused great harm [34].

5.1.8.6 THE UNCERTAINTY OBJECTION

Still other thinkers might make a fifth, or uncertainty, objection. How can physicians/scientists take action on DT when the science remains uncertain?

Although reasonable people can disagree about degrees of scientific uncertainty concerning DT, the uncertainty objection is invalid because it commits a logical fallacy, the appeal to ignorance. That is, it assumes that because something has not been proved harmful, it is harmless—that absence of evidence (e.g., for DT) is evidence of the absence (of DT). This objection also relies on at least three faulty assumptions. One is that doing nothing is the way to remain neutral/objective in science—a false claim, already rejected, in response to the neutrality argument. Another erroneous assumption is that the best evidentiary rule is to consider a known toxin innocent of health harm until proved guilty. However, this assumption has been widely challenged, partly through the precautionary principle, because waiting for certainty about a toxin's harm could cause massive death/disease. Consequently, to protect public health, arguably society should use a "preponderance of evidence rule," not a "beyond a-reasonable-doubt rule" to assess DT and possible action to prevent harm [27,28]. That is, the objection's third flawed presupposition is that the best health-science default rule, given scientific uncertainty, is the pure-science rule to minimize false positives. However, many physicians/scientists have shown that because welfare-affecting science must prevent serious harm/injustice, its default rule should be to minimize false negatives. After all, given uncertainty about fire/flood, one does not do nothing, but buys insurance. Given uncertainty about rain, one carries an umbrella. One gets medical check ups, balances her checkbook, exercises, visits the auto mechanic—despite uncertainty about harm. Analogous precautionary requirements also hold for uncertainty about more serious threats, like DT [34].

5.1.8.7 THE UNFAIRNESS OBJECTION

Even if scientists/physicians admit the importance of taking action, they may have a sixth, or unfairness objection. Is it fair for those—-who already have overwhelming research/healing/teaching duties—to have special duties to tackle DT?

Contrary to the unfairness objection, scientists/physicians have such special duties, as argued earlier, because of their special abilities, unearned advantages, greater wealth/consumption, etc. They also have knowledge that few others have and, as Bacon put it, knowledge is power. Those with more power have more responsibility. However, those who make the unfairness argument disagree, likely because of their false assumptions. One false assumption underlying the unfairness objection is that scientists/physicians have "earned" their privileges, hence should have no enhanced duties because of them. However, as already argued, scientists/physicians are not fully "self made." Because their high IQs (thus better income/ education/training/research funding, etc.) are partly unearned/undeserved, matters of chance—they have no right to full benefits from them. If not, as professional codes of ethics point out, scientists have special duties to "give back" to society [7,51], as through tackling DT. But if people ought not profit more than others, from largely unearned/undeserved benefits like high IQs, then fairness dictates scientists/physicians have greater duties to take action than many other people. Noblesse oblige. As the scientific research society, Sigma Xi, said: "Because the pathways that we pursue as research scientists are infinite and unfrequented, we cannot police them as we protect our streets and personal property. We depend on those other travelers...along such lonely byways of knowledge" to protect us [51].

Another false assumption often made in the unfairness argument is that, if others are doing little to tackle DT, fairness dictates that I also have little/no responsibility. However, while one's duties to help avoid societal harm may decrease if others fail to do their fair share, obviously others' behavior does not dictate ethics. Murder does not become morally acceptable, just because many people murder. To assume others' action/inaction justifies one's own action/inaction is to commit the logical fallacy of appeal to the people. Instead, only logic/facts/principles determine what is justified. After all, centuries of racism/sexism have not make them right.

5.1.9 SCIENTISTS/PHYSICIANS CAN TAKE ACTION

Citizens/physicians/scientists, however, have no duties to help protect others, in their areas of expertise, unless they are able to do so. "Ought implies can," as Kant [58,59] put it. How can scientists/physicians take action on DT?

At the group level, organizations like the Society of Toxicology or the American Public Health Association could issue recommendations for DT research/regulatory action. After all, a decade ago, the American Geophysical Union and the American Meteorological Society said we have "collective responsibility" to take action on climate change because we caused it [60]. An analogous claim holds for DT, as already argued.

Working with nongovernmental health/environmental organizations, both local and national—like the Environmental Working Group, or Physicians for Social Responsibility, both of which address children's health—physicians/scientists also can volunteer their time/expertise. The benefit of such group (and especially local) volunteering is that together, professionals can accomplish what no one, acting alone, could achieve. Recently, for example, the author and other university scientists failed to convince government not to permit a dangerous coal-gasification facility in our already-heavily-polluted area. However, once we gave our information to local doctors, the entire local medical association, hundreds of physicians, voted against the facility. Government was forced to do the same.

Individual physician/scientist action also is useful, such as writing popular essays/blogs on important health topics, whenever they publish analogous professional-journal articles. By "translating" their research for laypeople, scientists/physicians can help promote action on DT. They also can list themselves as media-friendly experts—through their universities, employers, and professional associations—so TV/radio/newspaper/internet reporters easily can contact/interview them. They can serve pro-bono, on local/state/federal advisory boards, such as that for the county health association, the local Sierra Club, or for national groups such as the US EPA's Science Advisory Board, or committees/boards of the US National Academy of Sciences (NAS). They can give pro-bono testimony in DT court cases. To promote consumer outreach/education on DT, they can speak at school-parent-teacher-association meetings, publish local op-eds, and advise citizens' groups. School-parent-teacher outlets are especially important because, regardless of people's politics, as parents they usually are deeply concerned about their children, hence likely to help take action on DT. Moreover, the effort needed for DT action is not great. If historians are correct, only about 14 percent of the early colonists supported the US revolution against England, partly because revolutions are not good for banks and businesses. Imagine the DT-awareness revolution that could occur if 14 percent of parents were mobilized.

At the university or medical-school level, scientists/physicians can encourage administrators, staff, and student organizations to work on phasing out pesticide-laden food, BPA-containing bottles, etc. from university facilities. Scientists/physicians in education can encourage students to do real-world environmental science/health projects, either for course credit or instead of exams. They can teach courses/parts of courses in which students learn to respond to draft health/safety regulations, environmental-impact assessments, and risk assessments—-thousands of which are released annually by the US government. In an annual biology course, the author's students typically receive up to four benefits from their pro-bono projects, responding to draft scientific/government/regulatory analyses. First, students often obtain publications from their work. Second, the victims/impacted communities receive free scientific assistance that helps protect and empowers them, although they cannot pay for help. Third, attorneys often can use this pro-bono student work to assist poor/minority communities harmed by pollution. Fourth, and most important, students who do this scientific work become "vaccinated by social justice," inspired. Once they realize they can make a difference, they often dedicate at least part of their lives to such pro-bono work, "liberation science," that helps protect vulnerable people [34].

5.1.10 POLICY SUGGESTIONS

In the policy arena, how might society take action on DT? One option would be banning all chemicals thought to be developmental toxins until they are proved reasonably safe. However, this strategy appears impractical. Funders of special-interest science probably would block such bans by using tactics like lengthy court challenges. After all, they have blocked most testing/regulation under the 1976 US Toxic Substances Control Act (TSCA). Despite massive growth in chemical production/use, since 1976, TSCA has required testing of only about 200—and has regulated only 5—of roughly 80,000 industrial-agricultural chemicals. Such failures suggest a more moderate strategy is needed.

Another option would be for government to request NAS to study DT and make regulatory/policy recommendations. Like the classic 1993 NAS report on pesticides in the diets of infants and children—which triggered passage of the 1996 US Food Quality Protection Act—a DT study might be the catalyst for protective legislation. The academy could assess DT triggers, criteria, and health consequences. It also could suggest default environmental-health recommendations, until the relevant science is clear—addressing product labeling, temporary exposure-limit safety factors/limits, DT research, testing, compliance assessment, etc. Although admittedly NAS reports take time, whereas taking action is urgent, relying on NAS expertise seems the best long-term strategy, given its credibility.

5.2 CONCLUSION

While important, deferring to NAS is not sufficient for taking action on DT. Individual citizens/scientists/physicians also must help. To motivate such help, this commentary has offered four main arguments. These focus on citizen duties to act, based on ethical theory, political theory, citizens' causing DT, and citizens' benefitting from it. Because of their special abilities/training/wealth/etc., scientists/professionals have heightened responsibilities, as both citizens and professionals, to protect against DT. After all, professionals have many unearned IQ/genetic/upbringing/income privileges from "the natural lottery of life" that have given them unintended but unfair advantages over others [31]. To help compensate for these unearned advantages, physicians/scientists can help level the scientific playing field and take action on DT. As Ghandhi put it, "Whenever I live in a situation where others are in need…whether or not I am responsible for it, I have become a thief" [61]. Like the Brazilian child, DT-threatened children are in need. We are partly culpable. We can be the light that helps banish the darkness around them.

REFERENCES

1.   Barouki R, Gluckman PD, Grandjean P, Hanson M, Heindel JJ: Developmental origins of non-communicable disease: Implications for research and public health. Environ Heal 2012, 11:42.
2.   Skinner MK, Manikkam M, Guerrero-Bosagna C: Epigenetic transgenerational actions of endocrine disruptors. Reprod Toxicol 2011, 31:337-343.
3.   United Nations Office on Drugs and Crime: Action against Transnational Organized Crime and Illicit Trafficking. UN, Geneva; 2011.
4.   Shimazono Y: The state of the international organ trade. Bulletin of the World Health Organization 2007, 85:901-980.

5. Grandjean P: We Have Only One Chance to Develop a Brain. Biomedical Research Park, Barcelona; 2012.

6. Boffetta P, McLaughlin JK, LaVecchia C, Tarone RE, Lipworth L, Blot WJ: False-positive results in cancer epidemiology: a plea for epistemological modesty. J Natl Cancer Inst 2008, 100:988-995.

7. Blair A, Saracci R, Vineis P, Cocco P, Forastiere F, Grandjean P, Kogevinas M, Kriebel D, McMichael A, Pearce N, Porta M, Samet J, Sandler DP, Costantini AS, Vainio H: Epidemiology, public health, and the rhetoric of false positives. Environ Health Perspect. 2009, 117:1809-1813.

8. Grandjean P, Eriksen ML, Ellegaard O, Wallin JA: The Matthew effect in environmental-science publications. Environ Health 2011, 10:96.

9. Landrigan PJ: Testimony before the Committee on Environment and Public Works, US Senate. Adelphi University, Garden City, NY; 2001.

10. Schierow LJ: The Toxic Substances Control Act, 7–5700. Congressional Research Service, Washington, DC; 2011. Hill AB: The environment and disease. Proc R Soc Med 1965, 58:295-3000.

11. Shrader-Frechette K: Randomization and rules for causal inferences in biology. Biological Theory 2012, 6:1-8.

12. Ross WD: The Right and the Good. Reprinted with an introduction by Philip Stratton. Oxford University, Oxford; 2002.

13. Kagan S: The Limits of Morality. Clarendon Press, Oxford; 1989:17n.

14. Bernal AJ, Jirtle RL: Epigenomic disruption. Birth Defects Res A Clin Mol Teratol 2010, 88:938-944.

15. Gluckman PD, Hanson MA, Low FM: The role of developmental plasticity and epigenetics in human health. Birth Defects Res C Embryo Today 2011, 93:12-18.

16. Grandjean P, Landrigan PJ: Developmental neurotoxicity of industrial chemicals.

17. Lancet 2006, 368:2167-2178.

18. Schug TT, Janesick A, Blumberg B, Heindel JJ: Endocrine-disrupting chemicals and disease susceptibility. J of Steroid Biochemistry and Molecular Biology 2011, 127:204-215.

19. Aristotle N: Ethics, editor and translator, D Ross. Oxford University Press, New York; 1925.

20. Aquinas T: On Law, Morality, and Politics, second edition, translator Richard Regan. Hackett, Indianapolis; 2002.

21. Sunstein C: Risk and Reason. University Press, Cambridge; 2002.

22. Morgenstern RD, Pizer WA, Shih JS: Jobs versus the environment. J Environ Econ Manag 2002, 43:412-436.

23. Dwoskin E, Drajem M: Regulations create jobs too. Bloomberg Businessweek 2012.

24. Kaplan GA, Pamuk ER, Lynch JW, Cohen RD, Balfour JL: Inequality and income and mortality in the United States. British Medical Journal 1996, 312:999-1003.

25. Trasande L, Landrigan PJ, Schechter C: Public health and economic consequences of methyl mercury toxicity to the developing brain. Environ Health Perspect 2005, 113:5990-96.

26. Beder S: Global Spin. Green Books, Glasgow; 2002.

27. Michaels D: Doubt Is Their Product. Oxford University Press, New York; 2008.

28. Wagner W, McGarity T: Bending Science. Harvard University, Cambridge; 2008:158.

29. Hahnel R, Sheeran KA: Misinterpreting the Coase Theorem. Journal of Economic Issues 2009, 43:215-238.

30. Mill JS: On Liberty and Other Essays. University Press, Oxford; 2008.

31. Rawls J: A Theory of Justice. Harvard University Press, Cambridge; 1971.

32. John L: Two Treatises of Government. University, Cambridge; 1960.

33. Shrader-Frechette K: Gene patents and Lockean constraints. Public Affairs Quarterly 2006, 20:135-61.

34. Shrader-Frechette KS: Taking Action, Saving Lives. Oxford University, New York; 2007. esp. pp. 129; 3–38, 113–149; 159–165; 156; 39–112; 159–165; 164–68; 182–210

35. American Association for the Advancement of Science: Principles of Scientific Freedom and Responsibility. AAAS, Washington, DC; 1980.

36. American Medical Association: Declaration of Professional Responsibility. AMA, San Francisco; 2001. http://www.ama-assn.org/resources/doc/ethics/decofprofessional.pdf

37. Shrader-Frechette KS: Ethics of Scientific Research. Rowman and Littlefield, Savage, MD; 1994.

38. European Environment Agency: Air Quality and Ancillary Benefits of Climate-Change Policies. EEA, Copenhagen; 2006.

39. Wahlin P, Palmgren F: Source Apportionment of Particles and Particulates (PM10) Measured by DMA and TROM in a Copenhagen Street Canyon. National Environmental Research Institute, Roskilde, Denmark; 2000.

40. Landrigan PJ, Schechter CB, Lipton JM, Fahs MC, Schwartz J: Environmental pollutants and disease in American children. Environ Health Perspect. 2002, 110:721-728.

41. Rabinowitz D: Climate injustice. Environmental Justice. 2012, 5:38-46.

42. Stern N: The Economics of Climate Change. HM Treasury, London; 2006.

43. World Health Association: Air Quality and Health. WHO, Copenhagen; 2011.

44. Bellinger DC: A strategy for comparing the contributions of environmental chemicals and other risk factors to neurodevelopment of children. Environ Health Perspect 2011, 120:501-507.

45. US Environmental Protection Agency: Technical Support Document: revision of December 2000 Regulatory Finding on the Emissions of Hazardous Air Pollutants from Electricity Steam Generating Units and the Removal of Coal and Oil-Fired Electric Utility Steam Generating Units from the Section 112(c) List: Reconsideration. October 21. US EPA, Washington, DC; 2005.

46. Rice G, Hammitt JK: Economic Valuation of Human Health Effects of Controlling Mercury Emissions from US Coal-Fired Power Plants, Northeast States for Coordinated Air Use Management. Harvard Center for Risk Analysis, Cambridge; 2005.

47. Grosse SD: How much is an IQ point worth? AERE Newsletter 2007, 2007(27):17-21.

48. World Health Organization: Childhood Lead Poisoning. WHO, Geneva; 2010.

49. Jaspers K: The Question of German Guilt. Edited by Ashton EB. Capricorn, New York; 1961.

50. Sartre J-P: What Is Literature? trans. Frechtman B. Methuen, London; 1950.
51. Jackson CI: Honor in Science. Sigma Xi, New Haven; 1986:33.
52. Koizumi K: R&D Trends and Special Analyses, AAAS Reports XXIX, XXVII. American Association for the Advancement of Science' 2005, Washington, DC; 2004.
53. Oreskes N: The scientific consensus on climate change. Science 2004, 306:1686.
54. Krimsky S: Science in the Private Interest. Rowman and Littlefield, Lanham MD; 2004.
55. Oreskes N, Conway E: Merchants of Doubt. Bloomsbury, New York; 2010.
56. Pichery C, Bellanger M, Zmirou-Navier D, Glorennec P, Hartemann P, Grandjean P: Childhood lead exposure in France. Environ Health. 2011, 10:44.
57. Gould E: Childhood lead poisoning. Environ Health Perspect 2009, 117:1162-1167. http://dx.doi.org/10.1289/ehp.0800408
58. Kant I: Lectures On Ethics, edited by Schneewind JB, translated by Heath P. University Press, Cambridge; 2001.
59. Kant I: Critique of Pure Reason, translated by Smith NK. St. Martin's, New York; 1965.
60. Leung L, Ruby L, Mearns F, Wilby R: Regional climate research. Bull Am Meteorol Soc 2003, 84:89-95. http://dx.doi.org/10.1175/BAMS-84-1-89
61. Goulet D: The Cruel Choice. Athenaeum, New York; 1971:133.

AUTHOR NOTES

CHAPTER 2

Acknowledgments

I thank A. Rowland, B. Lanphear, J. Matthews, W.K. Anger, and several reviewers for their many helpful comments. This paper is based on the Jakob Hooisma Memorial Lecture, 13th Meeting of the International Neurotoxicology Association, Xi'an, China, June 2011.

CHAPTER 4

Acknowledgments

We are grateful to the families of northern Manhattan who have so generously contributed their time and effort to the study.

Footnotes

This study was supported by the National Institute of Environmental Health Sciences (grants 5P01ES09600, P50ES015905, and 5R01ES08977), the U.S. Environmental Protection Agency (grants R827027, 8260901, and RR00645), the Educational Foundation of America, the John and Wendy Neu Family Foundation, the New York Community Trust, and the Trustees of the Blanchette Hooker Rockefeller Fund.

The authors declare they have no actual or potential competing financial interests.

CHAPTER 6

Footnotes

The authors declare they have no actual or potential competing -financial interests.

CHAPTER 7

Competing Interests
The author declares that they have no competing interest.

Author Contributions
AA performed the practical work and co-drafted the manuscript. LA provided samples and participated in the diagnosis of the autistic samples. AE designed the study and drafted the manuscript. All authors have read and approved the final manuscript.

Acknowledgments
This research project was supported by a grant from the research center of the center for female scientific and medical colleges in King Saud University.

CHAPTER 8

Acknowledgments
The authors appreciate the autistic subjects and their relatives for collaboration to this study. Hiroshi Yasuda conceived this review article and wrote the manuscript with the help of Toyoharu Tsutsui.

Conflicts of Interest
The author declares no conflict of interest.

CHAPTER 10

Acknowledgments
This study was supported by a Grant from Autism Speaks, Grant no. 5406, as well as Grants from the Taub Foundation, the Blanche Greene fund of The Pauline Sterne Wolff Memorial Foundation, the Verdant Foundation, and the Methodist Hospital Foundation. The authors acknowledge with gratitude the input of Marsha Widmayer and the first rate work done by Sophie Lopez who has maintained these cell lines with skill and dedication.

CHAPTER 12

Conflicts of Interest

The authors declare that there is no conflict of interests regarding the publication of this paper.

Acknowledgments

The authors would like to thank Andreas Sjödin, PhD. from the Centers for Disease Control and Prevention (CDC) for his assistance in the interpretation of the NHANES urinary PAH metabolite data. Zaynah Abid was supported by Yale University's Ruth and Milton Steinbach Scholarship. Julie B. Herbstman was supported by National Institutes of Health (NIH) R00-ES017051 and P30-ES009089. Adrienne S. Ettinger was supported by NIH K01-ES014907. The contents are solely the responsibility of the authors and do not necessarily represent the official views of the NIEHS, NIH, or CDC. The authors declare they have no actual or potential competing financial interests.

Institute of Diabetes and Digestive and Kidney Diseases (R01 DK077659) and the Wellcome Trust (WT087997MA). The latter also funded the salary of C.M-W. in relation to her work on this paper.

CHAPTER 14

Footnotes

This research was funded by the C8 class action settlement agreement (Jack W. Leach, et al. v. E.I. du Pont de Nemours & Company, no. 01-C-608 W.Va., Wood County Circuit Court, WV, USA) between DuPont and plaintiffs. Funds were administered by the Garden City Group (Melville, NY), which reports to the court. Our work and conclusions are independent of either party to the lawsuit. C.S. was supported by the National Institute of Environmental Health Sciences (K01 ES019156).

The authors declare they have no actual or potential competing financial interests.

CHAPTER 15

Competing Interests

The author declares she has no competing financial interests.

Author Contributions

The author drafted the first version of the manuscript, and the author revised the manuscript, based on reviewer's comments. The author read and approved the final manuscript.

Acknowledgments

The author thanks the US National Science Foundation (NSF) for research grant SES-0724781, "Three Methodological Rules in Risk Assessment," during which part of the research for this article was done. All opinions and errors are those of the author, not NSF. The author also thanks Philippe Grandjean for comments on an earlier version.

INDEX

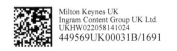
Milton Keynes UK
Ingram Content Group UK Ltd.
UKHW022058141024
449569UK00031B/1691